Adam Widdison was born in Nottingham and went to school at Dartford and Gravesend, Kent, England. He studied medicine at Oxford University, taught Anatomy at Cambridge University, undertook research at University College, Los Angeles, and trained in hospitals at Plymouth, Oxford, Norwich, Exeter and Bristol before being appointed consultant surgeon at the Royal Cornwall Hospital in 1995. In addition to a medical degree, he has an MA, DM, FRCS, a Hunterian professorship and a PGCE. Working in one of the busiest acute teaching hospitals in England gave him a wealth of experience, both clinically and as a teacher, and provided the inspiration for this book.

I would like to dedicate this book to my wife, Susan, my children, Nicholas and Natasha, and my parents, Ivor and Gill, who helped me with my career, put up with me arriving home late, working evenings and weekends for most of their lives; and to the healthcare professionals who work so hard to help their patients.

Adam Widdison

THE EXPERT CLINICIAN

Bridging the Clinical Divide

AUSTIN MACAULEY PUBLISHERS™

LONDON * CAMBRIDGE * NEW YORK * SHARJAH

ISBN 9781035831975 (Paperback)
ISBN 9781035831982 (Hardback)
ISBN 9781035831999 (ePub e-book)

www.austinmacauley.com

First Published 2024
Austin Macauley Publishers Ltd®
1 Canada Square
Canary Wharf
London
E14 5AA

I would like to thank the patients, colleagues, students, and other healthcare professionals from whom I have learnt so much over the years. I would particularly like to thank Dr Sanjeev Gupta and Dr Cara McLaughlin for their helpful and enthusiastic support for this book and to Holly (editor) and her team at Austin Macauley for their help in publishing this book. I would not have started on my medical career if it had not been for the love and support of my parents, Ivor and Gill, and the guidance and teaching of Mr. Ken Shorrocks, Mr. AJ Watson-Wemys, and the teachers at Gravesend School for Boys, who helped me get to university, and to Professors Peter Matthews and David Smith who offered me a place.

I am eternally grateful to the many dedicated, caring people I have worked with and learnt so much from over the years, but particular mention must be made of Messrs Michael Thompson, Alun Evans, Julian Britton, Dougie George, and Professor John Farndon who helped me with my career, and to Dr Harry Dalton, Paul Fortun, John Barnes, and Sanjeev Gupta who were some of the inspirational clinicians I worked with. Thank you.

Table of Contents

Preface

The Expert Clinician explains the skills and methods used by experienced clinicians to make the consultation meaningful and describes how these can be applied to the consultation. It is intended to bridge the divide between the traditional "clerking" taught to students and the approach used by experts and between a textbook knowledge of medicine and the basic sciences and clinical reality. *The Expert Clinician* is recommended for medical students, junior doctors and other health care professionals (HCPs) who want to become a better clinician and for the trainer who wants to help them on their journey.

Traditionally, trainee clinicians are taught to ask a sequence of questions and perform a complete examination using a standard format. It is then hoped that by the end of the consultation they will be inspired to think of a diagnosis and plan management. As a consequence, more often than not, the clerking is more of a checklist to complete a proforma rather than a consultation with purpose. It is inflexible and there is a tendency to rely on tests and guidelines to formulate a diagnosis and determine management. As the number and availability of guidelines and tests has increased, so the perceived value of the consultation has declined. This trend is self-fulfilling because, as the perceived value of the consultation declines, so the quantity and quality of the information learnt from the consultation declines.

The paradox is that as the number and availability of guidelines, tests and treatments increases and as patients become better informed the need for a meaningful consultation has never been greater. As trainee clinicians gain experience, knowledge and expertise, they realise the importance of the consultation in the care pathway and learn how to manage the consultation to maximise the value of the consultation. This led me to ask, what is different and what can be done to help trainees become experts?

The traditional format is well established. It has remained unchanged for more than a hundred years and is widely used and familiar to all. However, it is never used by experts. Experts determine the aims of the consultation and manage the consultation flexibly to ensure the outcome meets the aims and in response to the patient and the information learnt. Questions are asked and signs sought with purpose, usually to formulate a diagnosis or plan management, and the list of possible diagnoses or management options informs the questions to ask and signs to look for. Experts use method to help them apply their cognitive skills, clinical reasoning and a knowledge of medicine and the basic sciences throughout the consultation both to ask the right questions and look for signs and to understand and interpret the information learnt. As a consequence, the consultation is meaningful, and a meaningful consultation is more likely to be a successful consultation, both for the patient, who is reassured they are being cared for and will be helped, and for the HCP, who has to plan care.

I wrote *The Expert Clinician* to help you become a better clinician, to improve patient care and to improve the patient experience. In *The Expert Clinician* the methods available to make the consultation meaningful are described and how to apply them to the consultation explained. I recognise *The Expert Clinician* is a long book and if you are just starting on your clinical journey, it will seem a lot to learn. You may think a long book will be impractical in the time-constrained clinical context. However, the book is long so that the consultation can be short: in other words, the more you know, the quicker you will get. *The Expert Clinician* is a supplement to other textbooks, journals and internet articles, not a replacement, and a core knowledge of clinical practice is assumed.

Introduction

For millennia the consultation has been at the heart of the care pathway. It is the opportunity for the HCP to meet the patient, to learn and understand relevant information from the patient and for the patient to meet the HCP, to learn the opinion of the HCP, and for both to agree a management plan. Until recently, the information learnt when taking a history and examining the patient was the main method of formulating a diagnosis and determining treatment. However, in recent years, with the increased availability and choice of tests and guidelines the emphasis has changed. No longer do trainees and an increasing number of more senior doctors rely on the consultation to formulate a diagnosis and plan management, they now expect guidelines and tests to do that for them. As a consequence, the perceived value of the consultation has declined.

There is no doubt that the increased choice, accuracy and availability of tests and guidelines has improved patient care. Frequently, tests are essential to formulate a diagnosis and guidelines helpful for planning management. However, they are not always indicated, available or appropriate, they are not without risk and they are not infallible. A test or treatment may cause harm to a patient as a result of either a complication or side effect. A test result may lead to the wrong diagnosis being made and the wrong treatment being started or a false negative result to a false sense of reassurance and a delay in treatment. The predictive value of a test is strongly influenced by the prevalence of the abnormality in the sample studied. In other words, the diagnostic accuracy of a test is dependent on performing the right test for the right reason. Similarly, guidelines are very useful and are an important part of many care pathways. However, they are not always available and few are sufficiently comprehensive that they can be relied upon without considering the clinical context. Patients are a highly diverse group demographically, ethnically, socially and culturally and have an increasing number of co-morbidities making care more complex. Furthermore, patients are more knowledgeable and opinionated with increasing access to medical and pseudo-medical information. Therefore, as more guidelines, investigations and treatments become available and patients become more opinionated so it is more important, not less, to learn, understand and correctly interpret the available information from the patient to ensure the right management plan is undertaken for the right reasons and that it is appropriate for the patient. In other words, there is much more to patient care than simply following a guideline, ordering a test or starting a treatment.

> **As the demands and expectations of patients increases and more guidelines, investigations and treatments become available, so it is more important, not less, to learn, understand and correctly interpret the available information from the patient.**

Traditionally, trainee clinicians are taught to ask a series of questions and perform a complete examination before making a diagnosis or planning management. As a consequence, the effective aim of the traditional clerking is to complete a proforma or checklist. Experienced clinicians, on the other hand, determine the aims of the consultation at the start of the consultation and adapt the focus and format and the questions to ask and the signs to look for to ensure the outcome meets the aims. For some patients, such as a new patient, children or those with challenging behaviour, establishing a working relationship is the main aim of the consultation because it is a pre-requisite to learning about the problem. For most patients presenting with a new problem, a good working relationship is assumed and the aims of the consultation are to exchange information, to formulate a diagnosis and plan management. For other patients, such as those seen following an investigation, information about the problem and the diagnosis is known and the main aims of the consultation are to share information and plan management. Experts determine the aims of the consultation early and manage each consultation differently to ensure it meets the aims and to respond to the patient and the information learnt.

> **A flexible focus and format will ensure that the consultation meets the aims and responds to the patient and the information learnt.**

In the traditional clerking, the focus is on the "history of the presenting complaint". Trainees are taught to ask questions to learn about onset and duration, change, severity, location, character, aggravating and relieving factors and associated symptoms and then to examine the patient in a systematic way. The answers are pigeon-holed into sections with little attempt at understanding their meaning or interpreting the available information and formulating a diagnosis and planning management are left to the end, almost as an afterthought. Trainees hope that the symptoms and signs will match a textbook description they recognise. However, information from the patient is frequently presented in a chaotic or unstructured way, using language the patient is familiar with but not necessarily the HCP and rarely includes all relevant information. Similarly, a systematic examination undertaken in the hope of finding an abnormal sign is less likely to be successful. It is wishful thinking to expect that simply asking a set sequence of questions or systematically examining a patient will lead to the true diagnosis or to an appropriate management plan. Therefore, it is not surprising that the diagnoses suggested at the end of a traditional consultation are rarely supported by the clinical information or that "routine" or inappropriate tests are requested.

Experts, on the other hand, ask questions with purpose, to learn what is relevant and ensure they understand the information so that it can be interpreted correctly. Signs are sought based on information available and understood and interpreted together with other information available. Possible diagnoses and management options are considered pro-actively throughout the consultation, not reactively at the end. The aims and indications for a management decision are understood.

> **The information learnt should inform the diagnosis and management and the list of possible diagnoses and management options should inform the questions to ask and signs to look for.**

In the traditional clerking, "family medical history", "personal and social history", and "past medical history, drug history and allergies" are frequently included as an addendum. This may have been appropriate when patients fitted a socio-economic stereotype and few had ongoing or complex past morbidity but it is inappropriate now. Each patient is unique and many are clinically challenging because of their complex or special needs or significant co-morbidity, polypharmacy, safety concerns and risk factors. Experts recognise the importance of learning this information both to reassure the patient that it is being considered and because it is likely to inform the diagnosis and influence management so that it is in the best interests of the patient.

> **A person-focused format ensures that the outcome of the consultation is appropriate and in the best interests of the patient**

The traditional "clerking" may help the novice starting to learn to be a clinician or help the HCP complete a proforma but it is not used by experienced clinicians. *The Expert Clinician* describes the skills and methods used by experienced clinicians and explains how these can be applied to the consultation to make the consultation meaningful. It is intended to help trainees make the transition from novice to expert.

Change starts with the terminology. The terminology used in *The Expert Clinician* is different from the traditional terminology because the language used in the traditional format is out-dated and proscriptive. "Clerking" is no longer used because it implies the doctor is an administrator or a secretary taking notes. "Learning", the acquisition of knowledge, replaces "taking" because the consultation should be a conversation rather than an interrogation. Relevant information should be learnt to understand the problem rather than questions asked or signs sought as a ritual. The word "complaint" is replaced by the word "problem" because complaint implies the patient is making a fuss whereas a problem is something to be resolved. The word "history" is only used to refer to the past. The words "present", "current" or "ongoing" are used to refer to contemporary information. Therefore, "presenting problem" replaces "presenting complaint", "learning and understanding information about the problem" replaces "history of the presenting complaint" "learning and understanding information about the person" replaces "personal and social history" and "learning and understanding information about the person as a patient" replaces "past medical history". The term "drug" is no longer used to describe a medicine because "drug-taking" is associated with taking risky substances, including illegal substances, such as narcotics and is a risk factor for a medical condition.

> **Using the right terminology sends the right message to staff and patients**

In *The Expert Clinician*, there is an emphasis on establishing the aims of the consultation early and using these to determine the focus and format of the consultation, the questions to ask and the signs to look for.

> **The aims determine the focus and format, the questions to ask and the signs to look for**

For most patients and most consultations, formulating a diagnosis and planning management are the principal aims of the consultation. However, achieving these aims is dependent on the exchange of relevant information and information exchange is dependent on a good working relationship. These are the core aims of the consultation although the emphasis or principal aim will vary between patients and different consultations.

> **Establishing a good working relationship, information exchange, formulating a diagnosis and management planning are core aims of the consultation**

Meeting the aims of the consultation requires method. Method provides the roadmap for the consultation, ensuring direction and structure. Method enables the HCP to use their clinical skills, experience and a knowledge of medicine and the basic sciences throughout the consultation to know what questions to ask or signs to look for to learn, understand and interpret the available information. Method helps bridge the divide between the clinical features and "textbook" knowledge. The different methods available and skills needed to meet the aims of the consultation are discussed in the first section of *The Expert Clinician.*

> **Relevant information needs to be learnt, understood and interpreted using method and available medical knowledge to meet the aims of the consultation**

In section two, the application of method to the consultation is described. In *The Expert Clinician,* all consultations start with introductions and finish with a concluding conversation, documenting relevant information and agreeing and implementing a management plan. These are discussed in two separate chapters. The bulk of the consultation focuses on exchanging information relevant to meeting the aims of the consultation. Learning and understanding information about the person, the person as a patient, the problem and from the examination are described in separate chapters for convenience rather than to proscribe a set sequence: the focus and format will vary between patients and between consultations. For most patients with a new problem, asking questions to learn and understand the details of the problem or examining the patient to look for signs is the priority and takes up most of the consultation. For some patients, learning about their co-morbidity and any medications they are taking and the impact an ongoing illness has on the patient is the focus. For some problems, such as when a patient presents with a superficial abnormality, deformity or a mass, an examination of the abnormal part is the focus and is undertaken before learning about the problem. It is not uncommon for a consultation to switch backward and forward between topics during the consultation in response to the patient or information learnt (Figure 1). This is recognised by expert clinicians who use a flexible approach, different from the traditional format.

Figure 1: Illustrating a flexible approach to the consultation

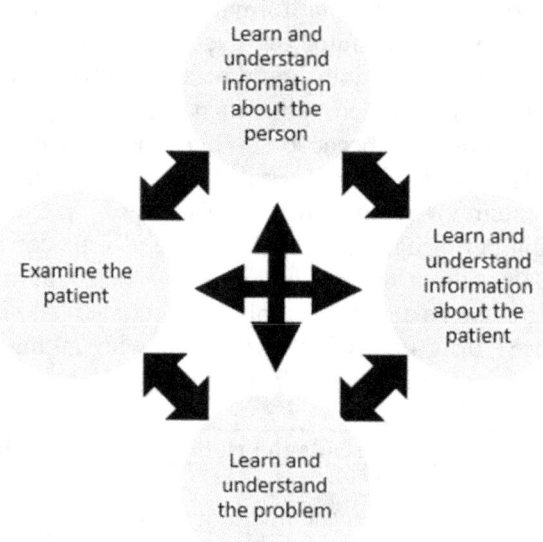

When the principal aims of the consultation are to formulate a diagnosis and plan management, learning about the problem and the examination are the principal parts of the consultation. The symptoms and signs may be pathognomonic or fit a classic pattern and the diagnosis apparent. However, as is more often the case, there is uncertainty. In which case, experts ask questions or look for signs with purpose, rather than as a routine. They know why they are asking a question or examining a patient and ensure they get the answers they need to learn and understand. Questions are asked and signs sought to formulate a diagnosis and plan management and possible diagnoses or management options are used to inform the questions to ask or signs to look for. Therefore, before asking the patient a question or examining part of the patient, it is necessary to ask yourself why you are asking the question or examining the patient.

> **A knowledge of medicine and the basic sciences should not only inform the questions to ask and the signs to look for but should also be used to understand and interpret the information from the patient**

Formulating a diagnosis is based on probabilities, pattern recognition and understanding the location and patho-physiology of the underlying abnormality. Relevant information, including important negatives, is co-located or linked to form an opinion and as evidence for a diagnosis and a management plan. In this way learning to understand bridges the divide between the clinical features and "textbook" knowledge.

Planning management in the best interests of the patient is not only dependent on learning and understanding information about the problem and identifying relevant signs but also on learning and understanding information about the person and the person as a patient. Each patient is unique, with their own thoughts, feelings and opinions, their own family, social and cultural relationships and their own medical background. The more information learnt during the consultation the more likely the diagnosis will be correct and the management appropriate. The right tests can then be requested and the results correctly interpreted. The right treatment can be given and the treatment will be appropriate for the patient.

> **Learning about the person ensures the patient is treated as a person with a problem and not just as a complaint. Learning about the person as a patient ensures co-morbidity, safety concerns and risk factors are considered**

The aims of the consultation, the patient and the information learnt from talking to the patient determine whether an examination is indicated and the aims, focus and format of the examination. When an examination is indicated the site of the problem is usually examined first and then, when indicated, other parts of the body are examined to look for associated or systemic signs. Usually, an examination should not be undertaken systematically as a routine in the hope that a sign will be recognised. Rather, signs should be pro-actively sought, understood and interpreted together with information learnt from talking to the patient.

> **The better the quality and the quantity of the information learnt during the consultation the more likely the diagnosis will be correct and the management appropriate**

A properly managed consultation will reassure the patient that they are being listened to and give the patient hope; hope that they will be helped and cared for. It will ensure relevant information is learnt, understood and interpreted correctly and appropriate and relevant information shared with the patient so that the patient can be managed properly and appropriately. It is the springboard to a pathway of care and to getting the right treatment for the patient. It will have lasting value not only because the agreed management plan is more likely to be appropriate for the patient but also because the patient is more likely to adhere and comply with future care.

Overview

Section 1: The methods available and skills needed for a meaningful consultation

Chapter 1: The methods available and skills needed to establish a working relationship

The consultation is the opportunity to establish a rapport with the patient, to enable the exchange of relevant and appropriate information. A well-prepared consultation organised by a functioning and effective team will lay the foundation for a good working relationship. It is then the responsibility of the HCP to use the consultation to maintain or build the relationship. The conduct of the consultation and, in particular, first impressions, are important. Giving the right impression, listening with empathy and understanding all help build a working relationship. A good working relationship is based on trust and gives the patient confidence; confidence to talk and confidence that they will be cared for. In a minority of patient's barriers need to be overcome and expectations managed. In this chapter the methods available and some of the skills needed to establish a working relationship are discussed.

Chapter 2: The skills needed and methods available to exchange information

Information exchange is about sharing relevant and appropriate information to meet the aims of the consultation. It is not enough to simply ask a series of questions or undertake an examination in the hope of learning something. Questions should be asked and signs sought to learn and understand the information to meet the aims of the consultation. This ensures the consultation is meaningful, so that it is not only a transaction, in which information is exchanged, but it is also transformational leading to an outcome that will help the patient.

Knowing what questions to ask or what signs to look for and understanding and interpreting the information is complex. Active deep listening skills are essential to learn all the available information from what is said, the way it is said and what is left unsaid. Conversational intelligence is needed to know what questions to ask and when and how to ask them and emotional intelligence to understand the patient's thoughts and feelings, wishes and expectations and the impact the problem is having on them. Examination skills are needed to know how best to identify, understand and interpret signs and to have the confidence to know when they are absent. Cognitive skills and a knowledge of medicine and the basic sciences are needed to know what questions to ask or signs to look for, to analyse, interpret and organise the information. Method makes best use of these skills. In this chapter the methods available and some of the skills needed to exchange information during the consultation are discussed.

Chapter 3: The methods available to formulate a diagnosis

Medical textbooks are usually organised anatomically, by tissue, organ or system, or by pathology, to explain the anatomical basis for disease, to demonstrate how pathology can arise and to explain the classic diagnostic symptoms and signs, investigations and treatments. Formulating a diagnosis is challenging because in clinical practice there is a need to reverse this process. Occasionally, the patient's description of their problem includes a pathognomonic or trigger symptom or sign that signposts a diagnosis or is consistent with a diagnostic pattern. Usually, however, the available information is presented in a chaotic or ambiguous way and the diagnosis is uncertain or the differential diagnosis long. In which case, relevant symptoms and signs need to be correctly learnt, understood and interpreted to formulate a diagnosis. For some patients, the symptoms or signs indicate a possible pattern or a short list of possible diagnoses. Sometimes, the combination of demographic information and the clinical features exclude many diagnoses and indicate a likely diagnosis. This then signposts the questions to ask or signs to look for to confirm or exclude a diagnosis. When uncertainty remains, learning and understanding the available information should be used to determine the location of the abnormality causing the problem and the type of problem. Linking information, including the symptoms and signs and information about the person, the patient and the problem can indicate a cause and a likely diagnosis or a short list of possible diagnoses. Formulating a diagnosis requires the right skills, method and medical knowledge to learn, understand and interpret relevant information. In this chapter the methods available and some of the skills needed to formulate a diagnosis are discussed.

Chapter 4: The methodology for planning management

Method and a knowledge of medicine should also be used to inform management. Planning management is a choice. A choice between reassurance and discharge, between different investigations or between different treatments, and whether to organise a follow up consultation or make a referral to another HCP. Choosing the right management option is determined by the aims, the indications, the benefits and risks, guidelines and MDT recommendations and, importantly, the opinion of the patient. Management options should be considered while learning and understanding available information so relevant information informs management and management options inform what needs to be learnt. To ensure management is appropriate it is important to learn about the person and about the person as a patient and to explain and discuss management recommendations. An agreed management plan should be the outcome of the consultation. In this chapter the methods available and some of the skills needed to plan management are discussed.

Section 2: Application of a clinical method to the consultation

Chapter 5: Starting the consultation

A consultation does not happen by chance and without purpose: every consultation needs to be organised and prepared. Before meeting the patient, the HCP should know the context of the consultation within the care pathway and the available information about the patient.

All consultations start with an introductory conversation and learning the headline information, which includes relevant demographic information, information known about the patient, the context of the consultation, first impressions and information about the problem. Introductions are an opportunity to welcome the patient, to check details, to make an initial assessment of the patient, to establish a rapport and to set the tone of the consultation. This is usually followed by asking the patient to describe their presenting problem or the HCP summarizing the reason for the consultation. This information determines the aims and the initial focus of the consultation. In this chapter the start of the consultation is discussed.

Chapter 6: Learn and understand information about the person

In *The Expert Clinician,* the emphasis is on caring for the patient as a person with a problem and not just as a "complaint". Each patient is unique, with their own thoughts, feelings, experiences, wishes, needs, hopes, expectations and opinions. Learning about the patient as a person with a problem and talking to them with respect, openness and honesty shows you care about them as an individual. This will help establish a rapport, build trust and put the problem in context, giving it an identity. For some patients, information learnt about the person will inform the diagnosis and management.

For most patients, learning about the person is undertaken as part of an "everyday" or "cosmetic" conversation during the introductions because it is unnecessary to learn detailed personal information about the patient. For a minority, it is appropriate to learn and understand relevant detailed personal information, such as about their home circumstances, lifestyle, close relationships, functional performance, quality of life or their personal views, beliefs and expectations. Personal information should only be learnt if it is relevant to meeting the aims of the consultation. In this chapter learning and understanding information about the person is discussed.

Chapter 7: Learn and understand information about the person as a patient

Learning about the person as a patient is both to document relevant ongoing and past medical conditions and their treatments, medications being taken, safety concerns and risk factors, and to inform the diagnosis and management. When a patient is "fit and well", learning about the person as a patient is simply a check and may be undertaken during the introductions. Nevertheless, the information, including important negatives, should be documented. On the other hand, when the patient has complex medical needs, learning and understanding information about the person as a patient may be the focus of the consultation because it is relevant to the presenting problem or management. In this chapter learning and understanding information about the person as a patient is discussed.

Chapter 8: Learn and understand information about the problem

Learning about the problem is the opportunity to learn the details of the problem, to understand the problem and to interpret the information to formulate a diagnosis and plan management. For most patients presenting with a new problem learning the details of the problem is the focus of the consultation. In this chapter learning and understanding information about the problem is discussed.

Chapter 9: Learn and understand information from the examination

An examination should be undertaken when it is indicated and it is safe and appropriate. The indications and the aims are determined by the context of the consultation, the patient and the information learnt from talking to the patient. The information learnt during the consultation should inform the signs to look for. Most examinations start by examining the site of the problem. Then, if indicated, the examination may include looking for associated or systemic signs. The examination findings may indicate additional questions to ask. In this chapter learning and understanding information from the examination is discussed.

Chapter 10: Concluding the consultation

The concluding conversation is undertaken with the aims of checking that all relevant information has been learnt and correctly understood, relevant information is shared with the patient and the recommended management plan agreed with the patient. For the patient, the concluding conversation may be as important as the rest of the consultation both because it is likely to be the only part the patient remembers and because it is when a management plan is finally agreed. In this chapter, the methods used to conclude the consultation and the next steps are discussed.

Section 1
The Methods Available and Skills Needed for a Meaningful Consultation

Chapter 1
The Methods Available and Skills Needed to Establish a Working Relationship

Abstract

A good working relationship is both a core aim of the consultation and a pre-requisite for a meaningful consultation. It enables the sharing of information, without which it is not possible to formulate a diagnosis or plan management. The quantity and quality of the information exchanged is dependent on a good working relationship: the better the rapport, the more likely the patient will talk freely and frankly and the more likely the outcome will meet the needs, wishes and expectations of the patient and the aims of the consultation. A good working relationship not only benefits the consultation but also the pathway of care.

A well-organised well-managed consultation will lay the foundation for a good working relationship. First impressions, the way the patient is welcomed and the introductory conversation set the tone for the rest of the consultation. A good start is likely to lead into a relaxed and meaningful consultation, whereas if the organisation or start are difficult or problematic the rest of the consultation is likely to be challenging.

A consultation that is managed well will give the patient the opportunity to talk about themselves, their medical background and the presenting problem. If we listen with empathy, we show we care and want to help. It will re-assure the patient that they have been listened to, that the HCP has understood their problem and that they will be helped. The patient should be and should feel that they are the focus of the consultation. Asking permission before discussing personal matters, such as a patient's thoughts or feelings, shows respect and empowers the patient. After all, they can say no. Behaviour, the words used, the tone and style can be very important. If we like someone, we are more likely to get on with them. If we trust someone, we are more likely to share personal information with them. If we respect someone, we are more likely to listen to their opinion.

For a minority of patient's, a concern or a barrier to a working relationship may be apparent at the outset or become manifest during the consultation. These need to be managed when they are relevant to the consultation or the pathway of care. Frequently acknowledging and listening to the patient's concerns and providing an explanation or an apology is sufficient to overcome a barrier. When the concern is more complex, an in-depth discussion may be indicated so that they can be addressed. Successfully managing concerns or barriers is dependent on a good working relationship, trust, respect and good communication.

The consultation is of particular importance in establishing a good relationship, although every aspect of the care pathway, from the time of referral to discharge should contribute. The start of the consultation sets the tone and expectations for the consultation and the concluding conversation sets the tone and expectations for the rest of the care pathway. A successful consultation is likely to ensure a reservoir of good which will benefit the rest of the pathway.

Introduction

"He cures most successfully in whom the people have the greatest confidence".
(Galen)

The consultation is dependent on a good working relationship in which the patient feels safe and comfortable and is able to talk freely in confidence about personal matters and the HCP is able to do their job. Establishing and maintaining a good working relationship is essential for a successful consultation and helps establish a reservoir of "goodwill" for the future. Without a good working relationship, a meaningful exchange of information will be difficult or incomplete and the consultation likely to be unsuccessful or unhappy with implications for the rest of the care pathway.

Building a working relationship is a process. It is always a work in progress that starts with the referral and continues throughout the consultation and the pathway of care.

Every aspect of the care pathway, from the time of referral to the end, should contribute to building a working relationship

We each have a unique identity and all want to be treated as an individual. Our personal thoughts and feelings, experiences and memories, beliefs, wishes, fears, expectations and desires influence our opinions, impressions and perceptions, including whether or not we like someone, trust and respect them. If we like someone, we are more likely to get on with them. If we trust someone, we are more likely to share information with them. If we respect someone, we are more likely to listen to them, believe them and follow their advice.

The aim of this chapter is to discuss the methods available to establish a working relationship.

Determine the Aims of Establishing a Working Relationship

Establishing a good working relationship is in itself a core aim of the consultation. However, it is an enabler, because the aim of establishing a good working relationship is to create an environment that enables the full and frank exchange of information. A meaningful exchange of information is more likely if the patient has a good rapport with the HCP, feels safe and relaxed, trusts the HCP, is able to talk freely and is confident the HCP will do everything they can to help them. A good working relationship established during the consultation is also likely to have benefits for future care, including adherence and compliance with management. In summary the aims of establishing a good working relationship are:

- To help the patient relax
- To build trust
- To ensure the patient feels they are being treated as an individual and that they are valued and respected
- To show the HCP cares and wants to help
- To enable information exchange
- To plan management
- To increase the likelihood of adherence and compliance with future care

Determine Whether Establishing a Working Relationship Is Indicated?

A good working relationship is a sine qua non for a successful consultation and care pathway. For most patients a working relationship is assumed but for some patients, such as some children, patients with special needs or people who have previously had a bad experience with health care, establishing a working relationship may be the primary aim of the consultation.

At all times the relationship should be professional; a "working" relationship. A more personal or friendly relationship between the patient and the HCP is contra-indicated and, if the relationship is already a close one, such as with another family member, the consultation is contra-indicated because there is a risk personal emotions, thoughts and feelings will influence care.

The Importance of the Pre-Consultation Organisation to Forming a Good Working Relationship

The process of establishing a good working relationship starts before the consultation happens, from the time the referral is made (Figure 2).

Scheduling a consultation, effectively communicating with patients, ensuring patients are seen in the right place by the right people at the right time requires competent staff, good cooperation and collaboration. A well organised, timely consultation has a positive impact on the patient. It not only ensures the patient and the HCP know when, where and why the consultation is occurring but also lays the foundation for a good working relationship. Problems with the organisation of the consultation are likely to have a negative impact on the patient and adversely affect the consultation and the working relationship. It is not uncommon for pre-consultation problems to undermine a patient's confidence in the health care system and the HCP and cause lasting harm to future care.

The HCP is but one member of a multi-disciplinary team working within a complex health care system. Potentially everyone has an impact on the working relationship either directly or indirectly. Good working relationships are required to ensure the pathway of care is efficient and responsive to change. Inter-personal difficulties between team members may not only adversely affect the organisation of the consultation but also the pathway of care, and are often detected by patients.

All consultations should be conducted in an appropriate setting, with the right staff and the right equipment available. The consultation should be safe for both the patient and the staff. The consultation should be private and not overheard by others. If the consultation occurs behind a curtain or partition there is privacy from sight but not sound. This should be remembered at all times.

Figure 2: Illustrating the organisation required for a consultation

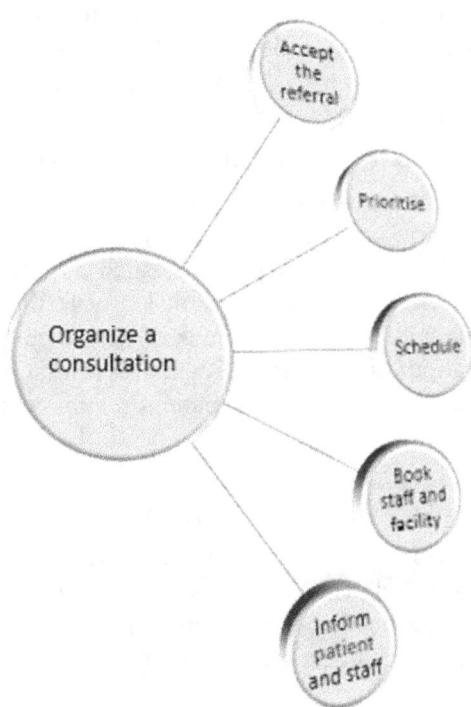

Use the Consultation to Establish a Working Relationship

The consultation should establish a working relationship to enable all relevant information to be exchanged with the aim of helping the patient. A consultation that is managed well will give the patient the opportunity to talk about themselves, their medical background and the presenting problem. It will re-assure them that they have been listened to, that the HCP has understood their problem and that they will be helped. A consultation that is well managed and successful will establish a reservoir of good will for the rest of the pathway of care. Every aspect of the consultation should contribute to establishing or maintaining a good working relationship (Figure 3).

Figure 3: Using the consultation to establish a good working relationship

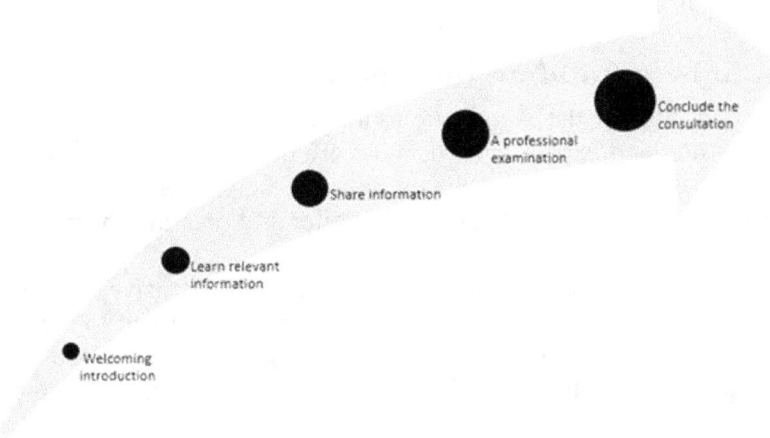

Use the introductions and headline information to establish a working relationship

The start of the consultation is very important for establishing a working relationship.

Introductions that are courteous and suit local convention show respect for the patient. A check of basic details, such as name and age and what the patient wants to be called ensures there are no misunderstandings that could undermine a working relationship. An initial conversation about something neutral and non-clinical will not only help the patient relax but also demonstrate that the patient is being treated as a person and not just as a problem.

The introductory conversation is not only an opportunity for the HCP to assess the patient but also is an opportunity for the patient to assess the HCP. How we appear and behave is likely to influence the working relationship. First impressions frequently influence trust, rapport and our willingness to share information.

Learn about the person to help build a working relationship

For most patients, a working relationship is assumed and learning about the person is undertaken only as part of an introductory social conversation. When nothing unexpected is revealed or is likely the focus of the consultation is on learning about the problem. However, for a minority of patients, such as when a patient appears very anxious or distressed or appears suspicious, angry or withdrawn, information learnt at the start or during the consultation may indicate a need to learn more about the patient as a person, to break down barriers and establish a working relationship. Learning about the person shows you care about them as an individual. It re-assures them that important aspects of their personal life are factored in. It also ensures the HCP and the patient's aims and expectations are aligned. This is an important part of informed consent.

Learn about the person as a patient to help build a working relationship

Learning about the person as a patient will ensure relevant medical information, including safety concerns are not only known by the HCP but also are documented. This is often very reassuring for the patient. Information about the person and about the patient together can be used to understand the impact illness is having on them. This will demonstrate empathy and may inform some of the questions to ask or signs to look for.

Learn about the problem to help build a working relationship

Most patients are reassured when someone listens to them. Listening with understanding and empathy demonstrates the HCP cares and re-assures them that they will be cared for. It is fundamental to a good working relationship. A good working relationship is seriously undermined if the patient believes the HCP does not care.

Share information with the patient

People usually want to know more about their problem and what the HCP thinks. This may include an explanation, a diagnosis or an assessment. People hope to be reassured that nothing is seriously wrong or that they can be treated. Some people are reassured when they are told the diagnosis, provided with an explanation for their symptoms and given some recommendations or advice for the future. If the diagnosis or nature of the problem is unclear to the HCP it is important to be honest and to tell the patient. Sharing information with the patient builds trust. On the other hand, withholding information may undermine trust.

Use the examination to help build on the working relationship

As with other parts of the consultation, the examination should be used to help build a working relationship. Talking with the patient, asking permission and explaining what you are going to do from the start of the examination and throughout the examination shows respect for the patient and will help a patient relax. A professional examination should give the patient confidence that they are being looked after and reassure them that the HCP is competent and thorough.

Even though most patients expect to be examined it is intrinsically intrusive and may be very embarrassing or uncomfortable for some. This should be recognised and the examination tailored to the individual. A chaperone will help but if the patient perceives an examination or a part of the examination to be unnecessary, inadequately or incompetently performed, inappropriately intrusive or caused them distress it may undermine the working relationship.

Use the concluding conversation to consolidate the working relationship

The concluding remarks may be the only things the patient remembers. Therefore, just as the start is important to establishing a working relationship to enable a meaningful consultation so the concluding conversation is important for the rest of the care pathway. A consultation should be concluded in a way that leaves the patient feeling reassured that they have been listened to, that their problem has been taken seriously and that something will be done to help them.

A successful consultation should leave the patient feeling better for having had the consultation. A good working relationship established during the consultation not only benefits the consultation but also the future pathway of care. Good documentation helps with future management. An incorrect, incomplete or inappropriate record that becomes apparent during a future consultation may compromise the relationship.

Impressions and Perceptions

For many patients' the impression we give the patient and how we are perceived profoundly influence the working relationship. Giving the right impression is important but how we are perceived is more important. Personal opinion is frequently more influential than the reality or facts. For example:

- We may be trustworthy, but does the patient trust us?
- We may command respect with our colleagues, but does the patient respect our opinion?
- We may try to be very nice, but does the patient like us?
- We may work very hard on behalf of a patient, but does the patient think so?
- If we are liked by the patient, they are more likely to tolerate things going wrong.
- The HCPs intended aim may be perceived differently; it may be misunderstood or misconstrued.
- When the expected outcome is achieved, yet it is not the outcome the patient expected and does not meet expectations.

We have our own thoughts, feelings and emotions, and this includes who we like and what we like. A good rapport or good inter-personal "chemistry" helps a working relationship: if we like someone, we are more likely to get on with them, we are more likely to believe them and we are more likely to do what they recommend. Although professionally, it is not essential for the HCP and the patient to like one another and competence, efficiency, organisation, trust and respect are probably more important, it does help if the HCP and patient like one another.

There is no magic formula to establishing a working relationship; it comes easily to some people but not to everyone. We each have our own style or method and our style needs to adapt to the patient, the problem and the context. The style that works is the right way. If it doesn't work then it was the wrong way. A good start to the consultation and a favourable first impression is important but so is the rest of the consultation. A consultation that is managed appropriately and professionally, conforming to the patients' expectations, is likely to build on the working relationship.

Learning about the person and the person as a patient shows the HCP is interested in them as an individual, learning about the problem and examining the patient with empathy and understanding shows the HCP cares and wants to help. Throughout the consultation the patient should feel they are being listened to and respected, that they are the focus of attention and that the HCP will do everything they can for them. The patient should recognise the questions asked are relevant and believe the answers are listened to. They should know the examination is relevant and appropriate. Together this builds trust. The content and conduct of the conversation and the examination, the words used, the tone, the behaviour, the timing and style are all very important. The wrong impression will undermine the working relationship.

There are many ways an HCP can give the wrong impression. For example, if the HCP appears rushed or seems distracted or is perceived as being disinterested, disorganised, arrogant or uncaring. For some HCPs, such as a specialist with a unique skill, or in some consultations, such as when the patient knows the HCP already or when the care goes well this may not have a negative impact. However, in general, when an HCP behaves like a prima donna or disregards the importance of developing a good working relationship it may be regretted later, particularly if the care does not go as well as hoped.

Build Confidence and Trust

Patients consult an HCP because they want help with a problem and hope that the HCP will be able to help them. The consultation is the opportunity to give them confidence that they can be helped and will be helped. A successful consultation is dependent on the patient being confident in the HCP and trusting the HCP.

Instilling confidence is a process which starts from the time of first referral and continues throughout the pathway of care. A well-managed referral and an organised consultation is the first stage in building confidence. A well-managed, professional consultation in which the HCP is self-assured, organised, thorough, competent and efficient, demonstrating understanding, care, empathy, knowledge, direction and authority, who commands respect is likely to instil confidence in the patient and their family that they are "in the right hands", in "safe hands", that they will be cared for and helped. A pathway of care which has the agreement and support of the patient, is efficiently organised and meets a patient's expectations further re-enforces confidence in the HCP and the health care system. Honouring commitments strongly influences confidence.

A good working relationship is dependent on mutual trust. The patient needs to trust the HCP and the HCP the patient. The HCP and the health care system trust that the patient will be open and honest with their information and cooperate, adhere and comply with management. The patient needs to trust that:

- The HCP and the rest of the health care team will do everything they can for them.
- The HCP will act in their best interests.
- The HCP has the necessary competencies.
- They will be treated with courtesy and respect.
- The HCP will listen.
- Any discussion will be in strict confidence.
- They will be informed of relevant information in an appropriate and timely way.

It takes a lot of trust for a patient to talk about personal matters, such as a personal problem or difficult and challenging personal circumstances, such as domestic violence, psychological, sexual or physical abuse. Trust also determines how much the patient believes and respects the opinion of the HCP, such as their ability to make a diagnosis, the importance of risk factors or predictions for the future. Adherence and compliance with recommendations, such as to change an aspect of their lifestyle, to have a risky invasive procedure or to take an unpleasant medication are all dependent on trust.

The ways the HCP can build confidence and trust include:

- Show respect.
- Share trust: "give trust to get trust".
- Show you care: show empathy.
- Be measured. Avoid appearing to rush the patient.
- Actively listen to the patient. Avoid interrupting the patient. Respond to the patients concerns.
- Show you understand. Do not make assumptions or appear to be biased.
- Show humility or vulnerability: admit when you don't know something or are wrong.
- Behave professionally. Avoid derogatory, flippant or off the cuff remarks. Avoid jokes or inappropriate humour. Do not try to be too clever. Avoid appearing selfish or arrogant.
- Keep the patient informed. Share information: explain what you think and why. Be honest.
- Plan management with the patient.
- Honour your commitments. Deliver on your promises. Avoid over-promising or making false promises.
- Take responsibility. Avoid blaming others or making derogatory remarks about others.
- Demonstrate teamworking.

Confidence and trust should never be taken for granted; they can be lost very quickly. Not only is it important to build confidence and trust but also to avoid pitfalls that may undermine confidence and trust. Examples of how confidence and trust can be compromised include:

- If the preparation prior to a consultation is disorganised, with excessive delays, changes, cancellations and miscommunication. Frustration, irritation and anger all undermine trust.
- When there are adverse external factors, such as adverse publicity, pre-conceived ideas held by the patient, or an unfavourable opinion or experience of family or friends.
- When the consultation is difficult or problematic.
- Failure to honour your commitments.
- When there is a perception, you do not care.
- Not keeping the patient informed.
- When the outcome is unexpected, unwanted or there are unexpected side effects or complications.
- When there is misunderstanding, confusion or disagreement during the pathway of care.
- When you forget. For example, forgetting important information about the patient or forget to organise a test.

When a patient has lost confidence or trust in the HCP or health care system it is difficult for it to be regained. If, during the consultation, it becomes apparent, or there is suspicion that confidence or trust is in doubt or has broken-down this should be recognised and managed. Recognising and acknowledging the concern is an important start to restoring confidence and trust. Managing a breakdown takes time and is frequently dependent on a consistent pattern of words and actions over time.

The importance and potential benefits of re-establishing trust are profound. The thoughts and feelings of the patient, the conduct of the consultation and engagement with the care pathway are all dependent on the patient having confidence and trust in the HCP and the health care system. Confidence and trust established during the consultation will be a reservoir of goodwill likely to benefit the rest of the care pathway.

Ask Permission

Permission is when the patient allows or authorizes something. Permission should be given voluntarily without undue pressure, coercion or manipulation. Permission empowers the patient because they are able to withdraw permission at any time. Asking permission shows respect for the patient's autonomy and helps build a working relationship. For some patients, a working relationship is necessary before they will give permission.

A meaningful information exchange is dependent on the permission of the patient. During the consultation a patient chooses what to say and what not to say, what information to divulge and what to keep secret. In other words, the patient only says what they want to reveal. Nevertheless, for some patients and for some topics, such as when asking about a thought or feeling, expressing an opinion or making a recommendation it is good practice to check the patient gives their permission.

If there is uncertainty about whether asking permission is indicated, then it is indicated

The questions to ask could include,

Is it OK if we talk about…?
Can I ask you about…?
Would you like to tell me about…?
Do you feel able to tell me more?

Medically, consent describes the process of obtaining permission from a patient. Consent not only protects the patient but also the HCP. It is part of shared decision making. Sharing ownership shares responsibility and will help the HCP have a clear conscience. Consent is not only needed for a treatment, such as an invasive procedure, but also during the consultation. For example, before examining a patient or undertaking a procedure. It is a "process" because, for permission to be valid, the patient needs to be given relevant information, be able to understand and consider the information and be able to remember the information. Patients should be given the information they need in a way they understand and the time and support they need to understand it. To ensure the information is appropriate, the HCP should try to find out what matters to the patient so they can exchange relevant information about the benefits and harms of proposed options and reasonable alternatives, including the option to refuse or take no action. Permission and consent are only valid within the scope of what was agreed: they are not transferable and can be withdrawn at any time.

Most adults have the capacity to make decisions about their care. When a patient lacks capacity, the care must be of overall benefit to them. In which case, decisions and consent should be made in consultation with those who are close to them or advocating for them and be in accord with legal requirements.

If there is uncertainty about whether the patient has the capacity to give their informed consent, prove they have the capacity

Verbal permission or "expressed consent" is usually sufficient but it has the disadvantage that there is no documented evidence that the consent process has been properly undertaken unless another HCP, such as a chaperone, is a witness. For many interventions, particularly if there is the potential for harm or distress written consent is indicated.

If there is uncertainty about whether verbal or written consent is indicated, then written consent is needed

Show Empathy

Professional knowledge and understanding, critical thinking, efficient organisation and decision making are important for a meaningful consultation but so is empathy. Empathy is a pro-social behaviour that demonstrates both inter-personal understanding and care. Empathy is the ability to recognise, to sense and share the thoughts and feelings of another. It is more than sympathy, when you feel sorry for someone, because it includes understanding and responding: understanding what it is like for them physically, emotionally and psychologically, and responding appropriately to their situation, their thoughts and feelings. For example:

- When a patient is in severe pain or very breathless validating the severity of their pain is important but going out of your way to initiate urgent treatment shows you care.
- Responding sympathetically to a patient's distress by not only showing appropriate emotions, such as sadness or concern, but also by being patient and giving the patient space and time.

All patients have a problem they are worried about and most are also worried about the consultation, the HCP and what they might think or what might happen. They may be slightly anxious or nervous or very stressed, even terrified. A few are defensive or wary and occasionally even angry or hostile. Such emotions may be obvious at the outset but some are only revealed during the consultation. Empathy is needed to recognise and understand these emotions and emotional intelligence is needed to acknowledge and manage them in an appropriate and timely way.

Appropriate body language, facial expressions and eye contact and asking meaningful questions shows you understand and care. It may be appropriate to make a comment or an observation such as:

That must have made [working] very difficult?
You must find it difficult [to get dressed in the morning]?

Showing you understand may include using meaningful comparisons. For example,

I expect the pain was as bad as a broken bone or child birth.
You must have felt as if you had lost a loved one.

Empathy includes not only an understanding of the severity and impact of the problem on the patient but also the impact the problem is having on their family. It may be appropriate to ask a question, such as:

How is this affecting your relationship?
Your [partner] must be very worried.

Sometimes, it is appropriate to give patient's the opportunity to share their thoughts, feelings and emotions. For example:

How does that make you feel?
You must feel very upset.

When there are obvious emotional issues, it is important to ensure the patient is given time to explain their thoughts and feelings. Listening carefully is an opportunity to connect with them. It shows you care and want to help. Thanking them shows you understand how difficult it is for them and how you appreciate them being open and honest.

To ignore a patient's emotions or to respond inappropriately risks aggravating a patient's distress, losing their trust and confidence and undermining the relationship. The patient may raise barriers, withdraw or become angry. Patients are left with a feeling of isolation, a loss of faith in the HCP, who clearly does not understand, and, if the HCP doesn't understand, the patient may question whether they will help them. A perception of being insensitive or uncaring will undermine any relationship no matter what the intention. Unfortunately, there are ways a normally caring HCP can appear to be uncaring, to lack empathy. For example:

- Appearing rushed.
- Appearing distracted.
- Being forgetful: repeating questions, or asking questions when the answer has previously been given.
- Lack of attention, such as when thinking about other problems.

- Interruptions during the consultation.
- Expressing inappropriate personal emotions.
- Downplaying or belittling the significance of a problem.
- Not recognising the significance of the emotion.
- Inappropriate behaviour or language, such as humour.
- Appearing to focus on the wrong issue.

The symptoms or consequences of illness, treatments and complications can be devastating for some patients. Emotional thoughts and feelings are natural for everyone but there is a fine line between empathy and emotional involvement by the HCP. As an HCP it is important to manage personal emotions, stresses and pressures associated with caring for others, without allowing them to adversely affect thought processes or performance. There are different strategies to help cope with difficult personal emotions arising from patient care including:

- Be professional at all times.
- Avoid becoming personally involved.
- Recognise the problem is their problem not yours.
- Focus on the patient not on yourself.
- Avoid putting yourself in their position or comparing their problem with your own.
- Maintain internal emotional barriers.
- Stay focused on the problem and the solutions rather than the emotions.
- Adopt a scientific approach.
- Do your best to help the patient. This ensures you will have a clear conscience.
- Discuss problems. Enlist support from other people, colleagues and other team members.
- Take breaks.
- Have relaxing distractions or hobbies, such as music, reading novels, a pet or exercise or practice an intervention such as meditation, yoga or mindfulness.
- Avoid getting tired, taking drugs or drinking alcohol to excess.

Being an HCP is not just a job, it is a way of life but it should not be a lonely one.

Sharing a problem helps manage a problem

Manage Barriers or Concerns

Barriers or concerns impact on the working relationship and impair the exchange of information. If during the consultation it becomes apparent that there may be a barrier or concern preventing a meaningful conversation it should be recognised and managed. A stepwise approach may help start the process (Figure 4).

Figure 4: A stepwise approach to managing a barrier or concern

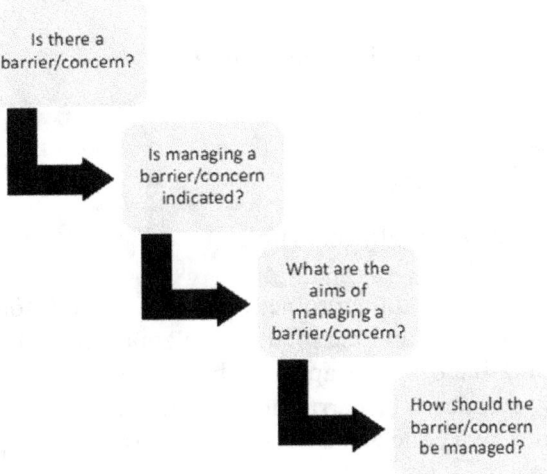

Ask yourself, is there a barrier or concern?

A barrier or concern may be expressed by the patient or suggested by the patient's behaviour, tone, facial expressions or body language. It may be apparent on first meeting the patient, such as when the patient is very frightened or anxious at the start of the consultation, or during the consultation, such as, when discussing management or the prognosis, benefits or risks.

Examples of barriers include:

- Children, teenagers and young adults are frequently suspicious and wary of strangers at first and are understandably initially reluctant to talk or cooperate.
- When a patient feels insecure or vulnerable it can be a barrier.
- Profound fear, anxiety or worry may be a concern.
- A patient's embarrassment may be a barrier.
- Some barriers are caused by ethnic, cultural or religious differences.
- When a patient is being threatened or intimidated it can be a barrier, particularly if they are victims of abuse or coercive behaviour.

Talking to the patient may signpost a problem. For example:

- The patient doesn't like the HCP specifically or health care generically.
- The patient doesn't trust the HCP specifically or health care generically.
- A patient may have a negative pre-conception about health care, such as when they have had a previous bad experience.
- The patient resents having to see an HCP or having a health problem.
- Some patients are very anxious about a risk or the risks.
- A patient may have inappropriate hopes and expectations. For example, some patients have an inappropriately optimistic or pessimistic expectation about their prognosis or life expectancy.
- A patient may be concerned about their age, life expectancy or quality of life. These are linked because our expectations change as we get older and our age and life expectation may influence expectations, such as about quality of life, and choices, such as risk-taking.
- A mental health condition can be a barrier to revealing the underlying cause of their condition.
- Some patients expect an investigation and are disappointed or concerned if one is not recommended.
- When a patient is upset if they do not get treatment for a problem or the treatment recommended is different from what they expected.

If a barrier or a concern is suspected,

Ask yourself, is managing a barrier or concern indicated and appropriate?

Managing a barrier or concern is indicated and appropriate when it is likely to affect:

- The patient. For example, causing disappointment or upset.
- The working relationship.
- Trust.
- The conduct of the consultation.
- The management planned.
- Future care, including adherence or compliance with care.

Information about the person, the patient and the problem can be used to inform whether managing the concern is indicated and to ensure the timing, the context and the method are appropriate. In general, talking about a concern or addressing a barrier is best done when it first becomes apparent because this is likely to be when the patient is receptive and ready to discuss it. Occasionally, a concern or barrier may need dedicated time in another consultation, a second opinion or specialist help from another HCP, such as a counsellor, a psychotherapist or a psychiatrist. In which case, this should be explained to the patient.

Before managing a barrier or concern:

Ask yourself, what are the aims of managing a barrier or concern?

The aims will be influenced by the nature of the barrier and the aims of the consultation. For example, they may include:

- Restore a compromised working relationship:
  - To restore confidence and trust.
  - To avoid a breakdown in the working relationship.
  - To reduce the risk of future disappointment or upset.
  - To maintain communication.
- Enable information exchange, such as when a patient is very shy or reticent about talking about their problem.
  - To formulate a diagnosis.
  - For informed consent.
  - To align expectations.
  - To help understanding.
- Inform management, such as:
  - To decide between options.
  - To agree on a plan.
  - To reduce the risk of a future problem.
  - Ensure compliance and adherence with future care.

When managing a barrier or concern is indicated:

Ask yourself, how should the barrier or concern be managed?

Managing a barrier or concern starts by recognising and then discussing the problem. Successfully overcoming a barrier or managing a concern does not happen by chance, it needs method (Figure 5).

If managing a barrier or concern is indicated, asking an open question will give the patient an opportunity to talk about the issue or to dismiss it. This is also a way of asking permission because a patient may not want to discuss the concern with the HCP at that time or stage in the consultation. It may be appropriate to ask:

Is there something you would like to talk about?
I sense there is something wrong, do you want to talk about it?
You seem very worried. Is that true?
Do you want to talk about what is worrying you?
Will you tell me what you are thinking?

There are many possible reasons for, or factors that may lead to, or influence, a barrier or concern. For example:

- An adverse previous experience may influence a patient's thoughts, feelings, opinions and expectations.
- A patient's hopes, fears or expectations about the likely outcome, such as whether or not they can be cured.
- The patient's personal goals or aspirations. For example, a patient may want to live long enough or be well enough to attend an impending marriage or birth.
- Personal values, faith, emotional, social and cultural opinions may influence the patient.
- The views of friends or family members may influence the patient. For example, it is not uncommon for elderly patients to want a treatment because that is what their family want for them.
- Psychological attitude to illness: some patients are optimistic, whereas others are pessimistic.

When listening to the patient's description of, or explanation for, the barrier/concern it is important to acknowledge the concern and show understanding.

Figure 5: A stepwise approach to restoring trust

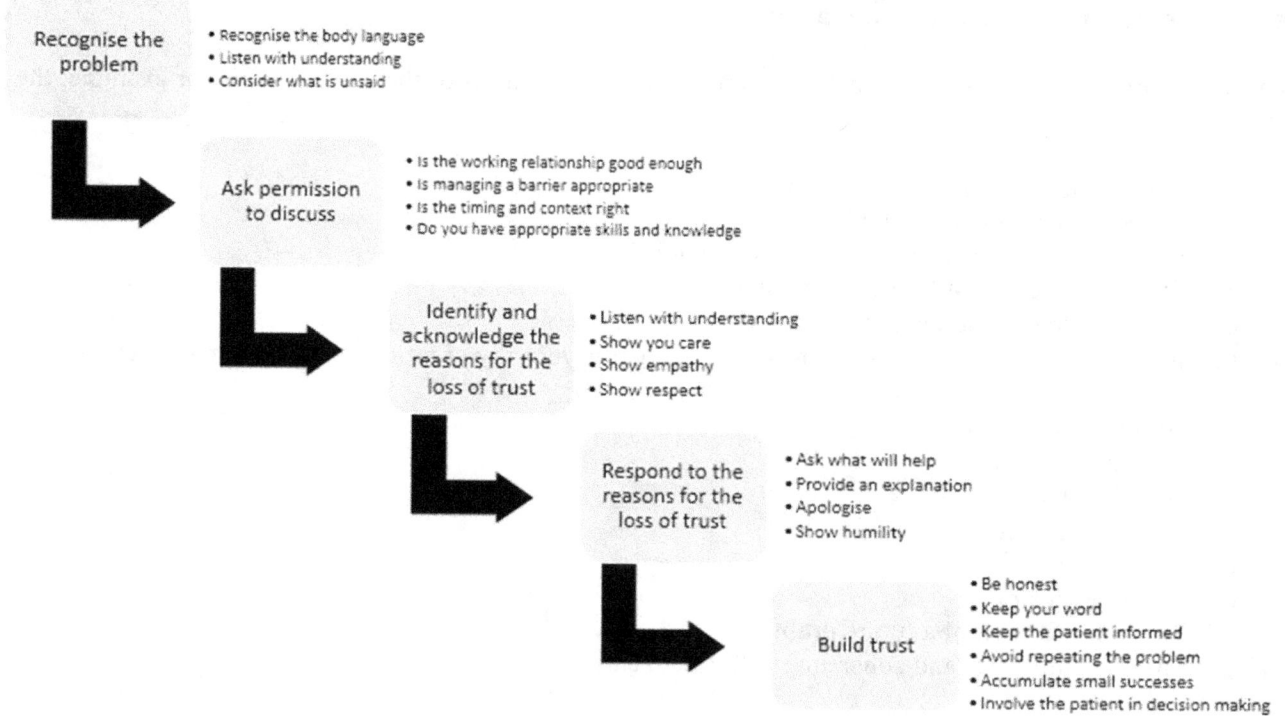

It is important not to assume the cause of their concern but to ask. For example:

Can you tell me why you think that?
Why were you expecting that?
What makes you think that?

It may be appropriate to ask leading questions. For example:

Do you think that because of your age?
Are you worried about the impact on your work/family?
Is it because of what happened to you before?

When listening, give the patient time to talk: silence is an opportunity for the patient to gather their thoughts and consider what to say. What you say is less important than listening to what they have to say. Listen in a friendly, supportive and caring way, showing appropriate empathy and understanding. Be respectful and avoid being judgemental or appearing to be dismissive and acknowledge their feelings. For example:

That must be very difficult.
I can understand your …
I am really sorry to hear …

It may be supportive to show gratitude that they have shared their thoughts and feelings with you. For example:

Thank you for telling me.
Thank you for trusting me
I'm glad you told me

Having learnt the cause for their concern or barrier the next step is to manage it. Before suggesting your own options, it may be appropriate to ask the patient:

What would help you?
I understand your concern, do you have any suggestions as to how I can help?

Sometimes, simply giving them the opportunity to talk about their concern is sufficient to manage a concern or break down a barrier. Sometimes acknowledging their concern and providing reassurance is appropriate. For example:

I know you are worried you have [cancer] but I want to reassure you that most people are cured with this treatment.
It is understandable to feel frightened, but I want to reassure you that the test only takes a couple of minutes and someone will be with you the whole time.

For some problems, an explanation is sufficient. Some patients are helped when mitigating measures are available. For example:

I know you were very sick after the last anaesthetic but treatments have improved a lot since then. If you tell the anaesthetist they will make sure you are given an effective treatment this time.

For some problems an apology is indicated. For example:

I am sorry you did not know you had to stop taking your [anti-coagulant] beforehand. It was re-assuring that this was checked so that you did not come to harm. I will re-organise the test immediately.

It may be appropriate to make a proposal based on the information learnt. For example:

- If there is misunderstanding, correct any misconceptions.
- If there is a lack of knowledge or understanding it may be appropriate to provide information in different ways. This may include providing written information, watching a video or talking to other patients.
- If there is a fear, provide reassurance. The patient may benefit from talking to another patient or another HCP.
- If there is choice, discuss the options.

If there is uncertainty, give the patient information and time to make a decision. A second opinion may be indicated.

Occasionally, a directive approach is indicated. For example:
- Telling the patient what they need. For example,
    You need a pacemaker.
- Telling the patient what is available. For example,
    This could be investigated by a colonoscopy or a CT scan
- Telling the patient what to expect.
    You will need to take medicine to clean your bowels

Managing a barrier or concern will help the working relationship both in the short term and the long term.

Chapter 2
The Skills Needed and Methods
Available to Exchange Information

Abstract

Information exchange refers to the HCP learning information from the patient and the HCP sharing information with the patient. It is both a core aim of the consultation and a pre-requisite to meeting the other aims of the consultation. Information exchange is meaningful when it is not only transactional, in which relevant information is learnt and documented but also transformational, in which information is understood and interpreted so that the outcome is of benefit to the patient. A meaningful exchange of information is likely to lead to a successful consultation and a successful consultation will reassure the patient and have lasting value later in the care pathway.

Conversation skills, examination skills and cognitive skills, method and a knowledge of medicine and the basic sciences are needed to learn, understand and interpret relevant information about the patient.

Conversation skills ensure appropriate and relevant questions are asked in a way the patient is likely to understand. Open questions give the patient the opportunity to talk about what they think is relevant, closed or leading questions focus on information the HCP thinks is important. Attentive listening ensures the information is learnt accurately and deep listening ensure it is properly understood and correctly interpreted. The consultation is not only the opportunity to listen to the patient but also to share information with the patient. Before sharing information, it is important to be well prepared. Knowing what and how much to tell patients is determined by the problem, the person, the context and timing.

When indicated, the examination is an important part of information exchange. The methods used should be appropriate to the sign and the part of the body being examined. Inspection and palpation are particularly useful when examining the limbs, face, neck, breasts and abdomen, whereas percussion and auscultation are most useful when examining the chest and blood vessels. Many signs are subjective and lack accuracy, being prone to inter-observer variation. Specialists often use tools to provide additional information when examining the patient. The accuracy of an examination is influenced by the patient, the skill of the examiner and the sign being sought. Some signs are reproducible with minimal inter-observer variation whereas others are more subjective and prone to inter-observer variation. The easier a sign is to identify, the lower the inter-observer variability and the more abnormal the sign is the more likely the sign is true.

Cognitive skills ensure relevant and appropriate questions are asked and signs sought so that the available information is not only learnt but also understood and interpreted correctly. Cognitive skills include the ability to critically analyse the information, organise the information and make decisions using the information. They enable diagnostic reasoning and management planning.

Method ensures information exchange is organised. It prevents the consultation from becoming chaotic, gives it direction and structure, ensuring all relevant information is learnt and appropriately linked to meet the aims of the consultation. The start of the consultation is the opportunity for introductions, to learn the headline information and to initiate the consultation. Learning about the problem is the key to understanding the problem, formulating a diagnosis and planning management. Learning about the person and the person as a patient ensures the person remains at the heart of the consultation and gives the problem an identity. Information learnt when talking to the patient should inform the focus and format of the examination and the signs to look for. The consultation is concluded with a conversation that includes recommending and agreeing a management plan. All relevant information should be documented.

Introduction

Information exchange refers to the HCP learning information from the patient and the patient learning information from the HCP. It is a means to an end: specifically, for the HCP to learn and understand information about the person, the patient and the problem and from the examination, with the aims of formulating a diagnosis and planning management and for the patient, to get an opinion and outcome that will help them.

"The less you talk, the more you are listened to."

Pauline Phillips

Information exchange is dependent on a good working relationship and a good working relationship is dependent on information exchanged. It is both an art and a science. The art is to facilitate the conversation or undertake the examination so that the patient trusts and feels comfortable with the HCP and feels able to share all relevant information. The science is to apply a knowledge of medicine and the basic sciences to know what to ask or what sign to look for, what is relevant and to understand and interpret the information to meet the aims of the consultation.

The HCP needs a range of different skills to learn and understand relevant information and to know what to share with the patient. These include conversation and examination skills, so that the relevant information is exchanged in a meaningful way, cognitive skills to know what questions to ask, what signs to look for and to understand and interpret the information correctly and method to ensure the consultation is efficiently managed, productive and not be chaotic, allowed to meander or be excessively long.

The aim of this chapter is to discuss the skills needed and methods available to achieve a meaningful exchange of information.

Determine the Aims of Information Exchange

Information exchange includes learning relevant and appropriate information about the person, the person as a patient, the problem and from the examination and sharing relevant information with the patient. Although information exchange is a core aim of the consultation, it is an enabler. This is because learning and understanding relevant information are with the aims of formulating a diagnosis and planning management. In addition, a meaningful exchange of information will contribute to a good working relationship, reassure the patient they are being listened to and will be cared for, inform the patient and is likely to help ensure adherence and compliance with future care. Therefore, before asking a question, examining the patient or sharing information with the patient:

Ask yourself, what is the aim?

In summary, the aims of information exchange include:

- To learn and understand available information.
- To document available information.
- To build a working relationship:
  - To inform the patient:
    - To explain symptoms or signs.
    - To suggest a cause, diagnosis or list of diagnoses.
    - About matters relevant to them. For example, lifestyle, risks and benefits.
    - The implications, risks and benefits, prognosis.
    - What to expect and what is expected of them.
    - As part of informed consent.
- To formulate a diagnosis:
  - To confirm a diagnosis.
  - To make a diagnosis.
  - To exclude a diagnosis.
  - To determine the location of the abnormality causing the problem.
  - To determine the type of problem.
  - To determine the cause.
  - To screen for:
    - Another abnormality.
    - A secondary abnormality.
    - A complication.
  - To assess:
    - Severity.
    - The impact on the patient.
    - Function.
    - Change, including to provide a baseline.
    - Future risk or prognosis.
- To plan management:

- Of the problem.
- Of the symptoms.
- Of the patient.
- Of the diagnosis.
- Of future risk.
- To share decision making and responsibility.

Determine Whether Exchanging Information Is Indicated

Indications and contra-indications are usually only considered in the context of investigations or treatment but they are equally relevant to information exchange. Before asking a question or examining a part of the body:

Ask yourself, is the question/examination indicated?

Asking a question or examining the patient is indicated when it meets the aims of the consultation, is relevant and appropriate and is not contra-indicated. An action is not indicated when it is unnecessary, inappropriate or the risks outweigh the benefits. For example:

- Learning the details of minor illnesses, such as an episode of chicken pox in the past, is unlikely to be relevant for most patients and is therefore not indicated. However, learning about previous chicken pox infection may be indicated when there is risk of exposure to an infected patient or for a pregnant female.
- Asking questions about a patient's sexual activity is not usually indicated. However, it may be indicated when the problem they are presenting with is likely to be a sexually transmitted disease.
- Examining an unaffected part of the body is usually not indicated. For example, performing a breast examination when a patient presents with abdominal pain. However, it may be indicated when cancer from a breast primary is included in the differential diagnosis.

Not asking a question or examining for a sign should be a deliberate decision, rather than an error of omission.
A question or an examination is contra-indicated when it should not be asked or undertaken. For example:

- Asking questions about clinically irrelevant private or intimate personal matters, a patient's finances or their political or religious beliefs is usually contra-indicated.
- Examining a patient when they have refused permission is contra-indicated.

Before sharing information with a patient:

Ask yourself, is sharing information with the patient indicated?

Sharing relevant information is almost always indicated. Patients own their problem: it is their problem not yours. Therefore, they have a right to know information about their problem. For example:

- Telling a patient what is wrong with them.
- Telling a patient how the problem came about.
- Demonstrating a sign.
- Telling a patient, the results of an investigation.

However, it is for the HCP to determine the details: sharing every detail is rarely indicated or appropriate.

Sharing information is contra-indicated when the patient refuses permission to be told. A relative contraindication is when the information may harm a patient.

Conversation Skills Needed for a Meaningful Exchange of Information

The conversation is usually the most important part of the consultation. It is the opportunity for the HCP to learn about the person, the patient and the problem and for the patient to learn from the HCP. For most problems, it provides most of the information needed to formulate a diagnosis, plan management and informs the examination. It ensures the problem is considered in context and relevant additional information is considered when formulating a diagnosis, planning management and undertaking an examination. It should be both transactional, in which information such as facts, reality, experiences, opinions, thoughts or feelings are exchanged and transformational because information is exchanged with purpose, to bring about change. In other words, it should be meaningful.

It is what is heard that is important, not what is said. In general, when talking to a patient:

- Speak clearly and speak to the person.
- Ensure your face can be seen while talking. Avoid turning your back to the patient or talking from behind a computer or a curtain.
- When a patient has difficulty with the local language an independent interpreter is needed.
- When a patient is unable to hold a meaningful conversation, such as patients with dementia or confusion, a guardian or advocate should be present.
- Use the right terminology. For example:
  o A "person with a disability" rather than a "handicapped person"
  o "Gay or lesbian" rather than "homosexual"
  o "Cross dresser" rather than "transvestite"
  o "Dual-heritage" or "bi-racial" rather than "half-caste"
  o "Black" rather than "coloured"
- Avoid:
  o Using non-inclusive language, such as "old man", "druggies", "alcoholics", "victim of", "suffer from", "black-list", "blind drunk", "able-bodied" or "deaf to our requests"
  o Avoid making personal or derogatory comments.
  o Avoid making personal or derogatory comments or criticising other professionals.
  o Avoid using technical or medical terms that the patient is unlikely to understand.
  o Avoid interrupting or finishing the sentence for the patient.
- Be patient; give the patient time to think and respond and time to say what they want to say. Don't rush or appear to rush the patient.

Often, it is not what is said that causes offence but the way it is said, what is not said and the context. Understanding and perception are influenced by many factors including a disability, a mental health condition, education, cultural and social background and previous experience, the context, the timing, the tone, the volume, facial expressions and body language. Facial expression and body language are non-verbal ways we communicate. Non-verbal communication, such as pupil size, gaze direction, blinking, eyebrows, facial wrinkles, lip movements, jaw or mouth opening convey many emotions including happiness/sadness, awareness/confusion, peace/anger, understanding/surprise, contentment/anxiety, contempt, desire, excitement or disgust. Enhanced processing skills are needed to correctly interpret facial expressions and body language because they are not always what they seem. For example

- A smile may be genuine, signalling happiness or approval, that they want to work with you, to be your friend, or may be a false happiness, sarcastic or cynical, or signal contempt or that you have fallen into a trap.
- A frown may signal misunderstanding and confusion or disapproval or unhappiness.
- A pout may be intended to show anger or annoyance, or to garner sympathy, to remedy an injustice or to look sexually attractive.
- Anger may be genuine or be used to make us feel defensive, to ensure we are taken seriously and the problem prioritised.
- Putting a hand up to cover the mouth may signal realisation or astonishment or be done to stifle a yawn or to hide an emotion.
- A clenched fist may indicate stress, anxiety, anger or be used to supress an emotion or to cope with pain, such as a wave of colic.
- Sitting up straight or leaning forward may signal interest and attentiveness but may be used to challenge or threaten.
- An open posture indicates friendliness and willingness to listen and cooperate. A closed posture, in which the arms and legs are crossed may be because that is how the patient feels comfortable, such as if they feel cold, or signal the patient feels insecure, defensive or threatened.

- Fidgeting and tapping fingers may be due to feeling uncomfortable in the chair or want to go to the toilet, or signal they feel excited, impatient, angry or irritated.

Misreading a patient's behaviour or emotions is likely to adversely affect the conversation and the working relationship. If there is uncertainty it may be appropriate to ask relevant questions.

The spoken conversation between the HCP and the patient is but one of many conversations taking place. In addition to the spoken conversation there are the unspoken conversations that go on in our minds when both the patient and the HCP are thinking about what they are going to say before it is said and thinking about what has been said afterwards. We may verbalise these thoughts or internal conversations or express them in other ways, such as silences, tone or through our facial expressions or body language or they may remain hidden.

A meaningful conversation needs both conversational and emotional intelligence.

Conversational intelligence is needed to know when to talk and when to listen, what to say and when, what questions to ask and how to ask them. It ensures the conversation is relevant and appropriate: sometimes factual and serious, sometimes light-hearted and friendly, sometimes sympathetic and understanding, but at all times professional, recognising and responding to the patients' thoughts and feelings. During the consultation most information is exchanged as fact with little emotion, but when there is a medical problem, it is natural to be emotional. Emotions may be expressed in many ways but when they are not expressed it does not mean they are not being felt. Emotional intelligence is needed to recognise and respond appropriately to emotions, even when they are not obvious. When they are expressed, the HCP needs to show professional empathy, when they are hidden, emotional intelligence and experience are needed to recognise their apparent absence. Listening to your own thoughts and feelings is an important start. Ask yourself,

What does your heart tell you?
How would you feel?

It may be appropriate to sensitively ask a leading question such as:

I expect you were very upset?
That must have caused you a lot of distress?

Conversely, the HCP should manage their own emotions and avoid becoming personally involved or allowing personal emotions to affect their judgement.

Ask the right questions

Throughout the consultation, the HCP should not only use method but also their knowledge of medicine and the basic sciences, experience and conversational and emotional intelligence, to determine what questions to ask. In other words, questions should be asked with a purpose and only when indicated. The HCP should know why they are asking a question and why they are asking that particular question. Questions asked should be appropriate to the context, use the right tone and show the right balance of factual knowledge, inquisitiveness and concern. Questions are more meaningful if they are concise; short and to the point. They should be asked in a way the patient is likely to understand and medical terms or abbreviations should be avoided. Open questions give the patient the opportunity to talk about the problem in their own words and to include what they think is relevant. An open question usually starts with, "*What...*", "*How...*", "*Are...*", "*Tell me...*" or "*Describe...*" For example:

What did you mean when you said...?
What makes it worse?
What helps?
How did it affect you?
Are there any aggravating/relieving factors?
Tell me what happened.
Describe what happened.

An open question may follow a statement, used to introduce the question. For example:

I heard you say you felt sick. What do you mean when you say you felt sick?

You said you felt hot and cold all over. Tell me more about what happened.

Open questions allow the patient to decide what information is relevant whereas with closed questions the HCP decides what is relevant. Closed questions may be indicated:

- To look for symptoms not mentioned.
- To confirm what has been stated.
- To exclude a symptom.
- To check understanding.
- To ensure the focus is on a topic the HCP thinks is important.

Closed questions usually start with *"Did you…"*, *"Do you …"*, *"Were you…"* or *"Have you…"*. For example:

Did you feel sick?
Do you mean you vomited?
Were you sick?
Have you ever been sick?

It may be appropriate to ask a seemingly unrelated question to complete a picture or exclude a symptom of diagnostic or management significance. For example:

Have you been abroad recently?
Have you eaten out?

A leading question may be indicated:

- When it is appropriate to show empathy or understanding.
- To confirm what has been stated.
- To focus on something the HCP thinks is important.
- To identify errors of omission or to exclude information.

A leading question may be a statement made with a rising tone or start with a statement, usually an opinion or a paraphrase of something the patient said, followed by a question. For example:

You must feel tired all the time.
That must have been very frightening.
That sounds really painful, you probably had to stop what you were doing.
You said you felt stiff. I expect you find getting up in the morning difficult.

Leading questions can mislead or introduce bias if a patient is inclined to agree rather than disagree.

It may be necessary to repeat questions at different times during the consultation or ask a similar question in a different way. The choice of words used, the gaps or silences, the context, their order, the emphasis, the delivery style, the volume, the tone and the associated facial expression and body language all contribute to a meaningful information exchange.

Patients should be given time to respond. Silence or gapping gives the patient time to answer a question, think of another piece of information or when a question resonates personally with the patient they may need time to consider it carefully. Gapping is an indirect way of asking a question because timely silences are frequently filled by the patient. It can be more informative than asking a question.

Listening to the answer is more important than thinking what to say next. It is not only important to ensure the words and phrases the patient uses are correctly understood but also that their meaning is understood. When a patient's response is ambiguous or unclear, it is important to ask questions to ensure understanding. This is particularly important when learning to understand. For example,

A patient may say "I can't swallow anything".

Ask yourself, what do they actually mean?

Swallowing is a complex process dependent on the desire to eat, the physical act of chewing and swallowing, a patent and functioning oesophagus, complex neuromuscular coordination, access to the stomach and gastric emptying. An open question could be asked such as:

What do you mean when you say you have "difficulty swallowing"?
Tell me exactly what happens after chewing your food.
What happens when you try to swallow food or drink?

Closed questions may be indicated, such as:

Does it affect both food and drink?
Does the food stick as it is swallowed? And if so, *where do you feel it sticks?*
Do you choke with some foods? Does it feel as if the food/drink has gone down the wrong way?
When the food is swallowed do you feel it go all the way down?
Does the food come back up? And if so, *when it comes back up, is it the same or different?*

Or a leading question such as:

That must make eating meat or vegetables difficult.
You are probably only able to eat soup or pureed foods?

- A patient may say they get a "sharp pain".

Ask yourself, what do they actually mean?

Does "sharp" indicate the character, as in a superficial cut or wound, i.e., a somatic pain, or does it refer to severity, a severe pain or to the onset, a sudden pain? An open question could be asked such as:

What do you mean by sharp?
Tell me more about your pain.

Alternatively, a closed question could be asked such as:

Do you mean the pain is severe?
Did the pain start suddenly?
Is it the same sort of pain you get when you cut yourself?

Or a leading question such as:

That must have been really painful.

Summarizing information is an important conversation skill. It can be used in many different ways:

- To focus on one particular symptom. For example:

You mentioned that you had a headache, felt sick and went hot and cold all over. Can you tell me more about your headache?

- To organise information. For example:

Can I check you first had abdominal pain, then your abdomen became bloated then you started to feel sick?

- To check for completeness. For example:
  You mentioned that you had a headache, felt sick and went hot and cold all over. Was there anything else?

- To check understanding. For example:

  Can I check you first felt a headache and then felt sick and went hot and cold all over?

- To restore focus to what is relevant when a patient's account includes irrelevant information such as who said what, or events, such as descriptions of what they or others were doing at the time.

  That's very interesting, but can you tell me more about...

Listening skills

For a meaningful conversation the HCP should ask relevant questions and listen carefully to the answers. Listen carefully to ensure all the available information is understood and there is no misunderstanding. Listen carefully to identify missing information or information withheld by the patient. Listen carefully to your own thoughts and feelings. Avoid distractions or diversions, such as thoughts about a family issue, a pressing work commitment, the time or a need to do other "jobs". Demonstrate an interest in what is said and show empathy; it is their time and their problem. Acknowledge the message and respond appropriately using facial expressions, eye contact, body language and reassuring, supportive or affirmative noises, such as "uh-huh", "yes" or "I understand". Listening is not only to learn information about the person, the patient and the problem but also to show understanding and compassion, to help build a working relationship.

Knowledge, experience and intelligence are used to critically analyse the information, to exclude the unnecessary or irrelevant, to understand and interpret the information, to look for patterns and associations, to prioritise, link and manage the information. It is also important to identify missing information. There are many reasons why not all the information is divulged including:

- It has been going on for a long time.
- It is not considered to be important or relevant by the patient.
- The patient has forgotten.
- The patient prefers to focus on another symptom. For example, a patient in severe pain may not include weight loss.
- The patient does not want to tell the HCP. For example, when the matter is embarrassing or of an intimate nature.

Gapping, volume, tone and their body language may indicate something is unsaid. Learning to understand, pattern recognition, checklists and asking questions to exclude a problem will help identify important omissions.

Share information with the patient

Information exchange is a dialogue. It is not only necessary for the HCP to learn relevant information from the patient but it is also important to ensure the patient is appropriately informed. Before sharing information with the patient ensure the context and timing is right. When the information is complex, meaningful, or may cause distress the patient should be accompanied by a friend or family member who is available to provide support for the patient and is more likely to remember what is said. Learn about the person to know about their background and potential barriers or challenges to ensure they have the knowledge and mental capacity to understand, retain and consider the information so that the content, the words, tone and empathy are appropriate. Ensure you have the skills to talk to the patient in an appropriate way. Know and understand relevant information so that you will be able to answer any questions. Decide on the aims and indications and consider the consequences.

Ask yourself, what is the aim?

The aims of sharing information with the patient include:

- To inform the patient.

- o   To help understanding.
- o   To explain symptoms or signs.
- o   To suggest a cause.
- o   About matters relevant to them. For example, lifestyle, risks and benefits.
- o   The implications, prognosis or future.
- o   What to expect and what is expected of them.
- o   As part of informed consent.
- o   For reassurance.
- To build a working relationship.
- To give an opinion.
  - o   An explanation.
  - o   The diagnosis or list of diagnoses.
  - o   The cause.
  - o   Risks and benefits.
- To make a recommendation.
- To share decision making and responsibility.

Sharing information done well will build trust and contribute to making the consultation meaningful. If it is done badly, the patient will remain uncertain, confused or even distressed, potentially causing harm, reducing trust and adversely affecting the working relationship.

Ask yourself, is sharing information indicated?

Sharing information may be indicated at any time during the consultation including during the examination. For example:

- Sharing the results of an investigation may be done at the start of the consultation or after learning about any change.
- Offering an explanation for their problem may be done after learning the details of the problem or during the examination.
- Giving an opinion may be done after sharing the results of an investigation, after learning about the problem or examining the patient, or at the end of the consultation.
- Giving advice, such as about their lifestyle, may be done after learning about the person.

Before sharing information with the patient consider the impact it may have on the patient. Conversely, when information is withheld from the patient, consider the likely consequences. As a rule, the default position should be to share information. Withholding information should be a deliberate decision undertaken in the best interests of the patient. The timing and detail of the information shared is likely to be influenced by many factors including:

- The context and timing.
- The nature of the information.
- The patient, their wishes, needs, expectations, vulnerability and resilience.
- Whether or not they are accompanied by a friend or family member.
- Their family or social support.
- The HCP, their self-confidence, knowledge and experience.

It may be appropriate to ask permission. The questions to ask could include:

Would you like to know what I think?
Do you want to know what I think the diagnosis is?
Can I tell you what I think?
Can I give you some advice?

For some problems and some patients, information is all that a patient wants or needs from the consultation. For example:

- When a patient presents with a minor problem, such as:
  o A minor viral illness.
  o A bout of gastro-enteritis.
  o A muscle strain.
  o A broken toe.
- When the patient wants reassurance that the problem is unlikely to be serious, such as:
  o IBS.
  o A tension headache.
  o Arthritis.
  o Anal pain from a thrombosed external haemorrhoid.

- When the patient wants advice, such as:
  o To stop smoking.
  o To reduce weight.

When this is the case, information is with the aim of providing reassurance.

Before sharing information with the patient:

Ask yourself, how should the information be shared?

It may be appropriate to check the patient is receptive to information being shared. This is best done by asking permission from the patient.

Not all information should be shared the same way. Factual information is evidence based and the same for all patients. It may be appropriate to discuss it with the patient first and then give them a handout or direct them to a website. For example:

- Giving the patient instructions.
  An endoscopy involves…
  You need to …

- Explaining risks and benefits.

  The risks of an operation are…
  The side effects of the treatment are…

- Explaining the results of an investigation.

  The test has shown…

A handout or a website is frequently better for providing factual information because the patient can read it at their convenience.

Opinions and recommendations are usually given verbally but may be followed up in a letter. Examples of opinions given include:

- Explaining symptoms or signs.
- Explaining the likely cause of the problem.
- Explaining the likelihood of a benefit or risk.
- Providing reassurance.

Examples of recommendations include:

- A change in lifestyle.
- An investigation.
- A treatment.
- Referral to another HCP for a second opinion or for additional or specialist information, such as dietary advice.

When talking to the patient it is important to state the source of the opinion or recommendation. Some are from the HCP, some from another HCP, such as the report of an investigation, some are from a guideline and others from an MDT. For example:

> *I think...*
> *In my opinion...*
> *I recommend you take...*
> *The radiologist has reported...*
> *The guidelines/ MDT recommend you have [a treatment/an investigation/an operation]*

When sharing information with the patient it is important to use language the patient is likely to understand and conveys the intended meaning. For example:

- If the patient is told the procedure is very safe and complications are rare, they are likely to understand, whereas telling a patient their risk of a complication is 20/100,000 is unlikely to be understood.
- Telling the patient that if they stop smoking the risk of a complication is halved is more meaningful than saying the risk of a complication is decreased to 10/100,000.

Avoid making predictions or forecasts. For example, saying "*you* have a 90% chance of surviving" is a prediction. It is factually more correct to say "The evidence shows that 90% of patients survive". Alternatively, give an opinion based on known information, such as "I am 90% sure you will survive". Care should be taken not to mislead the patient or introduce personal bias. For example:

- Telling the patient that if they stop smoking the risk of a complication is halved may be misleading if the risk is still very low, such as when the risk falls from 2/100,000 to 1/100,000
- Saying "*you* have a 90% chance of surviving" is more optimistic than saying "10% of patients die".

It is important to explain what is known and what is unknown, uncertain or pending. Be honest; information shared should be true and accurate even when it is incomplete. Sometimes patients misunderstand what is said or only hear parts of what is said. It is better to avoid a misunderstanding than try to correct a misunderstanding. Frequently, check that the patient has understood what has been said.

Examination Skills Needed for a Meaningful Exchange of Information

The examination should contribute to meeting the aims of the consultation. Usually, the aims are to formulate a diagnosis or inform management, and occasionally to help establish a working relationship. An examination is not always indicated and may be contra-indicated, such as when a patient refuses to be examined. When indicated, the examination is an important part of information exchange. For some patients, such as when a patient presents with a visible or palpable abnormality, it may be the most important part of the consultation and for others it adds to information learnt during the conversation. During the examination the patient should be in a comfortable position and the relevant part of the body exposed. The techniques used to examine a patient consist of inspection, palpation, percussion and auscultation. It is unnecessary to use each technique when examining every abnormality.

Use the right technique

The signs being sought and the part of the body being examined influence the technique. For example:

- Superficial abnormalities can often be seen and felt. Auscultation and percussion are rarely indicated.

- When examining the limbs, face, neck and back inspection and palpation at rest and during movement is usually sufficient. Percussion or auscultation are of limited value unless the peripheral circulatory system is being examined or a large mass palpable.
- When examining the abdomen and pelvis inspection and palpation at rest and during movement are the techniques of choice. Percussion can be used to assess resonance or peritonism and auscultation to listen to bowel sounds or for a bruit.
- When examining the chest percussion and auscultation are indicated whereas, inspection and palpation are of limited value except:
  - When there is a superficial abnormality.
  - To assess chest wall movements during breathing.
  - To palpate the apical cardiac pulsation.
  - To palpate for sub-cutaneous emphysema.
- Internal examinations are limited to palpation and inspection with the aid of specialist equipment, such as an auroscope, a speculum or proctoscope.

Each examination technique serves a different purpose and each should be used when appropriate. Therefore, when examining the patient:

Ask yourself, what examination technique should be used?

A brief description of the different techniques is included for completeness because there are many books and articles that describe the details of the techniques and methods available.

An examination usually starts with a careful inspection and palpation of the site of interest both at rest and during movement. Palpation augments inspection because they have greater value when considered together and when undertaken at rest and during movement. When inspecting and palpating compare sides or the area of interest with an equivalent but normal area.

Look, feel, move, look and feel again

Inspection and palpation are particularly useful when examining a superficial problem or a deeper problem affecting the limbs, face, neck, breasts and abdomen.
When inspecting the site, look at:

- The colour and texture, for example:
  - To detect jaundice
  - The conjunctiva as an indication of blood haemoglobin concentration.
  - To identify any surface abnormalities, such as scars, pits or ulcers
  - The change in colour on applying pressure to identify blanching erythema or measure capillary refill time.
- The contours, to identify a swelling, such as a hernia, ascites or a joint effusion, a mass, such as hepatomegaly, a deformity, such as a Swann neck deformity, a pulsation or guttering.
- The position. For example, when a joint is held partially flexed and any movement is exquisitely tender it is likely to be septic arthritis.

If an unexpected abnormality, such as a surgical scar is found, ask the patient:

Have you noticed [the abnormality]?
How long has it been present?
What caused this?

When palpating, feel to assess:

- Tenderness. When the site is likely to be tender, the periphery of the site should be carefully examined first, moving towards the point of maximal tenderness. The site should initially be gently palpated. If there is minimal tenderness the pressure can be increased.

Identify the precise location, extent and depth of any tenderness. In the abdomen, when there is tenderness, feel for guarding (an involuntary reflex abdominal wall muscle contraction in response to pressure). Guarding indicates parietal peritoneal inflammation. When moving, coughing or percussing the abdomen is very painful, peritonism is likely. When palpation of the abdomen while tensing the abdominal wall muscles is still very tender, the pain is likely to be from the abdominal wall itself.

- The local temperature. There is normally wide variation in temperature in different parts of the body so it is helpful to compare parts. When the abnormality is deep-seated, temperature differences may not be apparent. For example:
  - If the area feels relatively warm there may be underlying inflammation or a prominent superficial circulation.
  - If a limb feels cooler than normal it may be ischaemic.
- The texture of the skin and consistency of underlying tissues. There is wide variation so it is helpful to compare the abnormal part with a normal part. Feel for:
  - Excessive sweat, indicating a fever, severe pain or hypovolaemia.
  - Pitting oedema. It may be caused by inflammation or poor circulation.
  - An orange skin texture: "peau d'orange", may be caused by lymphoedema or cancer.
  - Decide whether it is appropriately hard, like bone, firm, like cartilage or soft, like fat, pulsatile or compressible?
  - To feel crepitus or a thrill.
  - When there is a mass to feel, assess the depth, proximity and fixity to nearby landmark structures, the shape, margins, consistency and response to pressure and any change in response to movement.
- Sensation. Assess sensation to light touch and, when indicated, to pin prick, temperature and vibration. When the sensation is abnormal decide whether there is:
  - Anaesthesia: a loss of sensation.
  - Hypo-aesthesia: a reduced sensation.
  - Paraesthesia: an abnormal sensation.
  - Hyper-aesthesia: when the sensitivity is increased.
- When an abnormality is near a named blood vessel, feel for pulsation, transmitted or expansile, or a thrill and compare it to other parts of the peripheral circulation. When a named arterial pulsation is easily felt, the artery may be aneurysmal or ectatic. When there is a thrill, there is likely to be a bruit.

Inspection and palpation should be undertaken at rest and during movement or in different positions. The examination method will depend on the site being examined or the signs being sought. For example:

- When peripheral ischaemia is suspected, assess a change in limb colour using Buerger's test, or look for venous guttering.
- When a neurological problem is suspected, assess movement against gravity or resistance to assess muscle power.
- When a joint is being examined, assess the range of movement.
- When examining the limbs, assess the impact on function, such as walking, dexterity or coordination.
- To assess pain, such as when moving a joint.
- To identify the precise location of an abnormality.
  - When there is a palpable mass, try to move overlying skin and subcutaneous layers, and conversely, try to move the mass over underlying or nearby structures.
  - Palpate the site while tensing or moving adjacent muscles. If the mass or tenderness is more pronounced it is superficial to the muscle, if it is more difficult to feel it is deeper, if it moves with the muscle it is associated with the muscle.
  - Palpate the site while nearby structures move or in different positions. For example:
    - A midline mass in the throat that moves on swallowing is likely to be attached to the trachea.
    - A mass associated with the liver or spleen may only be palpable during deep inspiration.
    - A right sub-costal tenderness, aggravated during deep inspiration, or associated with a "catch" on deep inspiration is likely to be associated with the liver.
    - A left sub-costal mass, more easily palpated during deep inspiration or while the patient lies left side up may be an enlarged spleen.

- A left flank mass palpated when the renal angle is balloted is likely to be associated with the kidney.
- An inguinal hernia may only be palpable in the upright position or during an activity such as coughing.
- A saphena varix may only be palpable in the upright position and a thrill palpable on coughing.
- The pain from a meniscal injury may only be demonstrated when the knee is moved while applying rotational torque to the lower leg.

Percussion is usually used to assess resonance, to identify a change in density. When the structure or abnormality is large enough, it can be used to distinguish between gas, which is resonant and fluid or solid, which are dull. Percussion can also be used to diagnose rebound tenderness or a tendon reflex.

Auscultation is used to listen for sounds associated with movement. For example:

- A wheeze or stridor during inspiration or expiration indicating upper airway air turbulence.
- Crepitations during inspiration or expiration indicating the opening and closing of the alveoli.
- A bruit indicating turbulent blood flow.
- A murmur indicating turbulent blood flow through a heart valve.
- Heart sounds caused by the closure of the heart valves.
- The noises made by the bowel during peristalsis. It should be noted that bowel sounds are rarely discriminatory, although very active bowel sounds (borborygmi) or a succession splash may support a diagnosis of obstruction.
- A pleural rub during inspiration or expiration caused by the movement of one pleural lining over another during ventilation.
- A pericardial rub caused by the movement of one pericardial lining over another during each heart-beat.

Auscultation and percussion are most useful when examining the chest and peripheral blood vessels. Specialist equipment is increasingly used during the examination. For example:

- An ECG and echocardiogram are used by cardiologists.
- Pulmonary function and spirometry tests are performed by respiratory physicians.
- An ophthalmoscope and slit lamp are used by ophthalmologists.
- An auroscope and audiometry are used to assess hearing.
- A duplex USS is used by vascular surgeons to assess flow in the peripheral circulation.
- Proctoscopy and sigmoidoscopy are used by colo-proctologists.
- Colposcopy is used by gynaecologists.
- Urine analysis and urodynamics are used by urologists.
- A magnifying glass, patch testing and punch biopsy are used by dermatologists.
- An USS and/or mammogram is part of the triple assessment in a breast clinic.

Examination accuracy

Just as with an investigation, it is important to consider the examination accuracy. Sensitivity and specificity are measures of accuracy:

> **The more sensitive an examination, the fewer the false negative results**
> **The more specific an examination, the fewer the false positive results**

When a sign is used to confirm a diagnosis, it should have a low false positive rate, i.e., a high specificity. When the absence of a sign is used to exclude a diagnosis, it should have a low false negative rate, i.e., a high sensitivity. Few signs are sufficiently accurate that their presence is diagnostic or their absence excludes a diagnosis and many signs are indeterminate. In general:

- Signs that are measurable and reproducible with minimal inter-observer variation are more likely to be accurate. This will include measurement of:
  - Height
  - Weight
  - Blood pressure

- o Temperature
- o The range of movement of a joint
- Subjective signs are prone to inter-observer variation and lack reproducibility and accuracy. For example:
  - o Pulses can be difficult to palpate in some patients and some people find it difficult to distinguish a patient's pulse from their own. The rate can be difficult to count when there is a tachycardia or an arrythmia and the pulse pressure difficult to assess if the arteries are calcified or small.
  - o Colour is difficult to assess. Some patients are naturally pale whereas others are normally flushed. Examining the conjunctiva is unreliable as a measure of anaemia except to demonstrate or exclude profound anaemia. The detection of jaundice may be influenced by the ambient light and décor.
  - o Bowel sounds are very variable. Bowel sounds differ between patients and are dependent on bowel activity and the listening time. Some can be very loud or frequent, or quiet and infrequent, yet peristalsis is normal. The absence of bowel sounds does not prove an ileus and the presence of active bowel sounds does not prove small bowel obstruction. The longer the time spent listening to the bowel sounds the more reliable the sign is likely to be.
- Body habitus affects many signs. For example:
  - o A deep-seated fullness or mass may be impalpable in an obese patient.
  - o A normal abdominal organ is easily palpable in a thin patient.
  - o Significant lordosis can highlight the kidneys or the aorta.
- Tenderness may be influenced by many factors, including the sensitivity of the patient or patient anxiety or the temperature of the examiner's hands.
- Signs that are obvious when examined are more likely to be accurately identified. For example, a visible abnormality is easier to measure than a palpable abnormality.
- Signs that are either present or absent are more reliably identified than signs that are dependent on gradation. For example, determining whether a pulse is present or absent is more reliable than assessing its rate or strength.
- The more obviously abnormal the sign, the more likely the abnormality is advanced.
- The accuracy of a sign is increased if it is consistent with the symptoms, associated information, such as risk factors, and other signs.
- A pattern of symptoms and signs is more accurate than a single sign. The more complete the pattern, the higher the probability the sign is true and conversely, the more signs that are absent the less likely.
- An absence of a sign does not always exclude a sign. For example:
  - o Fasciculation, paraesthesia and a positive Chvostek's or Trousseau's sign support the diagnosis of hypercalcaemia, but their absence does not exclude hypercalcaemia.
  - o Absent bowel sounds may be caused by an ileus, but the occasional bowel sound does not exclude an ileus.
  - o Being unable to feel a AAA or organomegaly in an obese patient does not exclude an abnormality.

Unlike investigations there is no quality standard for the examination. Quality control is frequently limited to self-assessment, peer comparison and self-reflection, when more is known about the problem. The reasons for a false negative examination include:

- The sign is not sought properly.
- The sign is difficult to elicit. For example:
  - o An early diastolic murmur.
  - o A tendon reflex.
  - o Splenomegaly.
- The sign is subtle either because it is not severe or the patient has presented early in the course of the illness. For example:
  - o A small hernia.
  - o A dense hemiparesis following a stroke is obvious whereas a slight weakness may be difficult to detect.
- The sign is intermittent and not apparent at the time of the examination. For example:
  - o A wheeze.
  - o A small rectal prolapse.
  - o An arrythmia.

- Patient factors, such as body habitus. For example, in a patient with central obesity, an impalpable bladder does not exclude the diagnosis.
- Sensory limitations of the HCP, such as reduced peripheral sensation or impaired hearing.

The reasons for a false positive examination include:

- Examiner error.
- Patient factors. For example:
  o An easily palpable aorta may be mistaken for an aneurysm in a thin patent with a pronounced lumbar lordosis.
  o A distended abdomen due to central obesity rather than an intraabdominal abnormality, such as ascites or a tumour.
  o A raised blood pressure in an anxious patient.

For measurable signs there is a reference range to represent a range of "normality". As a rule, the greater the deviation from the reference range the more likely the sign is abnormal. However, the reference range, sensitivity and specificity can be influenced by many variables. For example:

- The reference range for body temperature is 36.1-37.7°C. However, the measured body temperature can be affected by many factors including:
  o The site used to measure body temperature.
  o The instrument.
  o The age of the patient. The ability to generate heat and the activity levels decrease in older people so the normal core temperature is less.
  o The time of day. The core temperature rises during the day from >37.2°C in the morning to >37.7°C in the afternoon.
  o Ambient temperature.
  o Metabolic rate: exercise and a meal typically raise core temperature.
  o Hormones: pregnancy and ovulation.
- The blood pressure reference range is 90/60-120/80mmHg. However, the measured blood pressure can be affected by many factors including:
  o The age of the patient.
  o Activity.
  o Fitness.
  o BMI.
  o Body temperature.
  o Alcohol and caffeine intake.
  o Stress/anxiety.

Cognitive Skills Needed for a Meaningful Exchange of Information

The information should not only be learnt but also understood and interpreted to meet the aims of the consultation. Cognitive skills together with knowledge of medicine and the basic sciences and method are needed to acquire information, critically analyse the information, make decisions, organise and link information. Some of the cognitive skills needed include:

- Acquisition skills.
- Memory.
- Analytical skills or evaluative thinking.
- Decision making skills.
- Organisation skills.

Acquisition skills

Questioning, listening and the examining skills are key skills used to acquire information. Early on a trainee tends to focus on asking all the right questions and examining every part of the body in a predetermined sequence to ensure there are no errors of omission. A proforma or a checklist helps. As trainee's gain experience and knowledge learning is transformed. The emphasis is on asking the right questions, listening to the answers and pro-actively looking for signs, learning to understand, to meet the needs of the patient. Experts do it efficiently and effectively, often undertaking several acquisition tasks at the same time.

Some information consists of facts that are incontestable, such as age, gender, previous medical problems and their treatments and known safety concerns. Acquisition of such facts is usually done reflexively with little need for critical thought or deliberation. On the other hand, learning and evaluating descriptive or subjective information, such as symptoms and signs, is complex requiring a lot of thought. The HCP also needs to be able to acquire medical knowledge relevant to the information learnt from the patient. This includes knowing how to search the internet and electronic databases to find reliable relevant information and to be able to assess the quality of the information and clinical applicability.

Memory

Memory is the process of storing, maintaining and retrieving information on demand. It is essential for a meaningful consultation.

Many patients need help recalling relevant information because short term memory has a limited capacity and rapidly degrades. Our auditory memory degrades over minutes whereas our sensory memory lasts only seconds, unless it is significant. Only significant information is transferred to long term memory. In addition, with increasing age, stress and illness memory degrades. Information is more easily stored as a memory and recalled when:

- It is associated with an emotional or sensory experience.
- We feel well.
- We are in a good mood, not stressed or anxious.
- We are paying attention, not tired or distracted.
- The information is meaningful, not a list of facts.
- The information is organised, linked/associated or connected.
- If it can be visualised.
- The information is verbalised, repeated or reviewed.
- The information is anticipated.

We take a positive approach to learning rather than being negative: "I never remember what they said."
Patients frequently emphasise the present symptoms and current feelings rather than past symptoms, and feelings and symptoms associated with the strongest sensations or emotions are more likely to be remembered. However, such symptoms are not necessarily the most significant and other, less stimulating symptoms may be ignored or forgotten.

The methods available to help a patient remember include:

- Ask short precise questions.
- Ask questions in context and in sequence so that the association is apparent.
- Use words that will mean something to the patient. For example, reflect or paraphrase what the patient has said.
- Ask the patient to recount events in a sequence.
- Ask the patient, what were they doing at the time.
- Ask a leading or a closed question.
- Link information:
  o With the time of day, such as morning or night time.
  o With an everyday task, such as eating a meal.
  o With an event, such as while shopping.

Just as many patients need help recalling relevant information, so does the HCP. However, unlike the patient, most of the information is learnt as a fact without associated feelings or emotions. The information mentioned by the patient is often incomplete and presented in a disordered way using language unfamiliar to the HCP. Similarly, sensory experiences during the examination are limited and fleeting, such as feeling a pulse or palpating an abdomen. Therefore, the information is more difficult for the HCP to store and remember particularly when the HCP meets and cares for many patients. Therefore, it is important each HCP develops methods to ensure information is retained and can be recalled. The methods available to help the HCP remember include:

- A healthy lifestyle with regular exercise and a healthy diet, keeping the brain stimulated and challenged.
- Avoid being stressed or tired.
- Avoid distractions and multi-tasking.
- Listen attentively.
- Learning to understand. The main method of recording long-term memory is by remembering meaning ("semantic coding").
- Affirmation of expectations. It is easier to remember information that confirms what is already known, "an expectation" based on previous experience or knowledge ("top-down processing") than to learn new information ("bottom-up processing"). Paradoxically, when most of the information conforms to expectations, information that is unexpected is highlighted and more likely to be remembered.
- Combine information into groups ("chunking"). Small groups of related information are easier to remember. For example:
  - A previous medical condition and the treatment.
  - The presenting problem and a risk factor.
  - Disease pattern.
- Give the problem an identity: link information about the problem with the person.
- Link information learnt with familiar spatial, environmental or temporal landmarks to provide a route map that can be recalled or visualised. This can be achieved in various ways including:
  - Link information to objects in a familiar space, such as a room at home (the method of loci).
  - Link information with letters to form an acronym (a mnemonic). For example:
    - The causes of a sub-arachnoid haemorrhage "BATS": Berry aneurysm, Arteriovenous malformation, Trauma, Stroke.
    - The risk factors for oesophageal cancer "ABCDEF": Achalasia, Barrett's oesophagus, Corrosion, Diverticulitis, Oesophageal web, Family history.
- Ensure topics are separated and the information is not allowed to merge.
- Practice recall ("checking"):
  - With the patient: summarise the information.
  - To yourself:
    - Holding an internal conversation.
    - When completing documentation.
    - Reflecting on what has been learnt.
  - To another HCP by presenting or talking through the information.
- Other measures, such as mindfulness.

During the consultation, the brain has to combine short-term memories, such as what the patient says and the examination findings, and long-term memories, such as medical knowledge, into a working memory for meaningful recall.

Evaluative and analytical skills

Information needs to be evaluated to decide what is relevant and what is important before it can be analysed. Evaluation includes asking yourself questions, such as:

What does the patient mean?
What does it mean medically?
Is it relevant?
Is it significant?
Why did it occur: what is the cause?
How does it link with other information?

What is missing?

Analytical skills include the ability to form new ideas, to seek patterns, to use deductive reasoning to reduce a list of possible diagnoses or to determine the location of the abnormality causing the problem or the type of problem. Usually, acquisition, evaluation and analysis are done concurrently, throughout the consultation.

Occasionally, there is a need to reflect on the information or re-evaluate or re-analyse the information later.

When the symptoms and signs are classical and match the "textbook" description, information is processed in a sequential way, one step at a time ("serial processing"). Minimal analytical and evaluative skills are needed to understand the problem, formulate a diagnosis and plan management. For other patients and other problems, learning the symptoms and signs and using them to understand the problem, to formulate a diagnosis and plan management requires significant acquisition, memory, evaluative and analytical skills. This is a complex process in which several streams of information are processed at the same time ("parallel processing"). Method and experience help this process.

Decision making skills

Effective decision-making by both the patient and the HCP is needed to manage uncertainty throughout the consultation and during the succeeding care pathway. During the consultation, the patient decides what to tell the HCP and the HCP decides what question to ask or signs to look for, what the information means or what management option is indicated and most likely to help the patient and also the priority and timing of a management option. Decision making is complex and frequently a multi-disciplinary process which involves the patient and their family or friends and other HCPs. When many HCPs are involved, one usually remains responsible.

Shared decision making occurs when the HCP shares relevant evidence with the patient and, together, they agree on the best management option. When a patient makes a truly informed decision, the patient and HCP share responsibility for the decision and the consequences. The HCP is likely to feel more self-confident and the patient more satisfied.

Decision making is a stepwise process that starts with a problem and finishes when an outcome is agreed.

- Determine the decision to be taken.
- Acquire information.
- Evaluate and analyse the acquired information.
- Exclude irrelevant or unnecessary information.
- Consider the available options.
- Consider the details, the risks and benefits of each option.
- Make a decision or shortlist options. Some decisions are made on the basis of facts and evidence, others on the basis of personal opinions or experience.
- Explain the recommendation and the options, together with the evidence and ask the patient their opinion. The recommendation and the reasoning should be explained to the patient.

Decision making is not only about deciding what to do and when, it is also about deciding what not to do. There is often a tendency to want to do something or to be seen to be doing something.

> **Not doing something should be a positive decision rather than an error of omission**

Undoubtedly, for many patients, action is indicated, but occasionally, making a decision *not* to take an action is in the patient's best interests. This is summed up by a well-known surgical aphorism:

"Good surgeons know how to operate, better ones when to operate, and the best when not to operate"

Self-awareness: assumptions, preconceptions and bias

Everyone makes assumptions, has preconceptions and is biased. We make an assumption when we think something without having confirmed it is true. There is a tendency to make assumptions throughout the consultation and the care pathway. For example:

- We assume we know what a patient means when they are talking.

- We often assume we know the patient's wishes and views, what they need, their hopes, fears and expectations.
- We assume we understand their personal and social circumstances.
- We assume they understand the diagnostic implications of a symptom or sign.
- We assume we know the outcome a patient wants when planning management.

Making an assumption may be considered to be more efficient; avoiding the need to ask "an obvious question" or check a self-evident "truth". However, it can lead to error and misunderstanding, misguided care and undermine the relationship. Asking a question rather than assuming something avoids potential pitfalls and shows respect for the patient.

When we make an assumption before information becomes available, it is a preconceived idea. When this is used scientifically and leads to a meaningful enquiry it becomes a hypothesis but when it leads to negative thoughts it is prejudice. Proactively asking questions or looking for signs with an open mind tests a hypothesis. This can be a very useful tool to use during the consultation. For example, when:

- Looking for patterns.
- Formulating a diagnosis.
- Considering management options.

Bias occurs when we are influenced by opinions or beliefs that deviate from a neutral position. We are all prone to bias and we may all be perceived as being biased by others. Just as it is part of everyday behaviour so it is also prevalent in health care. We may be conscious we are doing it or do it inadvertently: unconscious or implicit bias. For example:

- Stereotyping.
- Gender bias.
- Conformity bias.
- Beauty bias.
- Affinity bias.
- Similarity bias.
- Halo effect, when we let a positive thought influence another thought.
- Horns effect, when we let a negative thought influence another thought.
- Contrast bias, when we compare people.
- Attribution bias.
- Confirmation bias.

Self-awareness of personal bias and checking or managing bias may prevent negative consequences.

Bias may influence clinical practice in many different ways. For example:

- Our relationship with the patient.
- The way we talk to them or how well we listen.
- Personal prejudices: if we like someone, we are likely to try harder on their behalf.
- Trust.
- Respect.
- Stereotypes.
- Our understanding and interpretation of the information:
  - Do we believe what they say?
  - Are they exaggerating?
  - Making assumptions.
  - Failing to consider all the available evidence.
  - Having pre-conceived opinions.
  - Favouring information that supports a pre-conceived diagnosis. and discounting or ignoring contrary information.
  - Making information fit a pattern.
  - Favouring familiar information.

- Over-reliance on subjective opinion and under-estimating objective evidence.
- Favouring information that is quickly available, the most recent information, a recent experience or information you are familiar with.
- Decision making.
- To influence, reduce or increase, the patient's expectation.
- To emphasise potential harm or benefit.
- To support what a patient wants or to challenge a patient.
- Discriminating between patients.
- Misdiagnosis.
- Delayed diagnosis.
- The recommended outcome.
- Fear of being wrong.

When it favours a patient to the disadvantage of others it is unfair or detrimental. When our bias is appropriate for the patient and aligns with the public opinion and "accepted practice" it is considered appropriate and beneficial. For example:

- When compassion influences priority.
- When compensating for an error or a misadventure influences priority.
- When clinical need influences priority.

Organisation skills

Organisation skills are needed both during the consultation, when acquiring, evaluating and analysing the information, and when recording the information so that it is an accurate record and details the evidence that supports an opinion.

The consultation needs to be organised and structured for it to be meaningful. Consultations start with introductions and learning the headline information and finish with concluding remarks including a summary of the information learnt, an opinion, a recommendation and an agreed way forward. The format and focus, i.e., the structure, of the rest of the consultation is determined by the aims, the patient and the information learnt during the consultation. The focus and format should be managed flexibly to ensure the exchange of relevant and appropriate information in a timely way. Usually, the focus of the consultation is on learning and understanding information about the problem and examining the patient with the aims of formulating a diagnosis and planning management. Additional information about the person and the patient may help establish a working relationship, contextualise the problem and may inform the diagnosis and management. Occasionally, they are the focus of the consultation. Organisation skills are essential to ensure the consultation has structure.

During the consultation it is not unusual for a patient to meander, to switch between topics, to deviate from the topic or to include irrelevant information. Similarly, it is not unusual for the HCP to jump from one topic to another and to ask seemingly unrelated questions or look of associated signs away from the site of the problem or to ask questions while examining the patient. Organisational skills ensure the HCP knows what they have covered, where they are in the consultation and where they want to get to. They ensure relevant questions are asked or signs sought, information is prioritised, linked appropriately and information is not missed. They ensure the consultation is managed efficiently, is productive and remains focused. Without organisational skills, the consultation will be chaotic.

Managing error

Everyone makes errors. It is the nature and frequency of the errors, the circumstances, consequences and how we respond and manage the errors that matters. Examples of errors that may occur during a consultation include:

- Errors of recall.
- Reasoning or decision-making errors.
- Transcription or execution errors.
- Errors of omission.

Diagnostic errors occur in 5-15% of hospital admissions and up to 40% of diagnoses are found to be different at autopsy. Management errors occur in up to half of all patients. Up to a third of prescribed medications are potentially unnecessary.

Managing error is a necessary skill. It starts with prevention. Good training, knowledge, method and communication skills, preparation, support systems, teamworking and a careful, safety-first approach will reduce the likelihood of error.

> **The more careful I am, the less likely I will make an error**

Errors may be caused by one or a sequence of circumstances and often follow a pattern. They may be a consequence of being emotional, stressed or tired, multitasking or under time constraints, excessive workload or when working in complex or unfamiliar circumstances or due to ignorance or incompetence.

> **When an error occurs, Recognise, Respond, Record, Report and Reflect**

A rapid response is indicated when an error is recognised. Always act in the best interests of the patient. Honesty, good communication skills and a good working relationship with the patient will mitigate the consequences of error both for the patient and for the HCP. Most errors happen for a reason. Self-reflection, being open to and responding to feedback, good working relations and a good working environment facilitating shared learning are all important to help learn from errors.

Conversation Methodology

Questioning, listening and cognitive skills are key skills but without method the conversation may become chaotic, information may be missed, forgotten, misunderstood or misinterpreted and the outcome may not meet the aims. Method is particularly important when using a flexible approach in which the conversation changes in response to the patient and the information learnt because it will provide a framework to ensure the information is complete, reducing the likelihood of errors of omission, to organise the information and link relevant information, and to maintain direction, momentum, and focus on meeting the aims.

All consultations start with an introductory conversation and finish with a concluding conversation. Following the introductory conversation, it is usual to discuss the reason for the consultation. This could include listening to the patient's description of their problem, learning about any change or sharing information with the patient, such as the results of an investigation. This, together with demographic information, information known about the patient from the medical records and other HCPs and the initial assessment of the patient constitutes the headline information (Figure 6) and determines the initial aims of the consultation.

Figure 6: Illustrating the information that makes up the "headline information".

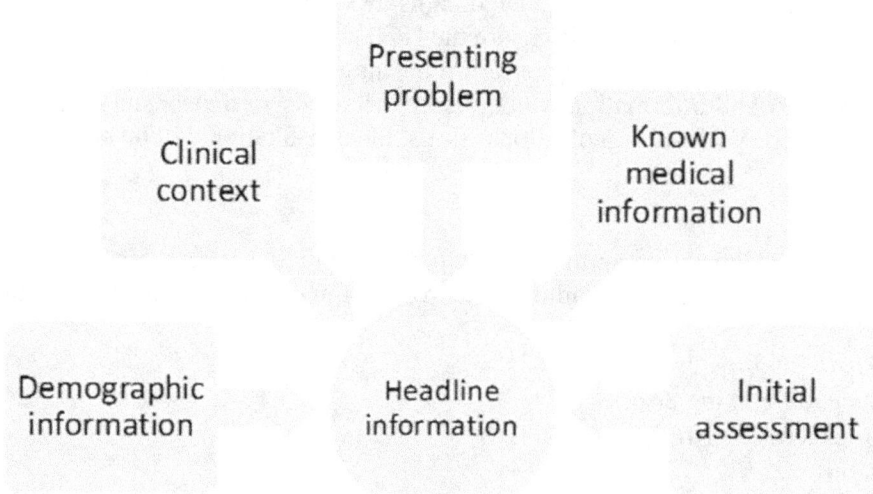

During the introductory conversation, use the available information to:

Ask yourself, what are the aims of the consultation?

Usually, the aims are to exchange information to learn and understand the problem, to formulate a diagnosis and to plan management or to share information with the patient and plan management. Occasionally, the aim is to establish a working relationship.

An initial conversation with the patient is always indicated. However, for some patients it is necessary to:

Ask yourself, is a detailed conversation with the patient indicated?

For most patients, a detailed conversation with the patient is indicated to learn about the person, the person as a patient and the problem. For a minority of patients, such as those with severe mental health problems, talking to the patient is unlikely to be meaningful and is not indicated.

Ask yourself, what is the focus and format of the conversation?

When a conversation is indicated, the aims, the patient and the available information determine the initial focus of the consultation. The subsequent focus and format will be determined by the patient and the information learnt. For example:

- When the patient presents with a new problem the main aims are to formulate a diagnosis and plan management. Learning about the problem is likely to be the initial focus of the consultation, and then learning about the person, the patient and the examination follow (Figure 7).

Figure 7: Illustrating the focus and format of the consultation when the patient presents with a new problem.

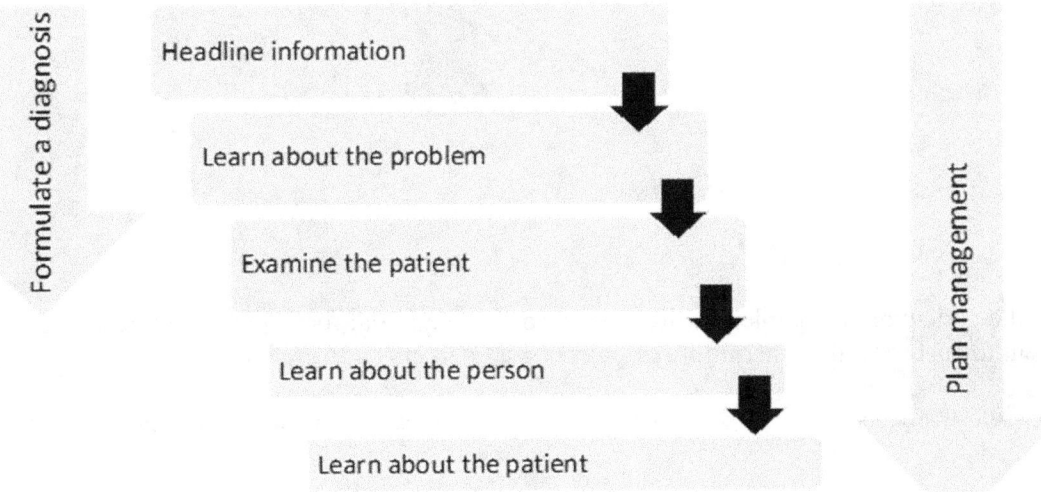

- When the consultation is a follow up the usual aim us to inform management. The initial focus may be on asking about a change in symptoms, re-examining the patient, or sharing the results of an investigation, then learning about the person and the patient (Figure 8).

Figure 8 Illustrating the focus and format of the consultation when the patient presents following an investigation when the diagnosis is known.

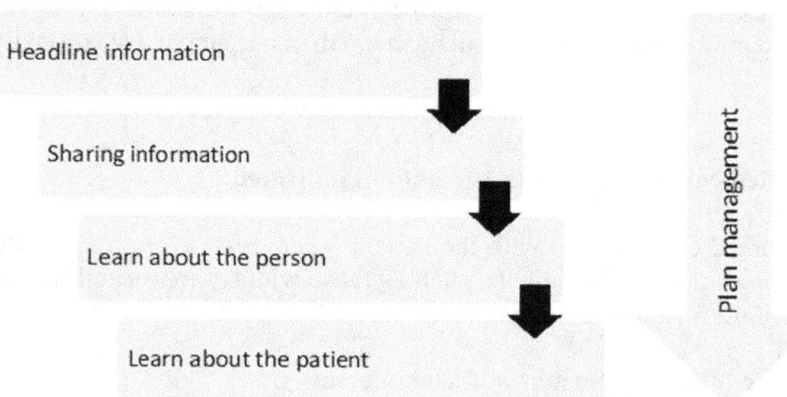

- When the patient has complex learning needs or challenging behaviour, the initial aim is often to establish a working relationship with the patient so the initial focus may be on learning about the person (Figure 9).

Figure 9: Illustrating the focus and format of the consultation when the focus is on establishing a working relationship.

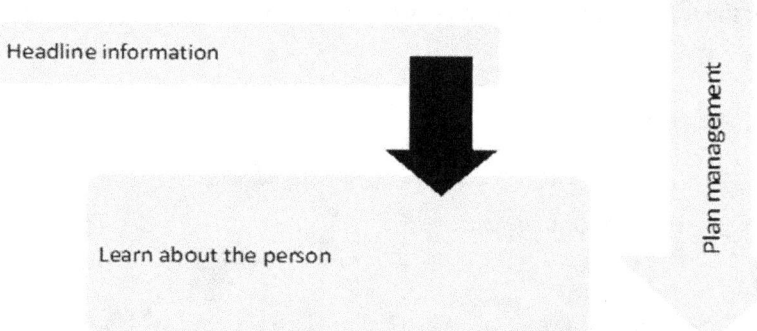

- When the patient has a complex medical background, the initial focus may be on learning about the person as a patient to ensure all the other information is considered in context (Figure 10).

Figure 10: Illustrating the focus and format of the consultation when the patient has a complex medical background.

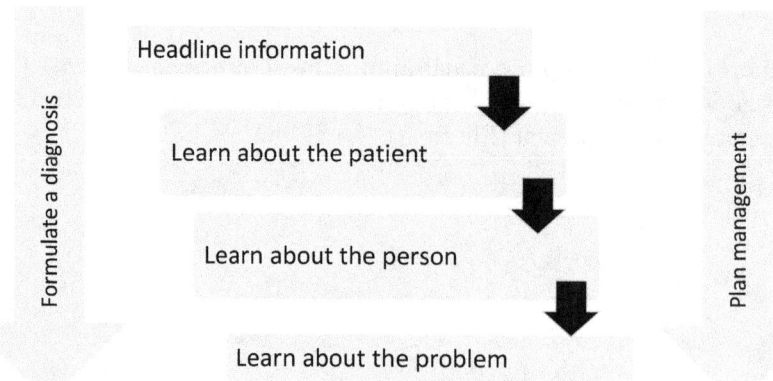

It is the responsibility of the HCP to manage the conversation to ensure all relevant information is learnt and understood, organised and documented to achieve the aims of the consultation. It is not unusual to switch backwards and forwards between different topics during the consultation (Figure 11).

Figure 11: Illustrating the interplay of the conversation with a patient.

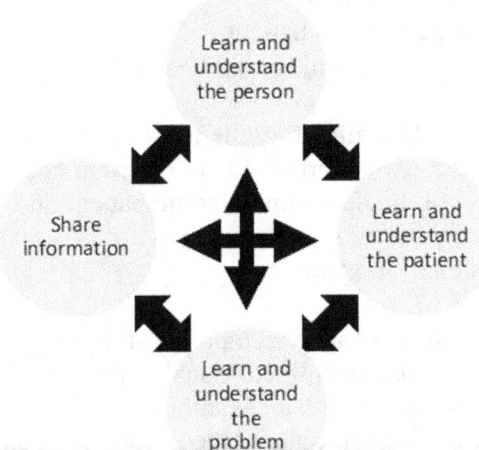

Examination Methodology

Examination skills and medical knowledge are important but, as with the conversation, method provides a framework to ensure the examination is complete and appropriate, the available information is organised, and the focus is on meeting the aims. Method also ensures information from the conversation and a knowledge of medicine and the basic sciences are used to inform the parts of the body to examine and the signs to look for and all the available information is learnt, understood, linked and organised. Before examining the patient:

Ask yourself, what are the aims of an examination?

The introductions, headline information, the patient and information learnt from talking to the patient will determine the aims of the examination. The aims of the examination may not be the same as the aims of the consultation but should align. Usually, the aims are to look for signs to help formulate a diagnosis. to plan management, to assess severity, determine the location of the abnormality causing the problem and the type of problem and/or to identify a cause. Occasionally, the aim is to screen for a complication or a secondary problem or to demonstrate something to the patient and help establish a working relationship.

Ask yourself, is an examination indicated?

When an examination is indicated, it is essential that the patient or their legal guardian give informed consent and the examination is conducted in a private setting and usually with a chaperone. For the examination to be informed the patient should know why they are being examined. When the examination follows a conversation with the patient this is usually self-evident. However, sometimes the reasons should be explained, such as when an examination of another part of the body is indicated. In some patients an examination is not indicated or not possible. For example:

- When the patient refuses to be examined.
- When an examination is not possible, such as a telephone consultation.
- When there are unlikely to be any relevant signs.
- When a test is going to be performed that is more accurate than the examination.

An examination is contraindicated when the patient withholds consent or the examination cannot be undertaken safely.

Ask yourself, what is the focus and format of the examination?

There are potentially four parts to the examination:

- Examine the site of the problem and, if it is different, the location of the abnormality causing the problem.
- Examine for signs associated with the problem.
- Examine to assess the systemic impact on the patient.
- Examine for signs of a complication or potential complication.

The initial focus of the examination is determined by the aims of the examination, the patient and the available information. It will vary between patients, between problems, in different contexts and in response to the information learnt. The subsequent focus and format will be determined by the patient and the information learnt. Not all parts of the body need to be examined and not all parts of the examination are of equal importance. However, an incomplete examination should be a deliberate decision. For example:

- When a patient presents feeling ill, with a pain or symptoms of deranged function, the initial focus is on learning about the problem and then the patient is examined. Usually, the aim of the examination is to help formulate a diagnosis and plan management and starts with an examination of the site of the problem. This is also often the focus of the examination. After examining the site of the abnormality, an examination of other parts of the body to look for associated or systemic signs may be indicated. In some patients, examining for a complication or an asymptomatic problem may be indicated (Figure 12).
- When a patient presents with a visible or palpable abnormality and the aim is to formulate a diagnosis and plan management the site of the abnormality is usually examined first. Learning about the problem is undertaken while examining the site of the abnormality or afterwards. After examining the site of the abnormality, an examination of other parts of the body to look for associated or systemic signs may be indicated. In some patients, examining for a complication or an asymptomatic problem may be indicated (Figure 13).

Figure 12: Illustrating the usual format of the examination when a patient presents feeling ill, in pain or with symptoms of deranged function.

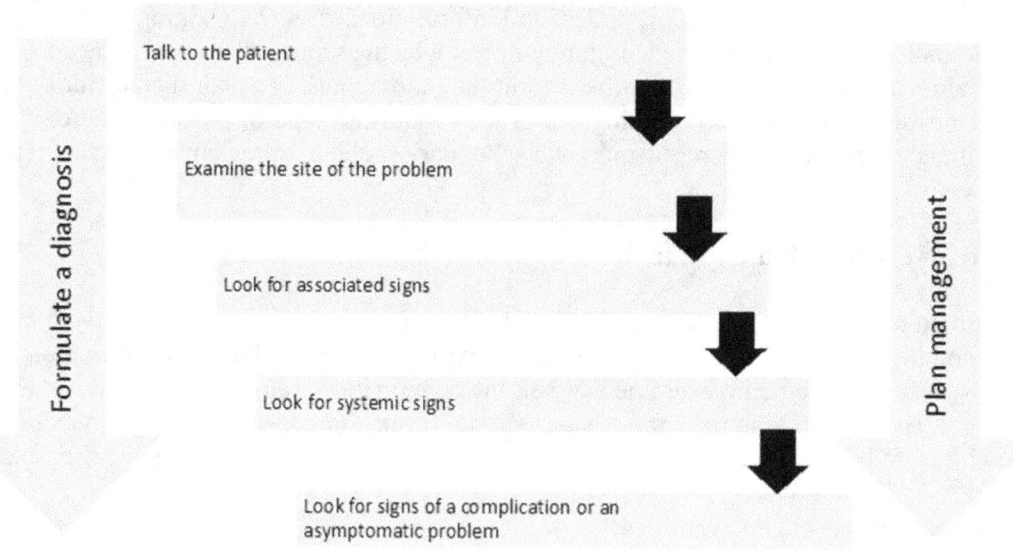

Figure 13: illustrating focus and format of the examination when a patient presents with a visible or palpable abnormality.

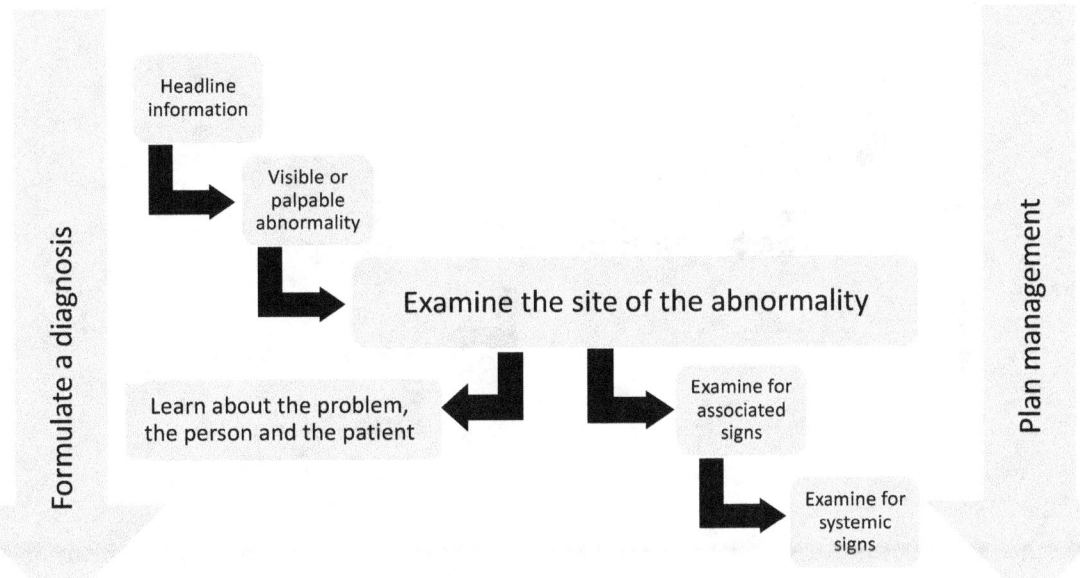

- When the patient is clinically ill, the initial aim of the examination may be to assess the severity of the illness, i.e., the impact on the patient, to inform emergency management. In which case, a systemic examination is the initial focus. In some patients, examining for a complication or an asymptomatic problem may also be indicated (Figure 14).
- When the patient is unable to give a meaningful account of their problem, the initial aim of the examination may be to look for abnormal signs. In which case, a systematic examination is undertaken (Figure 15).
- When the patient presents with a headache or a central neurological problem the brain cannot be directly examined, so the initial focus of the examination is on looking for associated neurological signs (Figure 16).
- When the aim of the examination is to screen for an asymptomatic problem, such as a complication or secondary problem, information about the problem or the person as a patient will inform the focus of the examination (Figure 17).

Figure 14: Illustrating the focus and format of the consultation when the patient presents feeling ill and the initial aims are to assess the impact on the patient and to inform emergency management.

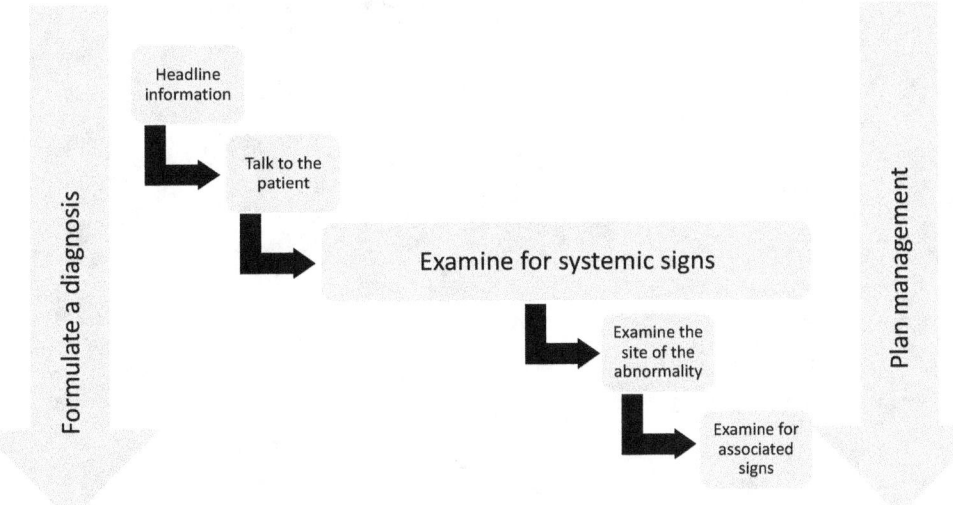

Figure 15: Illustrating the focus and format of the consultation when a patient is unable to give a reliable account of their problem and the location of the problem is unclear.

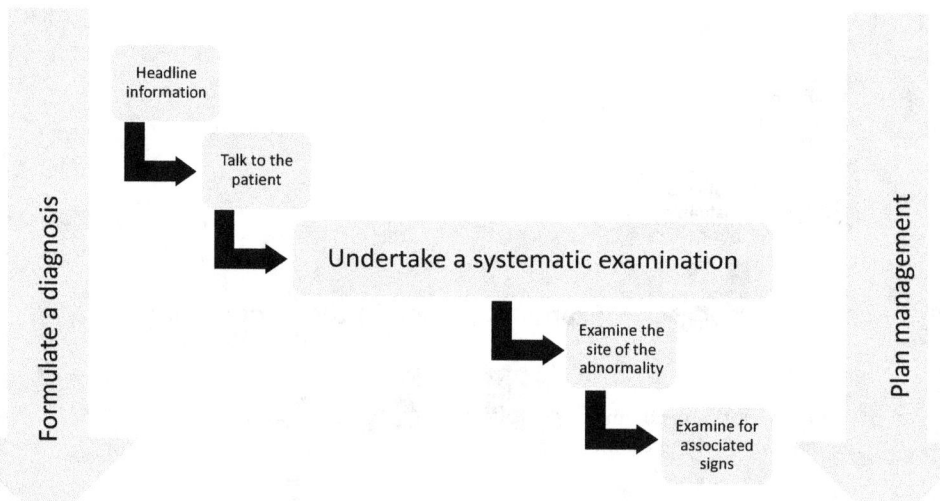

Figure 16: Illustrating the focus and format of the consultation when the patient presents with a headache or a central neurological problem. The brain cannot be directly examined so the initial focus of the examination is on looking for associated neurological signs.

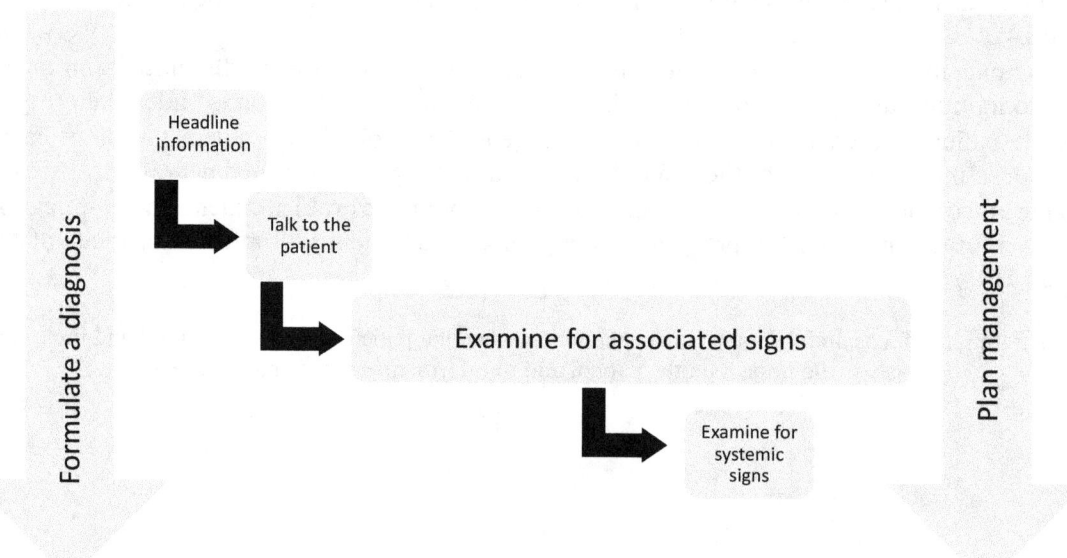

Figure 17: Illustrating the focus and format of the consultation when the aim of the examination is to screen for an asymptomatic problem

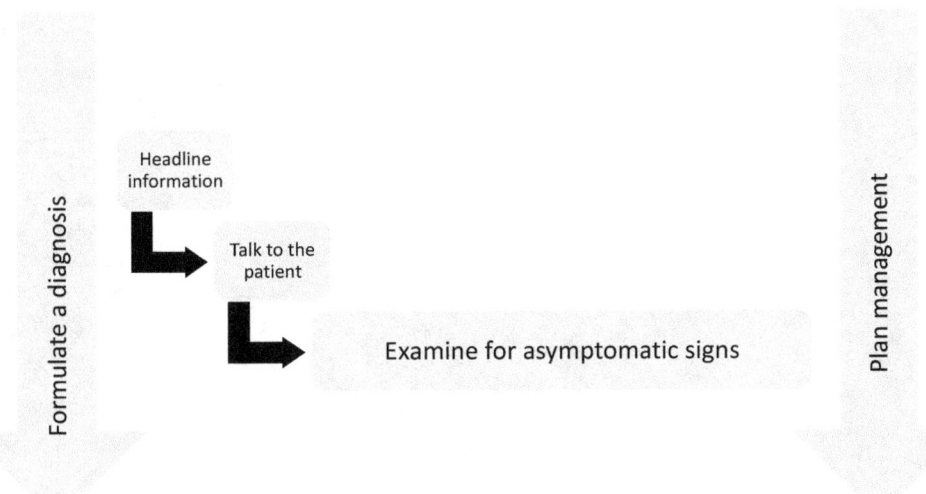

Document Relevant Information

As a rule, writing while trying to hold a conversation is likely to interrupt the flow of the conversation because the HCP will be focusing on what has been said and what to write rather than on what is being said, what it means and what to talk about next. Furthermore, it is distracting for the patient and may be considered disrespectful. Therefore, information should be recorded at an appropriate break in the conversation or at the end of the consultation unless it needs to be recorded contemporaneously to ensure it is not forgotten or mis-represented, such as background medical information, dates or lists. It is for the HCP to recognise what information needs to be recorded and when to ensure it is an accurate record.

The concluding conversation is an important part of the consultation because it may be all that the patient remembers and it confirms the plans and expectations for the next stage in the care pathway. At the end of any consultation the information learnt should be summarised, an opinion given, including a diagnosis or an explanation, and a management recommendation. It is important to check that the patient understands and agrees with the management plan and the next step. Relevant information, including the facts and important negatives, opinions and recommendations should be documented. It is often said that:

> **If it isn't written down, it didn't happen**

All documentation should include basic information about the patient, such as the patient's name, date of birth and a unique identification number, the date and time of the consultation and the name and signature of the HCP and, when available, a unique identifier for the HCP, such as a GMC number. Usually, the written record is a summary of what is known, including important negatives. It should be structured so that relevant information is co-located to provide the evidence underpinning the opinion and the recommendation. It should be clear what is fact and what is opinion and when the patient is quoted. Recording information about a person is not an opportunity to make an inappropriate comment and should not be used to give a personal opinion about the patient as a person.

Chapter 3
The Methods Available
to Formulate a Diagnosis

Abstract

There is little that is certain in medicine and that includes the diagnosis. A definitive diagnosis can be made when the cause of the problem is proven. A descriptive diagnosis describes the problem but the underlying cause is unknown. A working diagnosis is a provisional diagnosis within a list of diagnoses used to plan management. The main diagnosis is the primary diagnosis and other diagnoses are secondary.

Formulating a diagnosis does not occur by chance. It requires knowledge of medicine and the basic sciences and a clinical method. There are many different methods available. The simple methods include to ask the patient or to rely on intuition, a hunch or "wishful thinking". The internet, guidelines, diagnostic algorithms and checklists can be helpful and some HCPs rely on "routine" tests. However, more methods are available. Medical knowledge can be used to know what diagnoses are most likely or what diagnoses are unlikely based on probabilities. It can also be used to recognise pathognomonic symptoms or signs, trigger words, phrases or signs and identify diagnostic patterns that lead to specific questions to ask or signs to look for. A knowledge of medicine and the basic sciences can be used to understand the problem: the onset, the severity and to determine the location of the abnormality causing the problem, the type of problem and the cause. Understanding and interpreting the information will lead to a descriptive diagnosis or reduce the list of possible diagnoses. Additional information about the person and the patient, such as risk factors or co-morbidity, influence diagnostic probability and may suggest a likely cause or exclude some causes. Information learnt should be linked and interpreted together.

A clinical diagnosis is a proposition, it is an opinion and should be evidence based. The evidence will be affected by what is asked, what is included or excluded, prioritisation and understanding. There is always an element of uncertainty, at least initially. Diagnostic errors and bias are inevitable and not all diagnoses are true: some are incorrect, missed or incomplete and there is increasingly a risk of over-diagnosis. It is important to be aware of the potential for error and bias and to use measures to reduce the risk.

Formulating a diagnosis is a complex process in which all relevant information from the headline information to learning about the person as a patient should be considered. It depends on the HCP using a clinical method to pro-actively ask questions and look for signs. Leads should be followed and relevant information linked. The HCP should know why they are asking a question or examining a part of the body and how they will use the information learnt.

Introduction

The diagnosis of diseases constitutes the foundation of the Practice of Medicine.
Marshall Hall (On Diagnosis. In four parts. London: Longman 1817)

Formulating a diagnosis is a complex process which usually starts with the exchange of information during the consultation and finishes when the results of investigations are known or the efficacy of treatment proven. When a patient presents with a new problem or a change in a pre-existing problem the consultation is the opportunity to learn, understand and interpret information about the problem to formulate a diagnosis or to list possible diagnoses.

Learning, understanding and interpreting the available information requires the skills to talk to and examine the patient meaningfully, the knowledge to know what questions to ask, what signs to look for and what the answers mean and a clinical method to apply the skills and knowledge appropriately, effectively and efficiently. Occasionally, a diagnosis can be made with confidence on the basis of the information learnt during the consultation but frequently it is dependent on investigations, the passage of time or a trial of treatment.

The aim of this chapter is to discuss the clinical methods available within a consultation to formulate a diagnosis.

Diagnostic Definitions

A diagnosis is a medical term used to label the problem. The diagnosis is important because it has implications for the patient and, occasionally, their family, for management and prognosis. Not all diagnoses are the same. The different diagnoses depend on the level of evidence available and current medical knowledge. The main types of diagnosis include:

- A definitive diagnosis.
- A descriptive diagnosis.
- A provisional diagnosis.
- Primary and secondary diagnoses.

Definitive diagnosis

A definitive diagnosis is the true diagnosis. A definitive diagnosis can only be made when the fundamental cause of the problem is proven and the pathogenesis understood. Examples of a definitive diagnosis include:

- A broken bone caused by a fall.
- An infection caused by a known pathogen. For example, Haemophilus influenza pneumonia or HIV infection.
- A hypersensitivity reaction to a proven antigen.
- Cancer, when the primary is identified and the cause proven. For example, colon cancer caused by APC gene defects on chromosome 5 or MUTYH gene defects on chromosome 1.
- Poisoning, such as lead poisoning.
- A dietary abnormality, such as vitamin deficiency.
- An endocrine abnormality, such as diabetes insipidus or acromegaly.
- Acute intermittent porphyria caused by deficiency of porphobilinogen deaminase (or hydroxymethylbilane deaminase).
- COPD, vasculitis and liver disease caused by deficiency of the alpha-1 antitrypsin protein.
- Dark urine, skin and cartilage pigmentation and arthritis caused by the accumulation of homogentisic acid in alkaptonuria.

The evidence frequently used to make a definitive diagnosis includes one or more of the following:

- A characteristic set of symptoms and signs. This is a "clinical" diagnosis.
- Change over time. This is also a "clinical" diagnosis.
- The results of relevant investigations. The nature of the investigation describes the evidence available. For example, a "haematological" or "radiological" diagnosis or a "genetic" or "histopathological" diagnosis.
- The response to treatment: a "therapeutic" diagnosis.

Unfortunately, despite advances in medical knowledge, the cause and pathogenesis of many medical conditions remains uncertain and a definitive diagnosis is based on a combination of clinical features, the results of tests, a trial of treatment or the passage of time. For example:

- The cause and patho-physiology of osteo-arthritis is not fully understood. A definitive diagnosis of osteo-arthritis is made on the basis of the clinical features, radiological or arthroscopic appearance, the response to treatment and observations over time.
- The patho-physiology of cancer is increasingly understood but a lot remains unknown. A definitive diagnosis of cancer is made on the basis of the clinical features, radiological, endoscopic, histological or cytological appearances, the response to treatment and observations over time.
- The patho-physiology of many mental illnesses, such as depression or schizophrenia, remains unknown. A definitive diagnosis is made on the basis of the clinical features and the absence of radiological or laboratory abnormalities.

For many conditions, expert panels or professional bodies have used available research evidence to determine the combination of evidence sufficient for a definitive diagnosis. For example:

- The criteria accepted for a diagnosis of UC or Crohn's disease is a combination of:
  - Clinical features.
  - Colonoscopic appearance.
  - Histopathological appearance.
  - Exclusion of other causes, such as Cytomegalovirus
  - Response to treatment.
- Myalgic encephalopathy (ME), also known as chronic fatigue syndrome (CFS) is diagnosed on the basis of:
  - Persistent or recurrent disabling tiredness for >4 months.
  - Exclusion of other causes, such as a mental health condition, infections or auto-immune diseases.
- The criteria accepted for a diagnosis of IBS is recurrent abdominal pain or discomfort on at least 3 days each month, in the past 3 months, associated with 2 or more of:
  - Less pain after defaecation.
  - Pain associated with a change in frequency of bowel habit.
  - Pain associated with a change in consistency of stool.
- The Wells criteria is a "points" based probability assessment used to determine the likelihood of a deep vein thrombosis (DVT) or a pulmonary embolus (PE):
  - Clinical signs and symptoms of a DVT: long saphenous vein tenderness, unilateral swelling (>3cm), prominent collateral superficial veins, pitting oedema (1 point each). Risk factors. For example, immobilization for >3 days, surgery recently, previous DVT/PE, malignancy (1 point). A Wells score <2 has a high negative predictive value for a DVT.
  - A Clinical diagnosis of a PE or other diagnoses are unlikely (2 points), haemoptysis (1 point), heart rate >100 bpm (1.5 points). Clinical signs and symptoms of a DVT: long saphenous vein tenderness, unilateral swelling (>3cm), prominent collateral superficial veins, pitting oedema (1 point each). Risk factors including immobilization for >3 days, surgery recently, previous DVT/PE, malignancy (1 point each). A Wells score >4 has a high positive predictive value for a PE.

    NB there are different iterations of the Wells criteria and alternative diagnostic decision-making tools for a PE, such as the "Geneva score", "Charlotte rule", "Pisa rules" or the "PE rule-out criteria". Investigations, such as a D-dimer, a CT PA scan, a VQ scan or confirmation of a DVT on Duplex USS may be indicated.
- Framingham heart failure diagnostic criteria is based on 1 major and 2 minor criteria:
  - Major criteria:
    - Orthopnoea and Paroxysmal nocturnal dyspnoea (PND)
    - Acute pulmonary oedema
    - Pulmonary rales
    - Cardiomegaly
    - 3rd heart sound (S3 gallup)
  - Minor criteria:
    - Breathlessness on exertion
    - Nocturnal cough
    - Ankle oedema
    - Pleural effusion
    - Tachycardia (>120 bpm)
    - Hepatomegaly

Investigations, such as a blood atrial naturetic peptide (ANP) or an echo cardiogram are indicated for confirmation.

Descriptive diagnosis

Many clinically accepted diagnoses are descriptions of the patient's problem. Some simply describe the main symptom. For example, confusion, depression, schizophrenia ("split-personality") or mania. Some describe the signs. For example, anaemia, jaundice, multi-nodular goitre, kypho-scoliosis, erythema nodosum, rosacea, a naevus, mole, ingrowing toenail or a hernia. When pain or discomfort is the main symptom, the descriptive diagnosis may include the prefix, "dys" or the post-fix "-algia" or "dynia" or the type of pain together with the location of the pain. For example:

- Dys-pepsia: describing upper abdominal discomfort after eating a meal.
- Dys-phagia: describing an uncomfortable feeling while swallowing.
- Dys-pareunia: describing painful sexual intercourse.
- Neur-algia: describing an atypical superficial pain.
- Fibromy-algia: describing a widespread soft tissue pain.
- Mast-algia: describing breast pain.
- Proct-algia fugax: describing rectal colic.
- Cocci-dynia: describing pain in the coccyx.
- Head (location) ache (pain).
- Biliary (location) colic (pain).
- Ureteric (location) colic (pain).

Frequently a descriptive diagnosis is a composite of the location of the problem or of the abnormality causing the problem, and the type of problem. For example:

- When there is inflammation, a descriptive diagnosis usually includes the location of the abnormality and the type of problem represented by the post-fix "-itis" or the likely cause, "infection". For example, appendic-(location) itis, ulcerative col-(location) itis, olecranon burs-(location) itis, hip arthr-(location) itis, cholecyst-(location) itis, dermato-(location) myos-(location) itis, dermat-(location) itis, pruritis (type of problem) ani (location), urinary tract (location) infection, or chest (location) infection (type of problem).
- When there is a structural problem, a descriptive diagnosis usually includes the location of the abnormality and the type of problem or cause. For example, a ureteric (location) calculus (likely cause), obstructive (type of problem) jaundice (location), choledocho-(location) "lithiasis" (likely cause), perforated (type of problem) duodenal (location) ulcer (likely cause), inguinal (location) hernia (type of problem), obstructive (type of problem) uropathy (location).
- When there is a circulatory problem, a descriptive diagnosis usually includes the location of the abnormality and the type of problem. For example, ischaemic (type of problem) limb (location), popliteal (location) aneurysm (type of problem), ischaemic (type of problem) heart (location) disease/failure, or acute myocardial (location) infarction (type of problem).
- When there is a neurological problem, a descriptive diagnosis may include the location of the abnormality and the type of problem or be a description of the abnormality or the symptoms. For example, a stroke (location and type of problem), peripheral (location) "neuropathy" (description of the symptoms), or right sided hemi-(location) plegia (description of the symptoms).
- When there is a metabolic problem, a descriptive diagnosis may include the location of the abnormality and the type of problem or be a description of the abnormality or the symptoms. For example, renal (location) "failure" (type of problem), hyper-calcaemia (description of the abnormality) or DM (description of the symptoms).
- When there is cancer, a descriptive diagnosis may include the location of the abnormality and the type of problem. For example, carcinomatosis (type of problem) peritonei (location) or breast (location) cancer (type of problem).

It can be seen that clinically there are 6 different types of descriptive diagnosis.

Frequently a descriptive diagnosis also includes the onset or duration of the problem. Clinically, the onset is "acute" if the symptoms started suddenly, in a matter of minutes, over several hours or a few days or "chronic" if the symptoms have been present for many weeks or months (duration). For example:

- Acute (onset) kidney (location) failure (a metabolic type of problem).
- Acute (onset) confusional state (a neurological type of problem).
- Acute (onset) pericard-(location) itis (an inflammatory type of problem).
- Chronic (duration) heart (location) failure (a circulatory type of problem).
- Chronic (duration) obstructive (a structural type of problem) pulmonary (location) disease.

Some descriptive diagnoses are also called syndromes or the problem is eponymously named. Syndromes can refer to:

- A collection of diagnoses that present with similar clinical features. For example, acute coronary syndrome (ACS), adult respiratory distress syndrome (ARDS), carpal tunnel syndrome.
- A collection of symptoms and signs of uncertain aetiology. For example, irritable bowel syndrome (IBS) or chronic fatigue syndrome (CFS).
- Some abnormalities are eponymously named. For example, Asperger's syndrome, Tourette's syndrome, Angelman syndrome, Morton's neuroma, Peyronie disease or Dupuytren contracture.

Often, a descriptive diagnosis is a provisional or working diagnosis made on the basis of available information and informing management. When the cause is identified, it becomes a definitive diagnosis.

Provisional diagnosis

A provisional diagnosis is a proposition. There is insufficient evidence for it to be a definitive diagnosis. When there are a number of possible diagnoses, each one is a provisional diagnosis. When, a provisional diagnosis is used to plan management it is a "working diagnosis". For some patients a working diagnosis is sufficient for a trial of treatment. In others, it is an indication for an investigation. A provisional diagnosis that should be considered and confirmed or excluded as quickly as possible to reduce the risk of irreversible harm or further harm is a "high priority diagnosis". For example:

- A patient presenting with painful, tender perineal inflammation may have necrotizing fasciitis which is a high priority diagnosis that should be investigated and treated urgently.
- Unexplained weight loss of >10% over >6 months or unexplained iron deficiency anaemia are alarm or "red-flag" symptom for cancer. This is a high priority diagnosis that should be investigated urgently to confirm or exclude cancer.

The headline information can be used to draw up an initial list of provisional diagnoses: a "differential diagnosis". The list will change as more information becomes available during the consultation; some diagnoses become more likely and others unlikely. Each diagnosis on a list has its own probability of being the true diagnosis. The most likely diagnosis is the one with the greatest probability of being true. This is usually placed at the top of the list. However, the list order may be influenced by consequence rather than likelihood. Some diagnoses are unlikely but because delayed treatment may have serious consequences the priority may be to exclude them early. For example:

- In a 70-year-old man presenting with a sudden onset of colicky loin to groin pain the differential diagnosis includes ureteric colic, musculo-skeletal back pain or a AAA. Excluding a AAA is a clinical priority and may be the working diagnosis even though other diagnoses are more likely.
- A middle-aged patient presenting with a change in bowel habit that has persisted for a month may have colo-rectal cancer. The differential diagnosis is long and includes diverticula disease and colitis. The likelihood of it being caused by cancer may be only 5% but this diagnosis should be excluded because formulating a diagnosis early is a high priority.

A diagnosis remains provisional until there is sufficient evidence for it to be confirmed or excluded. As more information becomes available, more diagnoses can be excluded from a list of possible diagnoses and the likelihood of one of the remaining diagnoses being the true diagnosis increases. This is because the sum of the probabilities of all possible diagnoses is one or 100%.

Often the evidence includes information from the patient, the results of tests, the passage of time and/or the efficacy of treatment. Frequently, the nature of the evidence is used to qualify the level of certainty. When a diagnosis is made on the basis of the symptoms and signs it is referred to as a "clinical" diagnosis. When it is based on the results of laboratory investigations it is a "laboratory" diagnosis and when on the basis of imaging, a "radiological" diagnosis. For example:

- The differential diagnosis of a young man presenting with constant pain, tenderness and guarding in the right lower quadrant of the abdomen includes acute appendicitis. This is a clinical working diagnosis if it is used to plan management. The probability the diagnosis is true is increased if the patient presents with a classical pattern of symptoms and signs and blood tests confirm systemic inflammation. It is then a clinical and laboratory diagnosis. If the appearance on CT scan or USS are also characteristic of acute appendicitis it becomes a clinical and radiological diagnosis, but it is still a provisional diagnosis. For most patients this is sufficient evidence to inform treatment, usually an operation, in which case it is a working diagnosis. If the appearances at the time of surgery confirm acute appendicitis it becomes a surgical diagnosis. If the microscopic appearance confirms acute appendicitis, it is a histological diagnosis. However, this only becomes a definitive diagnosis when the cause is identified. Most cases of acute appendicitis are caused by a faecolith impacted in the base of the appendix. However, a few have other causes, such as a polyp or cancer at the base of the appendix, worms (usually ascaris) or a foreign body. Acute appendicitis becomes a definitive diagnosis when the symptoms and signs resolve after the patient has been treated and the histological result, including the underlying cause is known.

- A patient presenting with breathlessness, a productive cough, a fever and signs of right lower lobe consolidation is likely to have a chest infection. This is a clinical working diagnosis. For many patients this is sufficient evidence to start antimicrobial treatment. If the patient gets better, this is often considered confirmation of the diagnosis. If blood tests are taken and show inflammation and a CXR shows the characteristic features of pneumonia this is a clinical, laboratory and radiological diagnosis. To make a definitive diagnosis requires the culture of a pathogenic organism in the sputum or blood and resolution following antimicrobial treatment. This is microbiological and therapeutic evidence for the diagnosis.

- A patient who presents feeling unwell, with fatigue, diarrhoea, abdominal pain and anaemia may have coeliac disease. This is a clinical working diagnosis. A positive anti-trans glutamase antibody test, a laboratory or immunological diagnosis and/or the classic microscopic appearances of a duodenal biopsy, a histological diagnosis, are usually considered sufficient for a definitive diagnosis but the symptoms need to resolve on a gluten free diet and return when rechallenged by gluten for the diagnosis to be proven: a therapeutic diagnosis.

Predictions of a future diagnosis are "pre-diagnoses". This is a type of provisional diagnosis because the diagnosis has not yet arisen but is considered likely. Increasingly, health data sets, laboratory, imaging, pathological or genetic information are being used to predict the chance of a future diagnosis. When populations are studied this is presented as a hazard ratio but for the individual the level of certainty is usually described subjectively using terms, such as "highly likely", "likely", "unlikely" or "rare". This is because predictions are speculative, being influenced by many variables, including environmental and lifestyle variables, other risks and preventative or mitigating measures. As with other provisional diagnoses, the diagnosis can be discussed with patients and used to inform management, but with a "pre-diagnosis" caution is needed because speculation and screening tests can lead to over-diagnosis.

Primary and secondary diagnoses

When there is more than one diagnosis there may be two or more separate and unrelated diagnoses or, more frequently, a primary diagnosis and secondary diagnosis(es). The principal or primary diagnosis refers to the diagnosis of the main problem. This is usually the original problem. A secondary diagnosis refers to an additional problem that arises as a consequence of the primary diagnosis, such as a complication or a secondary problem. A complication, secondary problem or a second primary problem may be the reason for the patient presenting. For this reason, it is important to learn the symptoms at the start of the problem and the details of any subsequent change. This is best illustrated with reference to a number of examples.

- A patient who presents feeling unwell, with weight loss, polyuria and polydipsia is likely to have DM. The blood sugar level confirms they have DM. This is the primary diagnosis. While examining them they are also found to have retinopathy and peripheral neuropathy. These are both secondary diagnoses that are complications of the DM. If the patient, is found to be dehydrated on examination and the haematocrit, serum sodium and creatinine are raised, hypovolaemia is a secondary problem caused by the negative water balance.

- When a patient presenting with deteriorating vision is diagnosed as having retinopathy this would initially be the primary diagnosis. DM is one of a number of causes of retinopathy. If DM is confirmed, this would become the primary diagnosis and the retinopathy a secondary diagnosis.

- A stroke is frequently the primary diagnosis at the time of the presentation. However, there are many different causes of a stroke and these are "risk factors" until one is identified to be the cause. If the stroke was caused by an embolus and the patient has atrial fibrillation (AF), with mural thrombus in the right atrium confirmed on an echocardiogram, the stroke is a secondary diagnosis: a complication of an embolus from the mural thrombus caused by the AF. However, AF is a descriptive diagnosis and there are a number of causes of AF, including IHD. Once the cause of the AF has been identified this then becomes the primary diagnosis and AF is a complication and a stroke a complication of the AF.

- The likely diagnosis in a patient presenting with an acute onset of breathlessness, haemoptysis and pleuritic chest pain is a PE. This is initially the primary diagnosis. However, a PE is usually a complication of a DVT. If the patient is found to have an acutely painful swollen, warm and red calf indicating a DVT, the DVT is the primary diagnosis and the PE a secondary diagnosis, a complication. There are many risk factors for a DVT including prolonged immobilization, surgery, the oral contraceptive pill, thrombophilia or cancer. If a diagnosis, such as thrombophilia or cancer is the cause of the DVT this then becomes the primary diagnosis: the DVT was a complication and the PE a complication of the DVT.

When more than one problem is possible, this should be recognised early in the consultation and the details of each learnt.

Determine the Diagnostic Aims

When a patient presents with a new problem or a change in a pre-existing problem the ideal is to formulate a definitive diagnosis so that definitive treatment can be started. Unfortunately, this is rarely achievable during the consultation. In which case, the aim is to formulate a descriptive diagnosis, a list of provisional diagnoses or to learn sufficient information to determine the location of the abnormality causing the problem, the type of problem and a likely cause. Occasionally, such as when the consultation follows an investigation, the aim is to confirm a diagnosis or, when different diagnoses are possible, to exclude one or more diagnoses. Sometimes the aim of the consultation is to examine the patient to screen for an asymptomatic diagnosis, such as a complication, a secondary problem or another problem. In summary, the diagnostic aims are:

- To make a definitive diagnosis
- To make a descriptive diagnosis
- To make a list of possible diagnoses
- To confirm a diagnosis
- To exclude a diagnosis
- To determine the location of the abnormality causing the problem
- To determine the type of problem
- To determine the cause
- To screen for
  - Another abnormality
  - A secondary abnormality
  - A complication

Although formulating a diagnosis is a core aim of the consultation, it is an enabler. This is because learning and understanding relevant information and formulating a diagnosis is with the aim of planning management, to help the patient.

Determine Whether Formulating a Diagnosis Is Indicated

Formulating a diagnosis is indicated when it is necessary to plan management. It may also be indicated for information, such as to reassure a patient or to inform prognosis. Frequently, formulating a definitive diagnosis is not indicated and learning about the patient's main problem(s), determining a descriptive diagnosis or excluding a high priority diagnosis is sufficient. For example:

- Diagnosing the infecting organism causing a chest infection may not be indicated for treatment.
- When a patient presents with a change in bowel habit or a skin lesion, excluding a high priority diagnosis, such as cancer may be indicated rather than formulating a diagnosis.
- When a patient is at the end of their life and the diagnosis is unlikely to influence management, formulating a diagnosis may not be indicated. The consultation and management is usually aimed at alleviating symptoms.

When a patient does not want to know the diagnosis and does not want the HCP to know, and not knowing it will not affect management, formulating a diagnosis is contra-indicated.

The Clinical Methods Available to Formulate a Diagnosis

The methods available to formulate a diagnosis are:

- Inspiration, a "hunch", or "wishful thinking".
- "Straight to test".
- "Ask the patient".
- Recognise pathognomonic symptoms or signs.
- Recognise trigger words, phrases or signs.
- Pattern recognition.
- Probabilities.
- Exclude a diagnosis.
- Diagnosis-hypothesis testing.
- Learn to understand.
- Link or triangulate information.
- Use a diagnostic checklist.

The diagnostic methods are complementary. It is for the clinician to decide on the method to use at a given time in the consultation.

Inspiration, a "hunch" or "wishful thinking"

Traditionally learning about the problem involved asking a set sequence of questions and examining the patient systematically as a checklist in the hope that inspiration will lead to a diagnosis. However, this is little better than "wishful thinking". It is not a reliable or reproducible method.

"Wishful thinking" should be distinguished from intuition, an "inspiration" or a "hunch", when a diagnosis suddenly comes to mind. Although, it is often unclear what information leads to the "hunch" or why the diagnostic jump was made, it is not "wishful thinking" because the "hunch" is used as a hypothesis or a working diagnosis, to inform the questions to ask or signs to look for to confirm or exclude the diagnosis. Sometimes this will lead down a blind alley but it may be a short cut to a diagnosis. It is appropriate to use intuition or a hunch to inform the direction of a consultation or to plan management but it inappropriate to use it as the basis for a diagnosis because it may be biased, such as when an HCP is excessively influenced by recent experience or a significant event or persists with a belief despite evidence to the contrary.

To the casual observer, experienced clinicians appear to use this method a lot. Indeed, the tendency to be inspired increases with experience. However, in reality the hunch is based on a combination of pattern recognition and probabilities based on experience and knowledge. This means that inspiration is not a diagnostic method that can be taught.

"Straight to test"

"Straight to test" is frequently used in the emergency setting when it is important to exclude "high priority" diagnoses quickly. For example:

- Chest pain is investigated with a serum troponin and an ECG. If these are normal IHD is unlikely.
- Hypotensive collapse is investigated with an ultrasound scan (USS) or CT scan to exclude a ruptured abdominal aortic aneurysm (AAA).
- Severe breathlessness and pleuritic chest pain is investigated with a CT pulmonary angiogram (CT PA) to exclude a PE.

Some patients are eligible for screening tests. This is a form of "straight to test". Nationally, eligibility is determined by political, statistical, financial and resource risk-benefit assessments. Some tests are age dependent, such as AAA or bowel cancer screening. Some are age and gender dependent, such as cervical screening or breast cancer screening in women or prostate screening in men and some are restricted to high-risk subgroups, such as a chest radiograph (CXR) in asbestos exposed patients or a gastro-intestinal endoscopy in patients with familial adenomatous polyposis syndrome (FAP). Positive test results are managed according to standard pathways with rigorous governance arrangements for quality and time intervals. However, a negative result rarely excludes the condition and can give a false sense of reassurance. Furthermore, there are few opportunities for variance in a screening pathway, which can limit patient choice and compliance.

Unfortunately, many HCPs go "straight to test" following the consultation regardless of the information learnt from the patient. By ordering a test the HCP is seen to be "doing something" and for the HCP, it is hoped that an abnormal result will indicate a likely diagnosis and "tell" them what should be done next. Indeed, many patients are only satisfied when they are sent for a test and many HCPs and lawyers give greater weight to test results than clinical opinion. As the number and availability of tests increases it is not surprising that "straight to test" is increasingly used as a diagnostic method. However, there are significant risks when "straight to test" is used as a diagnostic method. These include:

- An unnecessary test may be performed. A test should be undertaken for the right reason. The aims of the investigation should be clear to both the HCP and the patient.
- The wrong test may be performed. A test should be performed because it is indicated not because it is available. There are specific indications for every test.
- A test may be performed that is not indicated. This reduces the pre-test probability and likelihood a test result is true.
- A test may be performed that lacks sensitivity or specificity. Negative test results can give false reassurance and positive results can be false or misleading. For example:
  o Breathlessness could be investigated with a CXR. It is easy to be reassured by a normal report but a pulmonary abnormality may have been missed. For example, up to 90% of small peripheral lung cancers are missed when a CXR is reported despite being visible on retrospective review.
  o Upper abdominal pain could be investigated with "liver function" blood tests and an USS. If these are normal biliary colic is considered unlikely. Biliary USS is very sensitive but will still miss a gallstone in 5-10% of patients with gallstones. The rate is higher in the obese or if the stones are small. Blood tests will only be abnormal if the stone migrates into the bile duct or there is inflammation.
  o A painful knee could be investigated with a knee arthroscopy. A normal arthroscopy may exclude an intra-capsular abnormality but does not exclude other joint and peri-articular abnormalities.
- A risk of reporting bias, error or misinterpretation. Some tests are considered "objective" when in fact they are subjective. Subjective tests, such as endoscopy, radiology or histopathology are susceptible to subjective bias, error or misinterpretation.
- Mis-understanding what the result means. For example, serum bilirubin, the transaminases and alkaline phosphatase are often collectively referred to as "liver function" tests despite the fact that changes are not specific to abnormalities in the liver.
- An incidental finding can lead to an overdiagnosis

Information about the patient is essential to determine the aims of the test, to ensure the test is indicated and when interpreting the results of tests. Choosing the right test for the right reasons increases the pre-test probability of a diagnosis which increases the predictive value of the test. This is discussed further in the chapter on methodology for planning management.

"Ask the patient"

Asking the patient what is wrong with them or what they think caused their problem may be helpful. It is indicated when there is the possibility that a patient may know the diagnosis, the cause of their problem or what led to the problem.

Some patients think they know what caused their problem and for some the problem is a recurrence of a previous problem. Other patients have talked to friends or family or have researched their symptoms. Their diagnosis may not be correct but, if nothing else, it informs the HCP what the patient is thinking. In addition, asking the patient what they think could be causing their symptoms shows respect and includes the patient in diagnostic decision making.

Recognise pathognomonic symptoms or signs

A pathognomonic symptom or sign is one that is well known, easily recognised and strongly predictive of a diagnosis: i.e., has a high positive predictive value. When listening to the patient's description of their problem it is important to listen for symptoms that may be pathognomonic. Examples of pathognomonic symptoms include:

- "Rice watery" stool is characteristic of cholera.
- Hydrophobia in rabies.

- Painless cloudy vision is characteristic of a cataract.
- Painful tunnel or halo vision is characteristic of glaucoma.
- Visual floaters or flashes of light suggest a retinal detachment.
- Vertigo and tinnitus are characteristic of Meniere's disease.
- Dark skin (hyperpigmentation) is characteristic of Addison's disease.
- Mid-cycle pain caused by ovulation.

When a patient presents with a visible or palpable abnormality the signs may be pathognomonic. Examples of pathognomonic signs include:

- Skin lesions, such as solar keratosis, psoriasis, hidradenitis, a pilonidal sinus, a BCC or an SCC.
- A soft smooth edged sub-cutaneous mass that slips to one side when being examined is likely to be a lipoma.
- Kayser-Fleischer rings are characteristic of copper deposition in Wilson's disease.
- Exophthalmos is characteristic of Graves' disease.
- Koplik's spots inside the mouth are characteristic of measles.
- A pill rolling tremor is characteristic of Parkinson's disease.
- Bull's eye rash is characteristic of Lyme disease.
- Rose spots on the abdomen are characteristic of enteric fever.
- Bronze skin pigmentation is characteristic of Addison's disease.
- Yellow sclera is characteristic of jaundice.
- Caput medusae is characteristic of porto-systemic shunt.
- Grey-Turner's sign is characteristic of retroperitoneal haemorrhage.
- Spinal deformity with increased curvature and rigidity is characteristic of kyphoscoliosis and ankylosing spondylitis.
- Hard palmar thickening and nodularity along the line of the flexor tendons to the index finger and adjacent fingers, tending to produce a fixe flexion deformity, is characteristic of Dupuytren's contracture.
- A barrel shaped chest with little change on inspiration or expiration is characteristic of emphysema.
- Coarse facial features are characteristic of Acromegaly.
- Moon face and buffalo hump is characteristic of Cushing's syndrome.
- A firm non-tender intra-abdominal mass is cancer until proven otherwise.
- Multiple small flat non-blanching petechiae are characteristic of thrombocytopaenia.
- A machinery murmur is characteristic of a patent ductus arteriosus.
- A firm smooth pulsating mass along the line of a major artery is likely to be an aneurysm.

However, it is rare for a symptom or sign to be truly pathognomonic. Most are indicative and additional information is needed to confirm the diagnosis.

The absence of a pathognomonic symptom or sign does not exclude one of these diagnoses.

Recignise trigger words, phrases or signs

The patient's description or the information learnt during the consultation may include trigger words or, on examination, there may be signs indicating a likely diagnosis. The focus is then on asking precision questions or performing a focused examination to pro-actively look for symptoms or signs to confirm or exclude the diagnosis. For example:

- A temporary loss of vision in one eye may be caused by amaurosis fugax. Are there any other symptoms or signs to support the diagnosis of a stroke?
- Pins and needles in the extremities indicates hypercalcaemia. Are there any symptoms or signs to support the diagnosis of hypercalcaemia?
- A reducible groin swelling is likely to be a hernia. Are the signs characteristic?
- A cyclical fever (a Pel Ebstein fever) is characteristic of Hodgkin's lymphoma. Are there signs of lymphadenopathy?

Pattern recognition

A pattern or cluster of information may match a "text book" description and indicate a likely diagnosis or their absence reduce the likelihood. For example:

- Crushing central chest pain, feeling sweaty and breathless indicating an AMI.
- Progressive dysphagia starting with solid food, progressing to soft foods and even liquids, associated with weight loss indicating oesophageal cancer.
- Sudden onset of loin to grain pain, which comes and goes in waves, causing the patient to move around to get comfortable, indicates ureteric colic.
- Thirst, excessive micturition and rapid weight loss indicating DM.
- Confusion, ataxia and visual disturbance in an alcoholic indicate Wernicke's encephalopathy.
- When a young adult presents with a fever that peaks at the same time each day, a sore throat, a non-itchy migratory rash and generalised aches the pattern fits adult-onset Still's disease.
- A sudden onset of severe constant and persistent loin to groin pain may be caused by ureteric colic, a AAA or testicular torsion:
  o If the pain is associated with a tender testicle in a young adult a testicular torsion is a likely diagnosis.
  o In a middle-aged patient, pain associated with tenderness in the loin or along the line of the ureter is likely to be ureteric colic.
  o If the patient is elderly, and they have collapsed or blacked out or have a tachycardia and low blood pressure, a leaking AAA is the likely diagnosis.

Questions can then be asked or an examination performed to complete a pattern and confirm or exclude the diagnosis.

The absence of a pattern may mean a diagnosis is unlikely but may not exclude a diagnosis, because, increasingly, patients present early in the course of an illness before all the classical "textbook" symptoms and signs are manifest.

Pattern recognition is an important method to use not only to formulate a diagnosis but also to determine the location of the abnormality causing the problem or the type of problem. For example:

- A headache can be caused by a primary brain problem or be secondary to a systemic illness. A headache that wakes the patient from sleep or occurs in the morning and is worse when coughing, sneezing or bending down fits the pattern expected if the ICP is raised.
  The signs to look for include hypertension, bradycardia and slow breathing (Cushing's triad) and swelling of the optic disc (papilloedema) on fundoscopy.
  The pattern of symptoms and signs would indicate a primary intracranial abnormality (the location) likely to be caused by a structural abnormality (the type of problem).
- Central abdominal pain can be caused by many different diagnoses. However, mid-gut colic, abdominal distension, nausea and sickness together fit the pattern expected for small bowel obstruction.
  A previous laparotomy scar, generalised tympanic mildly tender abdominal distension and active bowel sounds support the diagnosis of adhesional small bowel obstruction.
  The pattern of symptoms and signs would indicate the location of the abnormality is likely to be the distal small bowel and it is likely to be caused by adhesions, a structural abnormality.
- Upper abdominal colic or right upper quadrant colic, radiating round to the back on the right-hand side, associated with anorexia, nausea and a feeling of upper abdominal bloating is likely to be biliary colic.
  A tender right sub-costal region indicates cholecystitis, a palpable subcostal mass may be a mucocele of the gallbladder, a very tender ill-defined mass an empyema of the gallbladder or a localized perforation.
  The pattern of symptoms and signs would indicate the location of the abnormality is likely to be the gall bladder and it is likely to be caused by gallstones, a structural abnormality, with or without inflammation.
- Feeling ill with a fever, including pyrexia, peripherally flushed and sweating, breathless with tachypnoea and a sinus tachycardia indicate systemic inflammation. The problem first started with symptoms of dysuria and urinary frequency suggesting the source is a UTI.
  The pattern of symptoms and signs would indicate the systemic inflammatory response was secondary to a urinary tract (location) infection (type of problem).
- Feeling ill with weight loss and anorexia, may be caused by cancer.
  An atypical mole on the leg, with groin lymphadenopathy and hepatomegaly support the diagnosis.

The pattern of symptoms and signs would indicate the location of the abnormality is likely to be the leg and the abnormality a melanoma (type of problem).

The value of pattern recognition to formulate a diagnosis increases as medical knowledge and experience increases.

Probabilities

Probability is used as a diagnostic method throughout the consultation and the pathway of care. It is used to determine the likelihood of a diagnosis, to exclude a diagnosis, to determine the likely location of the abnormality causing the problem, the type of problem and the cause.

Probability is certainty quantified. Mathematically it is presented as a percentage or a ratio, whereas in clinical practice it is usual to use an adjective such as definite, probable, possible, likely, unlikely or rare. The quality and quantity of the evidence determines the probability and the reliability: the clinical information may indicate a particular diagnosis is likely but if the information is incomplete or inaccurate information the diagnosis may be wrong.

When a patient presents with a new problem, demographic information indicates the point prevalence of a diagnosis. The headline information, including demographic information, previous information known about the patient and an outline of the presenting problem will indicate likely diagnoses. Probability can also indicate the rank order of a list of possible diagnoses. As a general rule,

---

Common things occur commonly

Ockham's razor urges us to choose the simplest option

William Ockham (a theologian born around 1285)

For example, the common causes of feeling ill include:

- Common cold – 9%
- COPD – 4%
- Sinusitis – 4%
- Depression – 4%
- Hypovolaemia – 3%
- Pneumonia – 3%
- Anxiety – 3%
- UTI – 3%

Information from asking questions and examining the patient changes the probability of each diagnosis making some more likely and others less likely. For example:

- An acute fever is usually caused by a viral illness. However, recent travel to a tropical country increases the likelihood of a fever being caused by a tropical infection, such as malaria, Dengue fever or Rickettsia.
- Chronic breathlessness in a smoker is likely to be caused by COPD. However, if they have worked with asbestos the likelihood that the breathlessness is caused by pulmonary fibrosis or a mesothelioma is increased.

When management includes performing tests, the likelihood a clinical diagnosis is true is the "pre-test" probability. Tests, time and a change in clinical features provide more information and change the probability of a given diagnosis.

Probability, is also used as a measure of future risk: "potential morbidity". The likelihood a problem will arise for an individual tends to increase as the number of risk factors, the severity and duration of the exposure to the risk factors and the susceptibility of the individual to the risk increases. Treatment or change may reduce the risk. Absolute risk is the probability of the problem occurring, whereas relative risk is the comparative difference in probability between two samples. For example:

- The lifetime risk of a man developing bowel cancer is about 7% or 1 in 15 and for a woman approximately 6% or 1 in 18. Therefore, although the difference in absolute risk is only 1%, a man is 17% more likely to get bowel cancer than a woman. This is the relative risk.

- The risk of a 50-year-old man developing bowel cancer is 1.8% but when a first degree relative has bowel cancer it is increased to 3.4%. The relative risk is 178% greater.

The hazard ratio (HR) is another way of presenting relative risk. The absolute risk is set at 1. An HR of 0.5 means that the risk is halved and an HR of 2 means that the risk is doubled.

The variables that influence the risk for an individual include:

- The time course of the risk. Period prevalence is the proportion of the sample population that will get a problem over a period of time. In general, the likelihood of a condition developing is increased as exposure to the risk becomes more frequent, more severe, more prolonged or the risk is not managed. For example:
  o The greater the exposure to air pollution the higher the risk of developing lung disease.
  o The greater the severity of wound contamination the more likely a wound infection will occur.
  o The relative risk of a spouse developing coronary heart disease when exposed second-hand to <20 cigarettes/ day is 1.23, which increases to 1.31 when exposed to >20 cigarettes/ day.
  o There is individual variation in susceptibility. For example:
    ▪ A high alcohol consumption is associated with an increased risk of developing alcoholic cirrhosis. But not everyone who drinks a lot over a long time gets cirrhosis
    ▪ Air pollution is associated with an increased risk of lung disease in some people.
- The number of other family members affected.
- The published data may not be relevant to the patient, because the published data may be based on a different sample population or not all-important variables are factored in.
- Multiple risk factors may present a disproportionately greater risk together than they would individually.
- Mitigating factors may reduce a risk.

Diagnosis-hypothesis testing

The symptoms and signs together with demographic information may indicate a short list of possible diagnoses. This list can be used to inform specific questions to ask and signs to look for on examination to confirm or exclude each diagnosis.

Exclude a diagnosis

Excluding a diagnosis is part of "diagnosis-hypothesis testing" and is frequently based on "probabilities". However, it should be thought of as a separate diagnostic method because it is often deliberately used throughout the consultation to inform the questions to ask or signs sought.

Frequently, clinically, a diagnosis is "excluded" when the likelihood is very low. However, this may not be appropriate because, although the diagnosis is unlikely it is still possible. It is often more difficult to confidently exclude a diagnosis than to confirm a diagnosis.

When a diagnosis is excluded the list of possible diagnoses is decreased and the probability of the remaining diagnoses being true is increased (this is because the sum of the probabilities in a list is always equal to one or 100%).

Excluding a diagnosis starts with the demographic information. For example:

- Some problems are specific to only one gender. For example:
  o Pelvic inflammatory disease only occurs in females or testicular cancer in males.
- Some diagnoses are less likely in one gender. For example:
  o Males are less likely to get auto-immune disease and schizophrenia is less common in females.
- The likelihood of a diagnosis may be influenced by age. For example:
  o Ischaemic heart disease is less likely in the young.
  o Testicular torsion is rare in males >30 years of age.
- Some problems are less common in some ethnic groups. For example:
  o The prevalence of Sickle cell anaemia is low, except among people of African or Mediterranean descent.

Information in the patient's description of their problem, such as the onset, duration, severity or location of the problem excludes many diagnoses. As more information becomes available during the consultation more diagnoses are excluded. Excluding a high priority diagnosis early is important, to reduce the risk of irreversible harm.

Learn to understand

Formulating a diagnosis is difficult because there are many different diagnoses but relatively few ways they present. Therefore, when pathognomonic or trigger words or patterns are absent and the differential diagnosis long or uncertain, questions should be asked and signs sought to understand the problem. Traditionally, when the diagnosis is uncertain, a series of questions are asked to learn about the problem:

- How did the problem start and how long has it been going on: onset and duration?
- Has there been a change in the symptoms?
- Where is the problem?
- Are there any associated features?
- How severe is it?
- Describe its character?
- Are there any aggravating or relieving factors?

Then the patient is examined in a systematic way.

This approach will achieve the aim of filling in a proforma but is unlikely to help understanding. Learning to understand describes a diagnostic method in which questions are asked and the signs sought with the aim of determining the location of the abnormality causing the problem (the anatomy of the problem), the type of problem and the likely cause of the problem (the patho-physiology). Learning to understand is intended to bridge the divide between the clinical features and medical knowledge to formulate a diagnosis. The questions available are the same as those used in the traditional clerking. The difference is in the way the questions are used or the patient examined and the answers or signs understood and interpreted.

When learning to understand, questions are asked or a part of the body examined with purpose: the HCP should always know why they are asking a question or examining a part of the body and then they should ensure the question is answered or a specific sign identified or excluded. Therefore, when learning to understand, it is first necessary to ask yourself, why am I asking the question/performing an examination? In other words, what is the aim?

Ask yourself, what is the likely location of the abnormality causing the problem?

For many problems the location of the problem is the location of the abnormality. However, for others they are different. It is important to confirm or determine the location of the abnormality causing the problem because the differential diagnosis of the presenting problem is longer than the differential diagnosis when the location of the abnormality is known. For example:

- Breathlessness is a problem that affects the chest. However, it can be caused by a primary pulmonary abnormality affecting the airways, the lungs or the lung lining, such as a chest infection or pulmonary fibrosis, or be secondary to an abnormality affecting the mechanics or regulation of ventilation, such as a pneumothorax or a stroke, the circulation, gas transport, or demand, such as heart failure or anaemia.
- A headache is a problem that affects the brain. However, it can be caused by a primary neurological problem, such as a tension headache or migraine, a primary structural problem, such as a tumour, cancer, inflammation or a circulatory problem, such as a haemorrhage, or be secondary to a problem elsewhere, such as septicaemia, hypovolaemia, hypertension or hypercalcaemia.

Determining the likely location of the abnormality reduces the list of possible diagnoses. For example, when breathlessness is caused by an abnormality affecting:

- The airways, the differential diagnosis includes laryngitis, bronchitis or bronchospasm, cancer or a foreign body.
- The lungs, the differential diagnosis includes pulmonary consolidation, pulmonary fibrosis or oedema.
- The lung lining, the differential diagnosis includes a pleural effusion, a pneumothorax or cancer.
- The mechanics of ventilation, the differential diagnosis includes ankylosing spondylitis, severe kyphoscoliosis or motor neurone disease.
- Regulation, the differential diagnosis includes metabolic acidosis, medications or a raised ICP.
- The pulmonary circulation, the differential diagnosis includes heart failure, hypovolaemia, shunting or a PE.

- Gas transport, the differential diagnosis includes anaemia or carbon monoxide poisoning.
- Demand, the differential diagnosis includes sepsis or thyrotoxicosis.

When a patient presents with pain, symptoms of deranged function or a visible or palpable abnormality the location of the problem is usually the location of the abnormality. For example:

- When a patient presents with a headache, the abnormality is likely to be in the head.
- When the patient presents with haematuria, the abnormality is likely to be in the bladder.
- When a patient has a localized rash, the abnormality is likely to be affecting the skin.

However, the location of the abnormality should not be assumed, because the problem may be caused by an abnormality elsewhere. For example:

- A headache may be secondary to a systemic problem, such as hypertension.
- Haematuria may be secondary to a coagulopathy.
- A rash may be caused by an auto-immune reaction.

When a patient presents feeling ill, with a pain or deranged function, the patients description of the site of the problem should be considered together with information about the severity, onset, character, aggravating and relieving factors and associated symptoms to determine the likely location of the abnormality. When the location of the abnormality causing the problem is uncertain, a stepwise method should be used to determine the location of the abnormality. First determine whether the abnormality is likely to be at the site of the problem or referred from elsewhere. Then determine whether it is superficial or deep-seated, solitary or multi-focal, and then what tissue, gland, organ or part of the body is likely to be affected (Figure 18). This can then be used to inform the signs to look for to confirm or exclude the likely location. When a patient presents with a visible or palpable abnormality, such as cellulitis or a hernia, and the site is examined early in the consultation, a similar stepwise approach can be used to determine the location of the abnormality.

Ask yourself, what is the likely type of problem?

Clinically, patients present with symptoms and/or signs of an inflammatory type of problem, such as cellulitis, appendicitis, bronchitis, pneumonia, sepsis or rheumatoid arthritis; a circulatory problem, such as anaemia, heart failure, claudication or a PE; a structural problem, such as a sebaceous cyst, a hernia, choledocholithiasis, adhesions, COPD, a foreign body, pulmonary fibrosis, a pleural effusion, a pneumothorax or kyphoscoliosis; cancer; a metabolic problem, such as renal failure, DM or thyrotoxicosis; or a neurological problem, such as, migraine, peripheral "neuropathy" or motor neurone disease. Determining the type of problem is important because the type of problem together with the location of the abnormality may indicate a descriptive diagnosis or a limited list of possible diagnoses.

Figure 18: Illustrating a method to determine the location of the abnormality causing the problem.

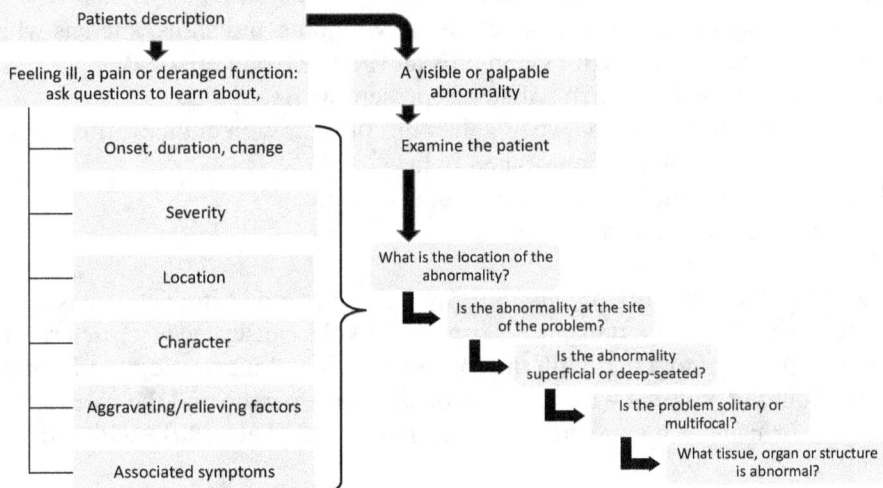

The type of problem may be obvious from the patient's description or from the signs on examination. For example, a fever is characteristic of inflammation and stridor indicates upper airway obstruction. If not, the available information should be used to determine the likely type of problem and additional questions asked or signs sought as required.

The location of the abnormality, will often limit the likely types of problem. For example:

- When the main presenting problem is breathlessness and:
  o The abnormality affects the airways, the type of problem is likely to be inflammation, such as laryngitis or bronchitis, a structural problem, such as bronchospasm or cancer.
  o The abnormality affects gas transfer between alveolar air and the blood, the type of problem is likely to be a structural problem, such as pulmonary fibrosis or a circulatory problem, such as pulmonary oedema or shunting.
  o The abnormality affects the blood, the type of problem is likely to be a circulatory problem, such as anaemia or a metabolic problem, such as acidosis or carbon monoxide poisoning.
  o The abnormality affects pulmonary perfusion, the type of problem is likely to be a circulatory problem, such as a PE or heart failure.
  o The abnormality increases oxygen demand, the type of problem is likely to be inflammation, such as sepsis or a metabolic problem, such as thyrotoxicosis.
  o The abnormality affects the regulation of ventilation, the type of problem is likely to be a neurological problem, such as from medications or a raised ICP.
- When the main presenting problem is a headache and:
  o It is a primary brain problem the type of problem is likely to be a neurological problem, such as a tension headache, migraine or a mental health condition, a circulatory problem, such as an aneurysm or an arterio-venous malformation, a structural problem, such as dementia, a tumour, hydrocephalus or an intra-cranial abscess, cancer or inflammation, such as encephalitis or meningitis, are uncommon causes of a headache.
  o It is secondary to an abnormality elsewhere, the type of problem is likely to be inflammation, such as an infection or auto-immune disease, a circulatory problem, such as hypertension, hypovolaemia, anaemia or heart failure, or a metabolic problem, such as renal failure.

Questions can then be asked and signs sought with the aim of confirming or excluding a type of problem. In this way, determining the type of problem is a stepping stone towards formulating a diagnosis.

It is not uncommon for a condition to present in different ways with symptoms and signs indicating different types of problem in different patients. For example:

- Cancer may present with characteristic symptoms and signs, such as a mass or with weight loss, or it may present with symptoms and signs characteristic of:
  o An inflammatory problem. For example, dermatomyositis and pyoderma gangrenosa.
  o A structural problem. For example, large bowel obstruction or jaundice.
  o A circulatory problem. For example, atrial myxoma, renal cancer, or a tumour embolus.
  o A neurological problem. For example, Eaton-Lambert myasthenic syndrome or encephalomyelitis.
  o A metabolic problem. For example, prostate cancer presenting with hypercalcaemia, Cushing's syndrome, insulinoma, neuro-endocrine tumours (carcinoid) or prolactinoma.
- A structural problem may present with characteristic symptoms and signs, such as when a gall stone presents with biliary colic, or it may present with symptoms and signs characteristic of:
  o A metabolic problem, such as when gallstones present with jaundice.
  o An inflammatory problem, such as when gallstones present with cholecystitis or ascending cholangitis.
  o A circulatory problem, such as a femoral embolus.
  o A neurological problem, such as an entrapment syndrome.
  o Cancer, such as large bowel obstruction.

Determining the location of the abnormality and the type of problem will indicate a descriptive diagnosis or a short list of possible diagnoses. It is then important to determine a likely cause because, determining the location of the abnormality and the type of problem together with the likely cause is a clinical bridge to formulating a diagnosis.

Linking information about the problem with information about the person and the patient may exclude some causes and, based on probabilities or using a diagnostic checklist, indicate a likely cause which then can be used to inform management.

When it is an inflammatory type of problem:

Ask yourself, what is the likely cause of inflammation?

Inflammation is the immune-mediated response to a variety of insults or abnormalities. In most patients, inflammation is caused by an infection (viral, bacterial, fungal, helminth and parasitic), but there are many non-infective causes of inflammation including:

- Trauma, such as healing following an injury or post-operative inflammation.
- A hypersensitivity reaction to an extrinsic allergen at the interface between the body and the environment, such as to pollen, gluten, peanut or latex, or to medications such as penicillin. When the onset is very fast, within minutes, it is caused by a type I hypersensitivity reaction. For example:
  o Asthma
  o Hay fever
  o A drug reaction
- An auto-immune reaction is a hypersensitivity reaction in response to a host antigen. The immune response may vary.
  o When a host antigen(s) stimulates a specific IgM or IgG mediated inflammatory response it is a type II hypersensitivity reaction. For example, auto-immune haemolytic anaemia, fibromyalgia, dermatomyositis, polymyositis, glomerulonephritis, atherosclerosis, cystitis, eczema, vasculitis, rheumatoid arthritis, sarcoidosis. rheumatic heart disease, thrombocytopaenia, Goodpasture's syndrome and sarcoidosis.
  o When the host antigen is a cell receptor it is called a type V hypersensitivity reaction. For example, Graves' disease and myasthenia Gravis.
  o When a host antigen(s) stimulates a T-cell mediated inflammatory response it is a type IV (delayed type) hypersensitivity. For example, contact dermatitis, chronic transplant rejection (through MHC and HLA antigens) and multiple sclerosis.
  o When immune complexes of IgG bound to circulating antigens are deposited in the organs, such as the kidneys and lungs, or joints causing chronic inflammation; disease it is a type III hypersensitivity reaction. For example, rheumatoid arthritis, glomerulonephritis, lupus erythematosus and alveolitis.
- "Chemical" inflammation. Inflammation may be caused by,
  o Fluid in the wrong place causing inflammation. For example, reflux oesophagitis, aspiration pneumonitis, a ruptured oesophagus, acute pancreatitis, a perforated peptic ulcer, biliary peritonitis or a ruptured ectopic pregnancy.
  o Extensive cell death or damage of a solid organ or gland. For example, alcoholic hepatitis or pancreatitis, hepatocellular damage following a paracetamol overdose, or sialadenitis.
- Degeneration can cause inflammation. For example, osteo-arthritis or diverticula disease.
- Radiation can cause tissue damage and inflammation. For example, radiation dermatitis or proctitis.
- Cancer inflammation is usually caused by ischaemia, when the tumour outgrows its blood supply, or an auto-immune reaction to tumour antigens.
- Ischaemic inflammation is usually due to cell death, such as torsion, reperfusion, such as compartment syndrome, or occurs at a boundary zone between healthy tissue and dead tissue.

The available information should be used to distinguish between infection and one of the many non-infective causes of inflammation.

When it is a structural type of problem:

Ask yourself, what is the likely cause of a structural problem?

Many organs, glands and tissues depend on their structural integrity for their function. The location and impact of the structural problem determine the presentation probability and indicate the likely cause. The available information should be used to distinguish between a tumour, which can be benign or malignant, primary or secondary, solid or cystic, and one of the many other types of structural abnormality including:

- Trauma. For example, haematoma, seroma, scarring, rupture, hemarthrosis or fracture.
- A foreign body.
- Degenerative changes affecting:

- o A solid structure. For example, pancreatic pseudocyst or osteoarthritis.
  - o A hollow organ, duct or tube. For example, calculi, bezoar, a stricture, scar tissue or adhesions.
- Metabolic changes affecting:
  - o A hollow organ, duct or tube. For example, calculi.
- A hernia.
  - o External. For example, inguinal, umbilical, incisional, femoral, Spigelian.
  - o Internal. For example, hiatus hernia or mesenteric hernia.
- Deformity.
  - o Congenital. For example, haemangioma, AV malformation, Riedel's lobe or a horseshoe kidney.
  - o Acquired. For example, Dupuytren's contracture or swan-neck deformity in rheumatoid arthritis.

When it is a circulatory type of problem:

Ask yourself, what is the likely cause of a circulatory problem?

The cells, tissues and organs are dependent on the circulation to function and for perfusion to increase in response to increased demands. Heart or circulatory failure, and anaemia or hypovolaemia affect the whole body, but, if perfusion of an organ or part of the body is significantly compromised then function of that part of the body is compromised and the associated ischaemia may cause pain and impaired function. Circulatory problems may be caused by a local or regional abnormality, such as arterial stenosis, an embolus, thrombosis, an aneurysm, an AVM, vasculitis or a varix, a cardiac abnormality, such as IHD or valvular heart disease, or a blood abnormality, such as anaemia, hypovolaemia, a clotting or thrombotic abnormality.

When it is a metabolic problem:

Ask yourself, what is the likely cause of a metabolic problem?

Metabolic problems disturb the body's homeostasis and affect the function of all cellular activities. They particularly affect nerve and muscle function and usually present with deranged function or cause the patient to feel ill. Metabolic problems may be caused by endocrine abnormalities, deranged organ function or a poison. The available information should be used to distinguish between the different causes.

- Endocrine disease. For example, DM, hypo- or hyper-parathyroidism, hyperthyroidism or myxoedema.
- Deranged acid-base balance. For example, renal failure.
- Abnormal water content and salt concentration. For example, from vomiting, diarrhoea, renal failure, or DM.
- Deranged "waste" management. For example, affecting bile, nitrogenous waste or urate excretion.
- Metabolism. For example, liver failure, porphyria or the mitochondrial diseases.
- Poisoning. For example, medication, drugs or lead poisoning
- Nutrition abnormalities. For example:
  - o An unusual diet.
  - o Abnormal digestion. For example, chronic pancreatitis or intestinal bacterial overgrowth.
  - o Absorption abnormality. For example, short gut syndrome.

When it is a neurological type of problem:

Ask yourself, what is the likely cause of a neurological problem?

Nerves regulate the function of every part of the body so a neurological problem can present with pain, symptoms or signs of deranged function or cause a patient to feel ill. Neurological problems can be caused by a central nervous system abnormality, such as migraine, a tension headache, mental illness, a stroke, or a raised intracranial pressure (ICP), a cranial nerve abnormality, such as Horner's syndrome, trigeminal neuralgia or Ramsay-Hunt syndrome, or a peripheral nervous system abnormality affecting, the spinal cord, a spinal root, such as sciatica, or a peripheral nerve, such as neuralgia or carpal tunnel syndrome.

When cancer is likely:

Ask yourself, what is the likely cause of cancer?

A consideration of the cause of cancer refers to both the likely origin or cell-type of the primary and the reason the cancer developed. Usually, histological or cytological information is needed to identify the primary. When the primary is identified, it is important to try to determine the cause. In 5% of patients there is a genetic risk, such as a genetic mutation or an affected first degree relative. Many other patients develop cancer as a result of their lifestyle choices, occupation or environmental risks. For example, smoking, drinking alcohol, sun-exposure, a low fibre diet or exposure to chemicals or asbestos.

Frequently, identifying the cause to formulate a definitive diagnosis awaits the results of investigations. For example:

- A chest infection is a provisional descriptive diagnosis until the infecting organism is identified. For example, microbiological evidence of a Haemophilus influenza or Corona virus infection.
- Ureteric colic is a provisional descriptive diagnosis until the cause is identified. For example, biochemical proof of urate stones.
- Heart failure is a provisional descriptive diagnosis until the cause is identified. For example, an angiogram demonstrating ischaemic heart disease (IHD), and echocardiogram cardiomyopathy, or immuno-histo-chemistry confirming thyrotoxicosis.
- Acute appendicitis is a provisional descriptive diagnosis until treated. The histology is likely to identify the cause.
- A unilateral pelvic mass is likely to be a tumour or a cyst. Identification of the origin of the mass, it's histological composition and the cause would be needed to formulate a diagnosis.

When research has yet to discover the fundamental cause of a problem, a descriptive diagnosis is medically accepted to be a definitive diagnosis. For example, ulcerative colitis (UC) or Crohn's disease, osteoarthritis, depression, CFS or IBS.

Link or triangulate information

In *The Expert Clinician* learning about the person, the problem, the patient and the examination are described separately to provide structure, whereas during the consultation it is usual to jump from one topic to another or for the examination to move from one part of the body to another so that leads or clues can be followed (Figure 19). Nevertheless, relevant information about the person, the patient and the problem and the signs should be linked so that it can be understood and interpreted to meet the aims (Figure 20).

Figure 19: Illustrating a flexible approach to the consultation

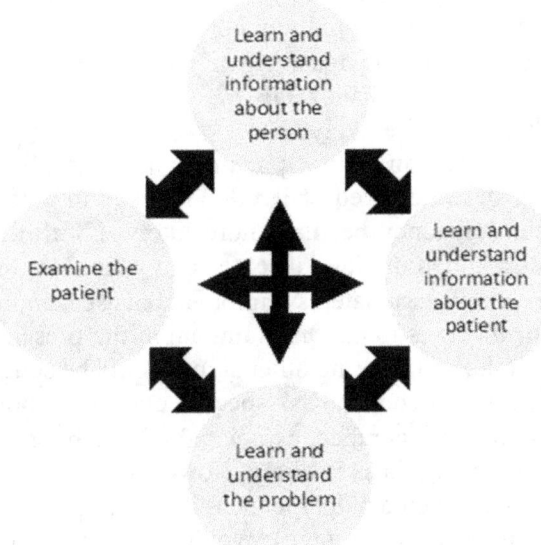

Figure 20: Illustrating how linking information can be used to formulate a diagnosis.

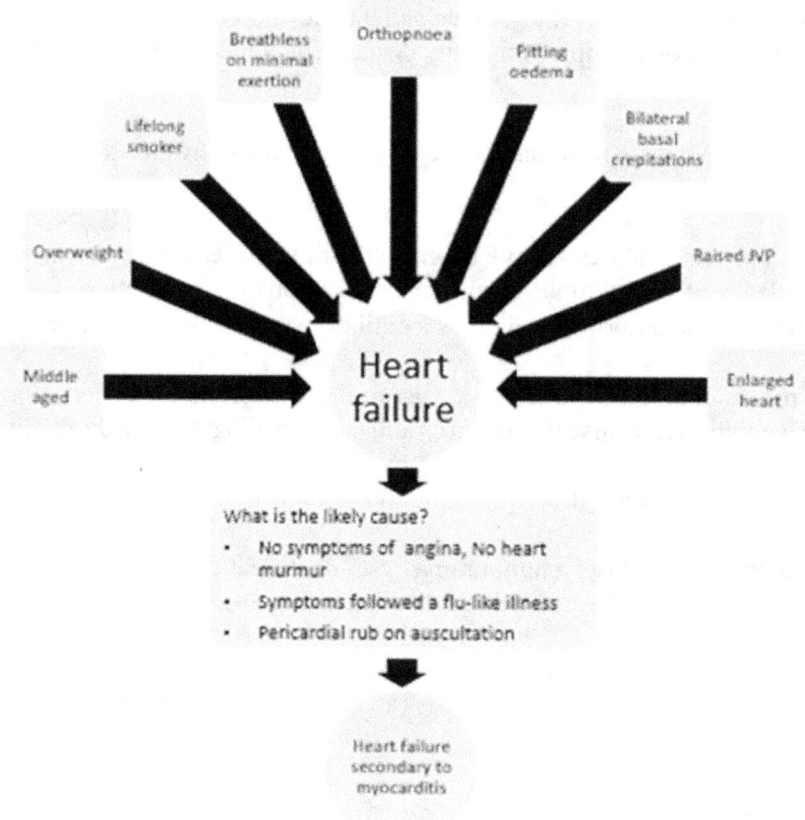

When used to formulate a diagnosis linking information can help identify a pattern, to confirm or exclude a diagnosis or to test a hypothesis. The likelihood a diagnosis is the true diagnosis is not only increased in proportion to both the quality and quantity of the evidence but also the consistency of the evidence. Linking information may highlight an inconsistency or an omission indicating additional questions to ask or signs to look for. If information is not linked, the wrong conclusions may be reached. For example:

- Headaches are common and are often caused by anxiety or stress. However, when a headache is associated with deep-seated neck and back pain, it may be caused by meningitis. Learning more about the headache and asking about other associated symptoms, such as photophobia or a rash, will inform the diagnosis.
- A patient who presents with breathlessness increasing over many years and associated with a chronic productive cough and bilateral crepitations is likely to have COPD.
  o If they are a lifelong smoker this is the likely cause.
  o If they have worked for many years in a mine, pneumoconiosis is a likely cause.
  o In a young patient who has never smoked or lived or worked in a hazardous environment, other causes, such as alpha-1 antitrypsin deficiency become more likely. If further enquiry revealed their father and grandfather, also non-smokers, died of "lung disease" at a young age this diagnosis becomes more likely.
- In a patient presenting feeling unwell, associated symptoms of nausea, anorexia, diarrhoea and fatigue are non-specific and the differential diagnosis is long. On examination the presence of a fine tremor would raise the possibility that they are an alcoholic and indicate other signs should be sought, such as palmar erythema, spider naevi, ascites and hepatomegaly and the need to ask specific questions about their alcohol consumption.
- When a patient presents feeling ill with jaundice, associated with itching, dark urine and pale stools, and there is sub-hepatic tenderness, choledocholithiasis is likely. However,
  o A well-defined non-tender pear-shaped palpable mass in the right upper quadrant of the abdomen, likely to be a palpable gallbladder (Courvoisier's sign), would be more consistent with cancer obstructing the common bile duct.

o Tender smooth hepatomegaly would indicate hepatitis.
o Non-tender, irregular hepatomegaly would be consistent with liver metastases.

Linking clinical features, including absent symptoms or signs may help determine the likely location of the abnormality, the type of problem and the cause. For example:

- When a patient presents with breathlessness it may be caused by a primary pulmonary problem, such as a chest infection or be secondary to, for example, a circulatory problem. Unilateral basal crepitations and dullness to percussion and the absence of a raised JVP, an enlarged heart and pitting oedema would indicate a pulmonary abnormality.
- When a patient presents with upper shoulder pain it may be a primary musculoskeletal problem or be secondary to cervical nerve entrapment or IHD.
  o When the patient is a competitive badminton player, the pain is likely to be from the shoulder.
  o When the pain followed a head on collision while driving a car it is likely to be referred from the neck following a whip-lash injury.
  o When the pain is brought on by walking up hills but disappears when stopping to rest it is likely to be caused by IHD.
- An agitated, irritable patient who has difficulty concentrating may be anxious and stressed; a neurological type of problem. However:
  o When the patient is hyper-active and the symptoms are associated with palpitations, weight loss, diarrhoea, a tremor and increased sweating, it is likely to be/ caused by a metabolic type of problem, such as thyrotoxicosis or withdrawing from a drug addiction.
  o When it is of acute onset and associated with a headache and a fever it may be caused by infection, such as encephalitis.

When information is linked its value is greater than the sum of the individual parts. Together the information becomes the evidence for an opinion and gives a power weighting to the opinion.

Use a diagnostic checklist

Occasionally, it may be helpful to work through a diagnostic checklist. Some of the many different checklists available are listed in Appendix 1.

- An anatomical checklist may help determine the location of the abnormality causing the problem.
- A checklist may help determine the type of problem and the differential diagnosis.
- A checklist may help determine the cause of a problem.

Diagnostic Error

A clinical diagnosis is an opinion, so there is an element of uncertainty and a risk of error. Avoiding or reducing the likelihood of diagnostic error is important both during the consultation and throughout the care pathway. At each stage, as more information becomes available the diagnosis should be reviewed. As the evidence in support of a diagnosis increases so the risk of error decreases.

Potential consequences of error

Every effort should be made to avoid diagnostic error because the consequences may be serious and irreversible. The consequences include:

- Additional or unnecessary investigations may be done. Not only do these expose the patient to a potential risk from the investigation itself but also there are financial consequences and consequences for other patients whose investigation has been delayed.
- Unnecessary or incorrect treatment. All treatments have side effects and risks. Patients on the wrong treatment are exposed to these unnecessarily. Inappropriate or incorrect treatment is also a waste of money.
- Delayed treatment for the true condition can affect the prognosis. When a diagnosis is time critical, delayed treatment may mean the opportunity for effective treatment is missed or risk an irreversible complication, such as cancer metastasising or septic shock developing.

- Physical and social consequences for the patient, including an impact on the patient's personal life and work.
- Psychological consequences, including anxiety and depression and reduced trust and confidence in the HCP or health care in general.
- Labelling. A diagnosis can be a label, with implications socially, financially and occupationally. This is particularly relevant to chronic conditions.
- Financial costs for the patient and the health care system.

Types of diagnostic error

Avoiding diagnostic error starts with being aware of the types of diagnostic errors possible. The potential types of error include:

- The wrong diagnosis: up to 5% of diagnoses are thought to be incorrect.
- An overdiagnosis. Overdiagnosis is the diagnosis of a condition that if left undiagnosed would not cause harm. It is a particular concern when performing screening tests or unnecessary tests. For the clinician and the patient, there is a tendency to over- rather than under- diagnose and this tendency is increasing as we strive to diagnose problems earlier to mitigate future risk. There are different forms of over-diagnosis:
  o Excessive use of descriptive diagnoses for which no diagnostic tests are available may lead to an overdiagnosis. Examples of "subjective" descriptive diagnoses include, irritable bowel syndrome, proctalgia fugax, depression, attention deficit hyper-activity disorder in children, restless leg syndrome or chronic fatigue syndrome.
  o Overdiagnosis can be a pre-diagnosis, a sub-clinical diagnosis or a risk factor that is a disease precursor. For example, pre-diabetes, "hypothyroidism unclassified", NASH, osteoporosis or heart disease.
  o Overdiagnosis can describe a true diagnosis in which treatment is unlikely to benefit the patient. For example, breast ductal carcinoma in situ, a focus of well-differentiated prostate cancer or a papillary thyroid cancer.
  o When tests reveal an abnormality unlikely to be clinically significant. For example, a liver cyst on CT scan, an adrenal "incidentaloma" or renal oncocytoma, an echogenic liver ("fatty liver") on USS, "hypertension" or a low eGFR in an older adult. It should be remembered that 5% of "normal" results are outside the reference range.
  o When the evidence is incomplete. For example, longstanding breathlessness with a persistent productive cough in a smoker is likely to be caused by COPD. However, there is a risk of over-diagnosing COPD unless spirometry testing is undertaken and demonstrates an irreversible reduction in FEV1/FVC to <0.7.
  o When there is a desire to make a diagnosis.
- A missed diagnosis. A missed diagnosis occurs when the diagnosis has not been made despite evidence being available. Most missed diagnoses become a delayed or late diagnosis because the diagnosis is made at a later date when the clinical features, the results of tests or a post-mortem examination are unequivocal and, with the benefit of hindsight, the evidence was available earlier. There are many reasons for a missed diagnosis including:
  o The original diagnosis was wrong.
  o The relevant symptoms and signs were not learnt or understood sufficiently to make a diagnosis.
  o The wrong test was performed.
  o Test results were falsely negative.
  o When a patient is seen or a test performed very early in the course of the illness.
  o When the condition progresses before a diagnosis is made.

    When a diagnosis is missed, treatment is delayed causing increased or more prolonged distress for the patient. Some delays are considered "acceptable" because delays waiting for tests are taken for granted or are inevitable. This includes awaiting the results of investigations before starting treatment. However, for some conditions delaying acting on the working diagnosis can be as consequential as a missed diagnosis. When the working diagnosis is a high priority time-dependent diagnosis a missed diagnosis is a missed opportunity for early treatment. This can have devastating consequences. For example, a missed diagnosis may delay the treatment of:
  o Sepsis, risking the development of septic shock.
  o Cancer, risking the opportunity for cure.
  o Stroke, risking additional irreversible brain damage.

o   Unstable angina, risking an AMI.
- A delayed diagnosis. It is not uncommon that a diagnosis is made at a later date, after a period of time has lapsed and when the patient is reviewed, i.e., the diagnosis is delayed. If sufficient evidence was *not* available earlier, it is not a missed diagnosis. There are many reasons why there may be a delay making a diagnosis, including:
  o   Patients present early in the course of their illness when the symptoms and signs are minimal or non-specific.
  o   Compensatory mechanisms mask the problem.
  o   The tests performed were insufficiently sensitive.
  o   The results of tests were not diagnostic.
  o   There was a delay reporting the test.
  o   There was a delay reviewing the patient.
  o   The patient delayed re-presenting, such as when they were falsely reassured.
- An incomplete diagnosis. Some diagnoses are incomplete. An incomplete diagnosis occurs when a provisional or descriptive diagnosis is accepted as the definitive diagnosis. As with a missed diagnosis, an incomplete diagnosis may delay when a patient receives the right treatment or receives preventative treatment affecting prognosis. For example:
  o   Making a diagnosis of "AF", without finding and treating the underlying cause.
  o   Making a diagnosis of obstructive jaundice, without proving the underlying cause.
  o   Making a diagnosis of intermittent small bowel obstruction, without finding and treating the underlying cause.

Potential causes of error

Reducing error starts with an awareness of the potential causes of error. These include:

- Information acquisition errors. Information acquisition not only refers to learning the relevant information but also understanding it. Information can be inaccurate, misunderstood, incomplete or over-looked leading to diagnostic error. This may be relevant to the consultation, interpreting the results of an investigation or when searching the internet.
- Process errors. Process errors not only apply to investigations but also to the consultations. Process errors can be caused by many factors including, haste, confusion, fatigue, distractions and multi-tasking.
- Knowledge errors. A knowledge of medicine and the basic sciences is essential to being able to recognise trigger symptoms or patterns or when learning to understand the problem.
- Interpretation errors. Misinterpretation or mis-representation can occur during the consultation, during the pathway of care or when searching the internet. There are many different interpretation errors including:
  o   Cognitive errors: misunderstanding or mis-interpreting information.
  o   Prioritisation or emphasis errors. It is important that the priority and emphasis is appropriate. It is possible to over- or under-estimate significance or ignore or dismiss a seemingly innocuous or less severe clinical feature and give too much emphasis on a less relevant aspect. For example, pain is an unpleasant symptom and can take priority over other symptoms such as dysphagia or weight loss, blackouts or palpitations that may be diagnostically more important.
  o   Incorrect associations. Assuming probability equals causation may lead to an error when assigning cause and effect. When an abnormality is obvious, it is likely to be the cause of the presenting problem. However, it is necessary to ensure the abnormality is the cause of the presenting problem and not just a co-incidental finding. For example:
    ▪   An inguinal hernia may be clinically obvious but is this the cause of vomiting? It is for the HCP to be confident that the problem is caused by the abnormality rather than assuming that because the abnormality is present, it is the cause of the problem.
    ▪   Even though alcohol is the cause of acute pancreatitis in approximately 50% of patients, it is also common for people to drink excessive amounts of alcohol. In a patient presenting with acute pancreatitis who drinks excessively, alcohol should not be assumed to be the cause.
  o   Correlation does not equal causation. Trends over time are particularly useful in clinical practice, such as changes in vital signs or serial blood test results. However, change needs to be interpreted with caution. For example, a falling blood pressure does not necessarily confirm bleeding or a climbing CRP, infection.

- Overdiagnosis errors. The causes of overdiagnosis include:
  - Broadening the definition of disease or lowering the threshold for disease.
  - The increased availability and use of tests. For example, the increased use of CT pulmonary angiograms has led to many more PEs being diagnosed and treated but there has been no change in mortality from PEs.
  - Excessive and inappropriate use of tests for ad-hoc "screening", such as measurement of blood "cancer markers".
  - Lack of understanding of what a test result means. For example, assuming a result outside the reference range or above a threshold level is abnormal.
  - A false positive investigation or mis-representing an incidental finding could lead to overdiagnosis.
  - Cognitive bias, including a tendency to look for an abnormality or to label the patient as having a condition.
  - Fear of missing a diagnosis: a perceived need to do something or to investigate.
  - Impatience and an intolerance of delay.
  - A desire to reduce future risk. The diagnosis of "pre-disease" conditions or precursor risks.
  - Over-reliance on tests regardless of the clinical features.
  - Over-estimation of the benefits of treatment.
  - Excessive and inappropriate use of, or over-reliance on the internet.
- Timing error. Some patients present early in the course of their illness when the symptoms and signs are minimal or non-specific. Some patients present late, when there are multiple abnormalities and it is difficult to distinguish between them.
- Bias occurs when we allow our opinions or beliefs to exceed, disregard or override the evidence. We may be conscious we are doing it or do it inadvertently. We are all prone to bias.

  Bias can affect decision making in many different ways. For example, we are more likely to believe a diagnosis if someone says they are 90% certain, rather than if they say there's a 10% chance, they are wrong. There are many potential causes of bias including:
  - Over-simplification. Complexity can be confusing. There is a tendency to over-simplify. For example, basing the diagnosis on one fact.
  - Making information fit a pattern. For example, asking questions to support a pre-conception.
  - Over-estimation of personal opinion or intuition. This can include being fixated on a diagnosis despite the evidence to the contrary.
  - Favouring information that supports a pre-conceived diagnosis and discounting or ignoring contrary information.
  - Favouring information, you are familiar with.
  - Favouring a diagnosis. Although, common conditions occur commonly and problems are usually caused by common diagnoses, the obvious diagnosis is not necessarily the right diagnosis.
  - Favouring information that is quickly available, the most recent information, or based on a recent experience.
  - Over-estimating your own intelligence or knowledge.
  - Personal prejudices.
  - Someone else "knows better". For example, hierarchy bias. In medicine there is a justifiable tendency to value the opinion of experts. Often, this is the best opinion available and should be followed. However, their decisions may be based on limited or inaccurate information or influenced by other considerations, such as resource, financial, social and political judgements. It may be wrong to disregard your own opinion particularly when you know more about the person, the patient and the problem.
  - Fear of being wrong.

  Investigations can also be biased. This can include:
  - Lead-time bias: when the diagnosis is made earlier but there has been no change in the end point (usually death).
  - Length-time bias: when the test detects more slowly progressive conditions that have a good prognosis.
  - Selection bias.

Measures to reduce error

Measures that reduce error include:
- Acknowledging error is possible and understand potential types and causes of error.
- Recognise when there is uncertainty.
- Keep an open mind.

- Training, including:
  - Awareness of diagnostic criteria.
  - Broad knowledge of diagnostic patterns and probabilities.
  - Good knowledge of medicine and the basic science.
  - Continuous professional development.
  - Method.
- Good communication and inter-personal skills.
  - Ask the right questions and listen to the response.
  - Examine the patient properly and pro-actively look for signs.
  - Learn the information correctly and check the information.
  - Repeat questions or a part of the examination if necessary.
  - Recognise there is patient diversity.
  - Avoid distractions during the consultation.
- Understand and interpret the information correctly.
  - Ensure the clinical features match the diagnosis thereby increasing the probability the diagnosis is true and reducing the false positive rate.
  - Common diagnoses are common. Know what diagnoses are prevalent in the population, i.e., the diagnosis is a frequent problem in patients with similar demographics and background.
  - Reduce the differential diagnosis, excluding as many alternative diagnoses as possible.
  - The more evidence there is, the higher the probability of a diagnosis.
  - Ensure the evidence is internally consistent. When the symptoms and signs are consistent, they are more likely to be reliable. If there is inconsistency, it is necessary to learn more about the problem or review the information. Check the time course of any inconsistent clinical features: it is possible that some clinical features are secondary. For example:
    - A patient presents with a head injury as the result of a trip while walking. Patients who trip usually hit the front of their head or the side of their head towards the front. If the head injury is on the occiput, this raises the question, why did they fall on the back of their head? It is important to ensure the nature of the injury is consistent with the mechanism of the injury.
    - An irreducible inguinal hernia is a common cause of small bowel obstruction, but not the only cause. If a hernia is present, it is important to ensure that the hernia is the cause of the small bowel obstruction, particularly in a patient who has had previous abdominal surgery.
    - A patient may present with an abscess on their back which they say started as an area of cellulitis a couple of days previously. On examination, there are signs of an abscess but it is associated with a firm well-circumscribed swelling consistent with a longstanding sebaceous cyst. It is likely the diagnosis is an infected sebaceous cyst.
    - A patient may present with acute breathlessness which they say has only been present for a few weeks. On examination, they have clubbing and a barrel shaped chest characteristic of longstanding emphysema.
- Use different sources of evidence.
- Multidisciplinary teamworking or a "second" opinion.
- Be alert to the misleading influence of a recent case, personal opinion, bias or prejudice, mood, illness or fatigue.
- Experience and familiarity.
- Reflection and review. Reassess the clinical features.
- If the outcome of the consultation is that the patient is reassured and discharged it may be appropriate to provide a safety net so that if symptoms persistent or progress, they can be reassessed to ensure the original diagnosis was not missed. If a patient is discharged having been falsely reassured it is likely they will delay re-presenting.

What to Do When the Diagnosis Remains Uncertain

Not formulating a diagnosis is not a failure when it is unlikely to cause harm or influence management. When the diagnosis is uncertain the challenges include deciding how important it is to formulate a diagnosis, how best to manage the problem, and how best to manage the patient and patient expectations. It is important to discuss the dilemma with the patient. Discuss what is known and where there are uncertainties or unknowns. It may be appropriate to discuss what diagnoses are possible or suspected but not confirmed and what diagnoses have been excluded. This will help the patient understand their problem and reassure them that it is being taken seriously. However, a conversation about uncertainty should be done carefully to avoid causing undue worry or undermining confidence in the HCP.

If the diagnosis remains uncertain at the end of the consultation and formulating a diagnosis is indicated, there are a number of management options available. Each option should be carefully considered and the benefits and risks discussed with the patient. Future management will be influenced by the person, the patient, their problem and the examination findings. Management options when the diagnosis is uncertain include:

- Organise an Investigation.
- Discuss the problem with a colleague or at an MDT.
- Use the internet, guidelines, apps or artificial intelligence to help formulate a diagnosis.
- Watchful waiting and timely review.
- Start a trial of treatment.
- Accept the absence of a diagnosis and manage the symptoms.

Organise an Investigation

Frequently, when the diagnosis is uncertain there is a desire or pressure from the patient to undertake an investigation. Requesting a battery of "standard" blood tests or a "benign" investigation, such as an USS is unlikely to do harm and the result may provide reassurance that vital organs and systems are functioning normally. Occasionally, it will reveal an abnormality that signposts a future management direction. Some investigations are organised to "exclude" a time sensitive diagnosis or to screen for an abnormality. However, requesting investigations for the sake of "doing something" is contra-indicated.

Some problems persist yet the investigations were "normal" and the diagnosis remains uncertain. A false negative result may occur for many reasons, including the investigation is undertaken early in the natural history of the condition, before an abnormality can be detected, or a reporting error has occurred. When relevant investigations are reported to be normal yet the problem persists or is deteriorating it may be appropriate to repeat an investigation after an interval, because an abnormality may be revealed at a later stage in the natural history of the condition.

Discuss the problem with a colleague or at an MDT

Occasionally a conversation with another colleague or at an MDT is indicated. The usual indications are when there is uncertainty about the most appropriate management option, such as discussing with a radiologist whether to request an USS, a CT scan or an MRI scan to investigate a liver abnormality, when there is diagnostic uncertainty, or to provide a "safety net" that nothing important is being missed. Some patients are re-assured if their problem has been discussed with another HCP or at an MDT. Similarly, some HCPs are re-assured when they have discussed a problem with other HCPs. However, when uncertainty remains, it is important to keep an open mind about the diagnosis and to beware a false sense of reassurance.

Use the internet, guidelines, apps or artificial intelligence to help formulate a diagnosis

Historically, reference books were the only repositories of medical information but now the internet is widely available and is usually the library of choice. The internet holds a vast store of data, an increasing number of diagnostic tools and numerous guidelines to help the clinician. These range from simple descriptions to complex algorithms or apps and are frequently linked to management recommendations. However, guidelines, apps and the internet should be used appropriately because there are many potential pitfalls. For example:

- There is a tendency to spend time with a computer rather than with a patient.
- There is a tendency to rely on the internet rather than on medical knowledge and method.
- There is a risk of divulging confidential information to a third party.
- Using the wrong keywords: lack of search specificity.
- Many choices in algorithms require "yes or no" answers. Unfortunately, medicine is rarely so simple and trying to fit the answer to the algorithm may result in the wrong diagnosis.
- The content may not be peer reviewed or standardised.
- The original source of the information may be unclear and potentially untrustworthy.
- A reliable, validated source may be unavailable or only available by subscription.

- The information may be misleading, incomplete, inaccurate or outdated.
- There may be too much information.
- Prioritisation may be compromised so that rare problems are highlighted.
- The information may not be relevant to patients with multi-morbidity.
- Advertising, marketing and money may influence content and ranking. Site ranking may result in relevant information not being seen.
- Lack of representation by all interested parties: a potential for subjective bias.
- Information may be based on an experts' personal view rather than expert factual evidence. Conflicts of interest may not be declared.

Measures to ensure guidelines and information are used appropriately include:

- Accurately learn and understand available information from the patient.
- Remain patient focused.
- Define the aims.
- Define the question being asked.
- Ensure patient confidentiality is maintained.
- Use trusted sources.
- Critically assess the source.
- Cross reference information.
- Ensure the information is internally consistent.
- Keep it simple.

Currently, "artificial intelligence" (AI) programs are not widely available in clinical practice but this will change. Undoubtedly, as AI becomes more available and accessible in "real-time" it will be increasingly used. It is likely to improve diagnostic accuracy because databases can store vastly more information increasing the likelihood that a pattern will be recognised or extending a list of possible diagnoses. However, increasing the number of diagnostic options may lead to more investigations and the risk of diagnostic error will remain. Furthermore, the introduction of AI to health care also raises many professional and ethical questions, including:

- The evidence and reasoning are likely to be hidden from the health care team and the patient. Who or what, decides on the decision-making methodology and the data used to make the decision? Who or what, decides which evidence to use or exclude, and the emphasis or weighting given to each piece of evidence?
- The outcome is dependent on reliable and representative data acquisition. Who is responsible for ensuring data acquisition is correct, complete, and representative? Can data entry be error checked?
- Who is responsible for interpreting the nuances of language? Will clinical options be restricted to a drop-down list with its associated constraints?
- Who is responsible for decisions made?
- Who is responsible for problems or errors that arise?
- What will happen to patient autonomy?
- Will the information be kept confidential?
- How will the information be protected from external interference?
- How will the AI be regulated?
- What happens when the AI is unavailable?

Watchful waiting and timely review

"Watchful waiting" or "masterly inactivity" is both a management option and a clinical method to formulate a diagnosis. It should be a positive decision based on the information available. However, it is often only considered when other options have been excluded because, it is more difficult to appear to do "nothing" than to do something. Watchful waiting is indicated:

- When there is uncertainty that there is a problem.
- When the problem is still evolving.

- When the symptoms or signs are early, subtle or non-specific.
- When there is diagnostic uncertainty, such as when a problem presents early.
- When a time-dependent high priority diagnosis, such as sepsis or cancer has been excluded.
- When the risk of delay is less than the potential harm caused by an investigation or a treatment.
- When there is management uncertainty or management options are not indicated.
- When it is likely the patient will get better without any intervention.
- When there is concern about performing another investigation. For example, it is not uncommon for patients to be subject to a cascade of investigations in the hope that something abnormal will be found or when an incidental abnormality has been identified.
- When there are delays before an investigation is undertaken. The interval may also be an opportunity for watchful waiting and subsequent re-assessment.

The potential risks of watchful waiting include:

- Delayed investigation or treatment leading to harm.
- Uncertain baseline, making interval comparisons unreliable.
- Choosing an inappropriate time interval.
- Bias when re-assessing the patient.
- A missed or delayed re-appointment.
- The patient is re-assessed by a different HCP without a reliable baseline for comparison.
- False reassurance.
- The patient may delay re-presenting when they have an appointment pending.

Watchful waiting frequently includes a re-assessment after an interval: a timely review, in the hope that there will be meaningful change or when investigation results are available. In some patients the problem resolves without investigation or treatment. In many, a follow up consultation will provide an opportunity to review the symptoms and signs and will increase the information available. A review is more likely to be meaningful if the problem is measurable, so that change can be assessed, and the time interval appropriate.

The period of watchful waiting determines the duration of the interval between consultations and should be determined by information about the patient and the problem. It should include a consideration of the severity and impact on the patient, their anxiety and expectations, a knowledge of the natural history of the problem, the duration of the problem and previous rate of change, the risk of a time-dependent diagnosis, a significant deterioration or of a complication rather than by external factors, such as consultation availability, work commitments or holidays. For example, it may be appropriate to review a patient:

- Every few minutes, such as when a headache is evolving or a significant postoperative complication suspected.
- After one to two hours, such as when there is concern that they may have early sepsis.
- After an interval of a few weeks, such as when they have a recent unexplained change in bowel habit.

When undertaking a review, it is helpful to:

- Review the symptoms at the start of the illness.
- Review the symptoms or signs to ensure nothing has changed or been missed.
- Reconsider whether the symptoms and signs align.
- Review the results of tests already performed. Ask yourself:
  o Are the results consistent with the clinical findings?
  o Were the right tests done?
  o Was a test performed too early?
  o Were the tests accurate enough to exclude an abnormality? Could the test lack sensitivity?
  o Could there have been a false negative result? A subjective investigation, such as an imaging investigation, may need reviewing or re-reporting.
  o Should a different test be performed?
- Consider if there could be two problems.
- Consider repeating a test after a reasonable interval.

- Consider whether the symptoms are a long term sequalae of a previous illness. For some patients, residual symptoms persist long after a problem is over. For example:
  - Chronic pain, neuralgia or reflex sympathetic osteodystrophy after an injury.
  - Persistent gastrointestinal symptoms after a gastrointestinal infection or broad-spectrum antibiotic treatment.
  - Weakness, lethargy and myalgia after a viral illness.
  - Long COVID.
- Consider whether a previous illness has relapsed.
- Consider a rare diagnosis or an unusual presentation of a common diagnosis. For example:
  - Could a neurological type of problem be:
    - Autonomic neuropathy.
    - MS.
    - Spinal arachnoiditis.
    - Spinal or brain tumours, spinal stenosis.
    - Fibromyalgia or chronic fatigue syndrome.
    - Irritable bowel syndrome.
  - Could inflammation be caused by:
    - Chronic infection. For example, TB, syphilis, EBV or HIV.
    - Non-infective inflammation. For example, SLE, coeliac disease.
  - Could abdominal symptoms be caused by adhesions, endometriosis or ovarian cancer.
  - Could it be a metabolic abnormality, such as:
    - Lead poisoning.
    - Thyrotoxicosis.
    - Porphyria.
    - Poly cystic ovary syndrome.

Consider whether the symptoms could be factitious or caused by an emotional, behavioural, social or a mental health problem. Rarely, it may be appropriate to consider a factitious disorder in which symptoms are feigned by the patient (syn Munchausen's syndrome). Factitious disorders are characterised by repeated presentations, often to different HCPs and different health care providers, with inconsistent symptoms, unsupported by the signs or results of investigations and without a desire to get better. Some patients are known to self-harm. Frequently, formulating a diagnosis of a factitious disorder takes time, investigations, repeat consultations and the opinion of other HCPs.

Start a trial of treatment

There are many indications for starting a treatment, including to help formulate a diagnosis. In which case, it is assumed that if a treatment is successful, it confirms the diagnosis. However, this may not be a valid assumption for many reasons including:

- There may be a placebo effect from taking the treatment.
- The resolution of symptoms is a coincidence.
- The natural history of the condition includes remission and relapse.
- The treatment may treat the symptoms but not the underlying problem.

There are many potential risks associated with assuming that a resolution of symptoms confirms a diagnosis, of which the most significant is when there is a false sense of re-assurance leading to irreversible harm.

Accept the absence of a diagnosis and manage the symptoms

Frequently, such as when a descriptive diagnosis is made, the cause is assumed and treatment started to relieve symptoms. This is usually a pragmatic clinical decision based on a knowledge of the patient, an understanding of the problem and the likely diagnosis. The assumption is that formulating a diagnosis is unlikely to change management which is likely to be aimed at relieving symptoms. For such patients it is important to have confidently excluded a time-sensitive diagnosis and to keep an open mind about the diagnosis and future management. Further review may be indicated to re-assess the problem and monitor change.

Applying Method to the Consultation

Different diagnostic methods are indicated at different times during the consultation (Figure 21).

Figure 21: Illustrating the different diagnostic methods

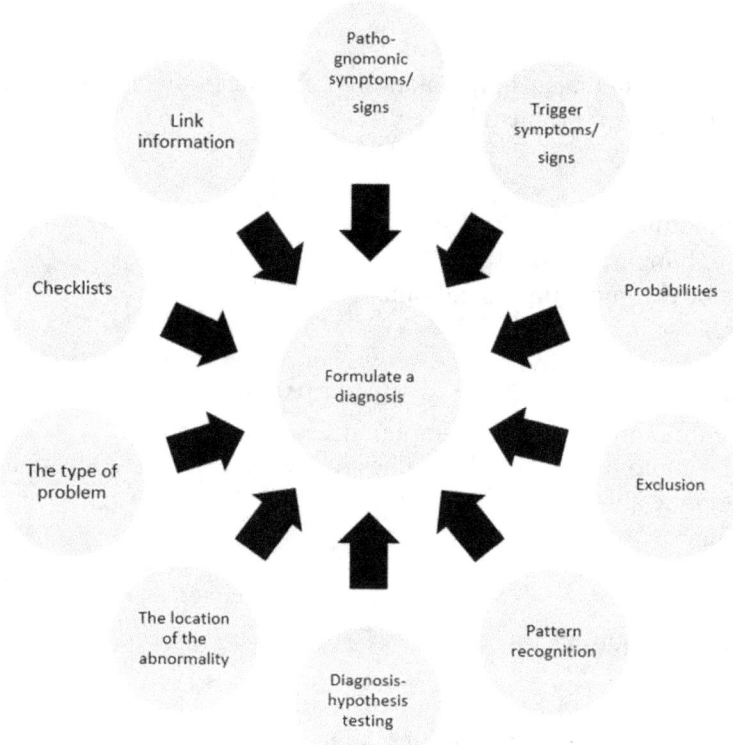

Diagnostic methods used when learning headline information and during the introductory conversation

In most patients, presenting with a new problem, the patient's description of their presenting problem together with other headline information provides the first insight into possible diagnoses. Indeed, occasionally the patient's appearance and what they say will "inspire" a diagnosis, reveal a pathognomonic symptom or sign, a trigger symptom or suggest a diagnostic pattern. In which case, this will signpost the questions to ask or signs to look for to check that the clinical features match a "text-book" description: diagnosis-hypothesis testing (Figure 22). In summary, while listening to the patient's description, ask yourself:

Are there any trigger or pathognomonic symptoms?
Do the symptoms fit a diagnostic pattern?
What diagnosis(es) is/are likely (probable) and what can be excluded?
What questions should be asked or signs looked for (diagnosis-hypothesis testing)?

When the differential diagnosis is long or the diagnosis uncertain it is necessary to learn and understand information about the problem.

When a patient presents as an emergency, a standard battery of tests is often organised while talking to and examining the patient: i.e., "straight to test".

Figure 22: Illustrating the questions to ask yourself during the introductory conversation.

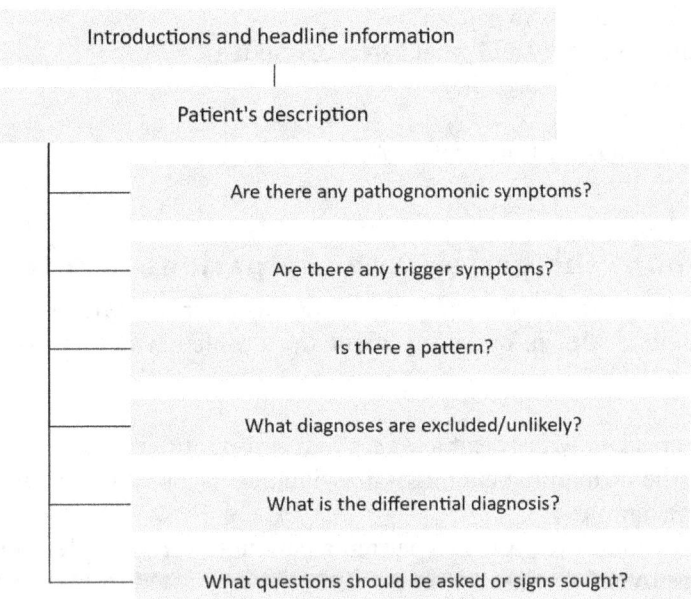

Diagnostic methods used when asking questions to learn and understand the details of the problem

It may be appropriate to start by asking the patient if they know the diagnosis or what may have caused or brought on their problem. Usually, if they think they know the diagnosis or the cause it will have been mentioned in their description of the presenting problem.

When learning to understand, questions are asked to determine the location of the abnormality causing the problem, the type of problem and the cause. As before, while talking to the patient, probabilities, excluding unlikely diagnoses, pattern recognition and diagnosis-hypothesis testing are used to inform the questions to ask to understand and interpret the information and inform additional questions to ask. This information will lead to a descriptive diagnosis or a limited list of diagnoses. Checklists may help determine the likely location of the abnormality and the possible cause. Relevant information should be linked (Figure 23).

Figure 23: Illustrating the questions to ask yourself while learning about the problem.

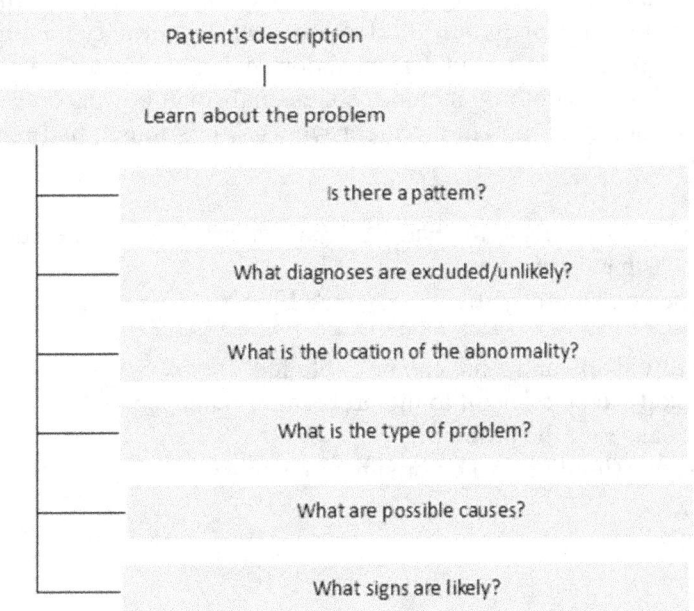

In summary, while listening to the patient, ask yourself:

Do the symptoms fit a diagnostic pattern?
What diagnosis(es) is/are likely and what can be excluded?
What is the location of the abnormality?
What is the type of problem?
What are the possible causes of the problem?
What signs should be looked for?

Use information about the person and the patient to inform the diagnosis

Occasionally, linking information about the person, such as their lifestyle or about the person as a patient, such as an ongoing medical condition, with information about the problem will indicate a likely diagnosis or cause. For example:

- When the patient presents with breathlessness and information about the problem indicates it is likely to be caused by asthma, the differential diagnosis may include air pollution. Learning about the person may indicate a likely cause. For example:
  o Frequent and prolonged exposure to particulate matter. For example, from diesel exhaust, open fireplace or wood-burning stove.
  o Frequent and prolonged exposure to volatile compounds and gases, such as from cars, trucks and buses, cleaning products or "air-fresheners".
  o Frequent and prolonged exposure to mould in a damp and poorly ventilated building.
- When the patient presents feeling ill:
  o With a headache in the evenings after work or at weekends, learning about the person may reveal they heat their home with an old gas heater. If so, carbon monoxide poisoning should be included in the differential diagnosis.
  o With headaches, abdominal pain and constipation, learning about the person may reveal they live in an old house with lead pipes. If so, lead poisoning should be included in the differential diagnosis.
  o With weight loss, learning about the patient may reveal they have just finished a course of cancer treatment. They may have recurrent cancer.
  o Agitated and confused, feeling sweaty and tremulous, learning about the person may reveal they are in the habit of taking drugs. They may be withdrawing from drugs.
- When the differential diagnosis of the presenting problem includes a condition known to be a complication of an ongoing or pre-existing medical condition. For example:
  o The differential diagnosis of feeling ill in a diabetic may include a metabolic abnormality, such as ketoacidosis or renal failure, or an occult infection, such as a urinary tract infection.
  o The differential diagnosis of recurrent central abdominal colic, bloating and a feeling of nausea in a patient who has had a previous laparotomy includes adhesional small bowel obstruction.
  o Recurrent urinary tract infections in a patient who has previously had renal stones may be caused by a recurrent calculus.

Linking information about the person and the patient is particularly useful when determining or excluding a cause or when prioritising a list of possible diagnoses.

While learning about the person and the patient ask yourself:

What diagnosis(es) is/are likely and what can be excluded?
What information is likely to be relevant to the problem or management?
What are the possible causes of the problem?
What additional questions should be asked or signs looked for?

Figure 24: Illustrating the questions to ask yourself while learning about the person and the patient.

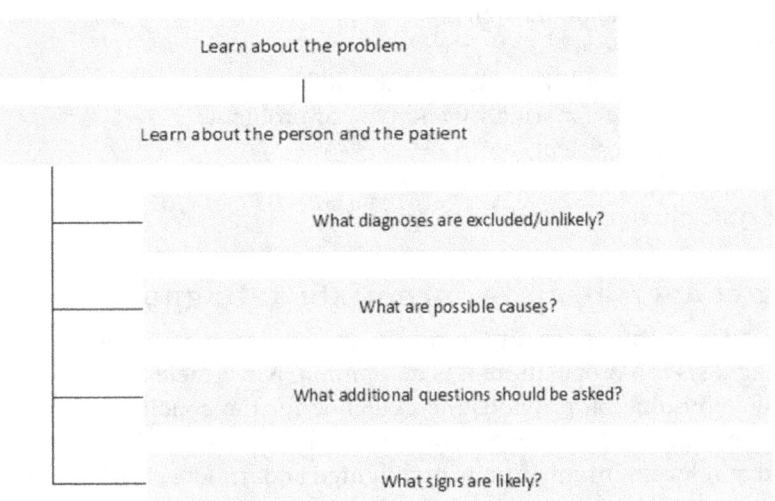

Diagnostic methods used during the examination

For many patients, and particularly when the patient presents with a visible or palpable abnormality, the examination is important to formulate a diagnosis. Information from talking to the patient will indicate the signs to look for when examining the patient. When the patient presents with a visible or palpable abnormality, the signs on examining the site of the problem together with other headline information provide the first insight into a likely diagnosis. Occasionally, the signs will "inspire" a diagnosis, reveal a pathognomonic sign, a trigger sign or suggest a diagnostic pattern. In which case, this will signpost addition questions to ask or the signs to look for elsewhere.

While examining the patient, use probabilities, pattern recognition and diagnosis-hypothesis testing to understand and interpret the information available and to inform the signs to look for to determine the likely location of the abnormality, the type of problem and the cause to formulate a descriptive diagnosis or a short list of possible diagnoses. Symptoms and signs should be linked to ensure they are internally consistent. Checklists may be helpful (Figure 25).

Figure 25: Illustrating the questions to ask yourself while examining the patient.

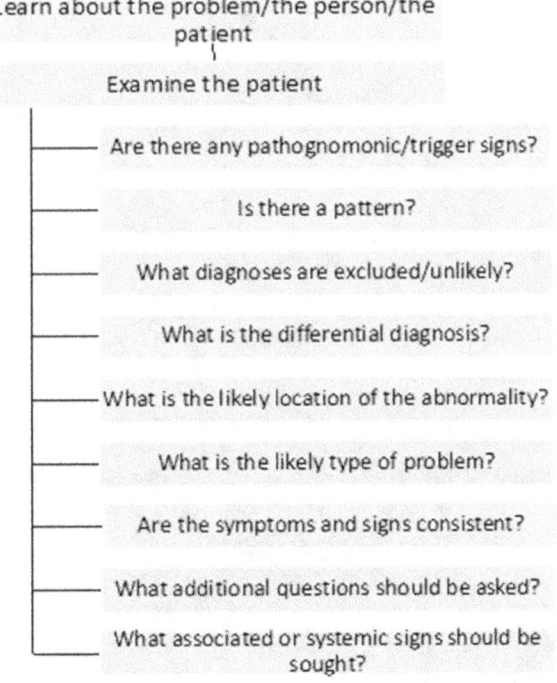

In summary, while examining the site of the problem ask yourself:

Are there any trigger or pathognomonic signs?
Do the signs fit a diagnostic pattern?
What diagnosis(es) is/are likely and what can be excluded?
What is the likely location of the abnormality and type of problem?
Are the symptoms and signs consistent?
What additional questions should be asked?
What associated or systemic signs should be sought?

Use the concluding conversation to formulate a diagnosis

The concluding conversation is an opportunity to review the evidence, to ensure it is correct, internally consistent and complete. A clinical diagnosis is a proposition, it is an opinion. Nevertheless, it should be evidence based. Linking information learnt during the consultation provides the evidence for the conclusions reached. The information learnt depends on the questions asked and the signs sought, but the evidence is dependent on understanding, interpreting and sorting the information so that relevant information is highlighted and irrelevant information excluded. The quality and quantity of the evidence constitutes a "power weighting" similar to that used in medical research. The closer the evidence matches recognised diagnostic criteria the more likely the clinical diagnosis is a true diagnosis. Additional information, such as the results from investigations, will add to the evidence and increase the "power rating" of the opinion. In general, the predictive value of laboratory or imaging evidence is increased if it aligns with the clinical features. In clinical practice, the power rating is highly subjective. It is usually described using adjectives such as definite, probable, possible, likely, unlikely or rare. When there is diagnostic uncertainty ask yourself:

Is it safe to wait?
Should the problem be discussed with a colleague?
Is additional information, such as from a textbook or the internet likely to be helpful?
Is a test likely to be helpful?
Is a second opinion indicated?

Chapter 4
The Methodology for
Planning Management

Abstract

Management planning is the process of determining and agreeing with the patient the care that follows the consultation. The ultimate aim is to help the patient, but how this is best achieved will vary between patients, between consultations, at different stages in the pathway of care and may be different for different problems. Management may be as simple as providing a treatment at the end of the consultation or involve a complex series of management options, each with a different aim.

Management options should be considered from the start of the consultation and throughout the consultation while learning about the person, the patient, the problem and while examining the patient. All available information should inform management planning, and possible management options should inform some of the questions asked or the signs sought to ensure management is not only indicated and meets the aims of the consultation but also that it is appropriate to the patient and timely.

As a rule, the HCP chooses the management option to recommend and the patient chooses whether or not to consent to it. For most patients, the choice is between requesting an investigation, and if so what investigation, and starting a treatment, and if so what treatment, changing a life choice, discharging the patient or arranging a follow up consultation, and if so when, or making a referral to another HCP. The management decision is determined by the aims of the consultation, the indications, and what is available and appropriate for the patient. It is necessary to balance the expected benefit with the potential risk and timing. Benefit-risk assessment is strongly influenced by what is deemed acceptable to the patient, the HCP and to the health care community. It is important to consider the consequence and likelihood of a risk, the time frame and what can change the risk. This process may be helped by guidelines or the recommendations from an MDT.

Once management is agreed, responsibility for planning management is with the HCP but responsibility for compliance and adherence rests with the patient. At the end of the consultation the information considered and the rationale used to agree on a management plan should be recorded.

Introduction

"By failing to prepare, you are preparing to fail"

Benjamin Franklin

Management planning is the process of determining and agreeing with the patient the care that follows the consultation. Traditionally planning management was reactive, frequently left to the end of the consultation. This may have been appropriate when medical knowledge was limited, patients were less complex and few management options available, but it is not appropriate now. A lot more is known about disease and disease processes, there are many management options available, including numerous tests and treatments and patients are better informed and frequently want to be involved in planning their health care. Therefore, planning management should be undertaken pro-actively from the very start of the consultation, when first meeting the patient, and throughout the consultation while learning about the person, the patient and the problem, and examining the patient. This is so that the information is not only used to formulate a diagnosis but also to inform management, and management options can be used to inform some of the questions asked or the signs sought. Information learnt during the consultation should be understood and interpreted in the context of published evidence, guidelines, recommendations from an MDT, the likely benefit and possible risk, and a knowledge of the available management options.

The aim of this chapter is to discuss the methodologies available to help plan management.

Determine the Management Aims

The primary management aim is to help the patient, and all management should work towards achieving this aim. However, determining the best way to help the patient is a complex process which involves careful consideration of the problem and the examination findings together with information about the person and the patient, such as their wishes, needs and expectations, safety concerns and co-morbidity. Often there are a number of steps undertaken before achieving the primary aim, and each step will have a different aim. Therefore, for most patients, management is a process, or a journey, which starts with the consultation, the point of contact with the patient, and finishes when the patient is helped. Sometimes, this can be achieved following the first consultation, sometimes after a long pathway of care.

It is important to be clear on the management aims before making a recommendation to the patient. Often, initial management includes starting a treatment for a clinical diagnosis or to alleviate symptoms, help function or to prevent or slow disease progression. For some patients and some problems this is sufficient and the patient can be discharged. For other patients, investigations are indicated with the aim of formulating a diagnosis, or to confirm or exclude a diagnosis, to screen for or exclude a diagnosis, to assess severity, to learn more about the problem or the patient, or to inform treatment. Occasionally, the aim of management is to reassure the patient and the HCP. Therefore, before asking a question or examining the patient:

Ask yourself, what is the management aim?

In summary, the management aims include:

- To formulate a diagnosis:
  o To confirm a diagnosis.
  o To make a definitive diagnosis.
  o To exclude a diagnosis.
  o To understand the problem:
    ▪ To determine the location of the abnormality causing the problem.
    ▪ To determine the type of problem.
    ▪ To determine the cause.
  o To screen for:
    ▪ Another abnormality.
    ▪ A secondary abnormality.
    ▪ A complication.
  o For assessment of:
    ▪ Severity.
    ▪ The impact on the patient.
    ▪ Function.
    ▪ Change, including to provide a baseline.
    ▪ Future risk or prognosis.
- To provide treatment:
  o Definitive treatment.
  o To alleviate symptoms.
  o To help the patient.
  o To help function.
  o To slow the rate of disease progression.
  o To reduce the risk of a future problem.
  o To prevent a future problem.
  o As a trial to formulate a diagnosis.
- To help build a working relationship:
  o To provide information or reassurance for the patient.

Decide What Management Option Is Indicated

When learning information about the patient it is also necessary to consider which management option is indicated to best achieve the aims of the consultation. A management option is indicated when it meets a specific aim that contributes to meeting the overall aim of the consultation.

The indications are different for different management options. For example, the indications for a CT scan will be different from the indications for a blood test. Information already known about the patient and learnt during the consultation, such as the result of a previous test, indicate whether or not a management option is indicated. As more information becomes available, the indications for a management option change. For example:

- A patient presenting with a slowly enlarging soft sub-cutaneous lump is likely to have a lipoma. If the lipoma is asymptomatic and small it is unlikely to affect the patient or cause harm, so there is no indication for investigations or treatment. Some patients, will only be "reassured" if an investigation such as an USS, is performed. The test is not diagnostically indicated but may be clinically indicated with the aim of reassuring the patient. Some lipomata arise at an inconvenient site for the patient or cause symptoms. In which case, excision may be indicated with the aim of relieving symptoms. Occasionally lipomata are intra-muscular or in close proximity to an important structure, such as a major nerve or blood vessel. In which case, an USS, CT or MRI scan is indicated to understand the anatomy. If excision of the lipoma needs to be performed under a general anaesthetic, additional investigations such as blood tests, a CXR and an ECG may be indicated with the aim of screening for other abnormalities, as part of a pre-operative assessment. A minority of lipomata are atypical and it may be difficult to distinguish a benign lipoma from a liposarcoma or another lesion, such as a lymph node. In which case, further investigations with an USS, CT or MRI scan are indicated with the aim of formulating a diagnosis or excluding a diagnosis. If uncertainty remains serial investigations may be indicated to assess change over time.
- When a patient presents with a recent onset of feeling ill with a cough, breathlessness and a fever and a chest infection is the working diagnosis an absence of chest signs would suggest it is a viral infection and no specific treatment is indicated. The patient can be reassured that they will get better. On the other hand, a fever and signs of right lower lobe consolidation would suggest a bacterial infection and antibiotics may be indicated. When the symptoms or signs are severe, the diagnosis or the cause uncertain, investigations including blood tests and sputum for microbiological assessment and a CXR may be indicated with the aims of confirming the diagnosis, excluding other diagnoses, to assess severity or to plan treatment. Sputum cytology and a chest CT scan may be indicated if cancer is suspected. If uncertainty remains serial investigations may be indicated to assess change over time. If the problem is recurrent in a patient who has smoked all their life pulmonary function tests may be indicated to screen for COPD.

Management options such as discharge, referral to another HCP or whether or not to organise another consultation are binary choices: they are either indicated or not indicated. On the other hand, there are many different investigations and treatments to choose from, and, although the indications and contra-indications for each is published, choosing the most appropriate for a given patient with a given set of symptoms and signs is often at the discretion of the HCP, and is influenced by opinion. When clinically there is little to choose between a number of management options, patient related factors should be considered and these should be discussed with the patient. For example:

- When a patient presents with a change in bowel habit an investigation is usually indicated to exclude a diagnosis, such as cancer or colitis. Having decided an investigation is indicated, it is necessary to decide which investigation to recommend: should it be a flexible sigmoidoscopy, a colonoscopy, a barium enema, a CT colonoscopy, a CT enema or a standard CT scan with or without contrast?
- When a patient is diagnosed with prostate cancer treatment may or may not be indicated. When treatment is indicated, it is necessary to determine which treatment to recommend: should it be hormone treatment, radiotherapy, chemotherapy or a resection?
- When a patient is on different treatment pathways, one may influence the other, such as whether an investigation or a treatment is indicated and the timing of the different investigations.

For some patients, a management option is not indicated. If there is insufficient information, uncertainty about the information or conflicting information a management option may not be indicated. It also may not be indicated if it is inappropriate. For example, many medications are not licensed for use in children, during pregnancy, or in some other patient groups and are therefore not "officially" indicated. This does not mean they are contra-indicated, because experience may have shown that they are likely to be effective and unlikely to cause harm and so are recommended with caution and an explanation.

For a minority of patients, a management option is contra-indicated. Information about the person and the problem usually determine when an option is contraindicated. For example:

- A management option, with the exception of discharge, is contra-indicated without the consent of the patient.

- In patients with an iodine allergy, intravenous contrast for a radiological investigation is contra-indicated because it may cause an untreatable anaphylactic reaction.
- Performing an MRI scan on a patient with a ferro-magnetic metal implant is contra-indicated because the implant may be moved by the magnetic field.

Many contra-indications are relative and there is a balance between benefit and risk and what mitigation is possible. For example:

- In children and fertile females at risk of being pregnant, exposure to ionizing radiation is relatively contraindicated because exposure risks future harm to the child or to the unborn baby. However, the contraindication is relative because there are occasions when there is an immediate risk from not doing the Xray.
- Mental health conditions and disability may be a relative contraindication for some tests or treatments. For example, claustrophobia and an MRI scan or paraplegia and a colonoscopy. There are usually ways of mitigating the risks.
- On examination, a patient may be found to have a very high blood pressure or an untreated arrythmia that is a contraindication to an invasive procedure. Appropriate treatment would mitigate the risk.
- In a patient with renal failure, intravenous contrast is a relative contraindication because it may cause a deterioration in renal function. It is a relative contraindication because the risk can be mitigated by prehydration or the risk of not doing the test may outweigh the risks of the test.
- An immunosuppressed patient is at increased risk of acquiring an infection. This may be reduced by increasing aseptic precautions or prophylactic antibiotics.
- Medications may be a relative contraindication. For example, anti-coagulant treatment is a relative contraindication to an invasive procedure that has a bleeding risk. This can be mitigated by stopping the anticoagulant in advance or taking the risk and treating the bleeding risk should bleeding occur.
- Fasting a patient taking diabetic medication is a relative contra-indication due to the risk of hypoglycaemia. Converting to intravenous insulin prior to an invasive procedure will mitigate this risk.

Link or triangulate information to inform management

Management is usually determined by linking information about the problem and from the examination. In addition, different and diverse information is learnt throughout the consultation. Some information is revealed at the start, when first meeting the patient, and other information is learnt when asking questions about the person, the patient and the problem, or during the examination. Linking relevant information ensures it is used to inform management planning (Figure 26).

Figure 26: Illustrating how triangulating different information can inform management.

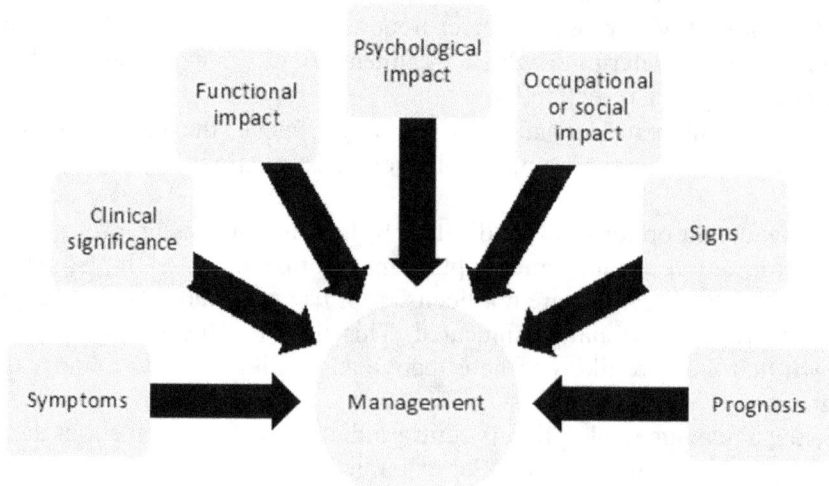

In most patients, information about the person and the patient will not change the recommendation. However, in some patients, it will affect the management plan, such as when there is a contraindication or safety concern, or to determine the priority and whether or not a management option is inappropriate. Linking information may highlight additional questions to ask or signs to look for and will ensure the management plan is indicated, appropriate and evidenced.

During the consultation there are many different occasions when linked information is used to inform management. For example:

- Link problems and information about the patient with demographic information, such as age.
- Link information about severity with the impact on a patient's function to validate a severity assessment and management priority and planning.
- When a patient has had different treatments or is on various medications, including preventative treatments, or awaiting treatment the condition and the treatment should be linked, to avoid uncertainty and ensure internal validation.
- A relevant safety concern or its absence should be linked to a management plan.
- Risk factors should be linked with a descriptive diagnosis to highlight a likely cause or exclude a possible cause.
- Link evidence with an opinion or recommendation.

Use information from guidelines to inform management

Guidelines are recommendations, whereas a protocol is a set of rules or instructions that *must* be followed. Protocols are widely used in clinical practice, particularly when there is a health and safety risk. For example, when managing radioactive agents, or in the vicinity of the powerful magnets of an MRI machine. However, it is uncommon for patient management to be determined by a protocol, because they are too restrictive. For this reason, the term "guidelines" is generally used.

Guidelines can be as simple as a recommendation for a certain investigation or treatment or as complex as diagnostic algorithms linked to treatment. For example:

- When a patient presents with a sudden onset of chest pain/tightness or discomfort acute coronary syndrome (ACS), either angina or an AMI, is a likely diagnosis. An immediate ECG is indicated. If the chest pain is atypical or the ECG non-diagnostic serial serum troponin levels are indicated. If the working diagnosis based on the clinical picture or ECG changes is stable angina a CT coronary angiography is indicated. Regional ST segment elevation or new left bundle branch block on an ECG indicates an AMI.
Treatment for an AMI includes intravenous opioids for symptom relief and 300 mg of aspirin orally. If there is ST elevation emergency percutaneous coronary intervention (PCI) or intravenous thrombolysis is indicated. In patients with a non-ST-elevation AMI and a mortality risk >3% (measured using the "Global Registry of Acute Coronary Events" risk score) PCI within 72 hours is indicated.
Following an AMI patients should be treated with dual anti-platelet medication for 12 months and preventative measures, including statins, beta blockers or angiotensin converting enzyme inhibitors considered.
The management of an increasing range of problems is set out in published guidelines.

> Sources of Published Guidelines
>
> - National Institute for Clinical Excellence (NICE)—www.nice.org.uk
> - Scottish Intercollegiate Guidelines Network (SIGN)—www.sign.ac.uk
> - Specialist association guidelines. For example, https://www.britishcardiovascularsociety.org/resources/publications-reports
> - Journals. For example, Guidelines in Practice www.eguidelines.co.uk
> - Centre for reviews and dissemination—www.york.ac.uk/inst/crd

In addition, there are many local guidelines and an increasing number of MDTs that make recommendations regarding patient care. The HCP needs to either know the relevant guidelines or know how to access them when needed. Published guidelines are appropriate for most patients and help management planning in many ways including:

- Inform and reassure the patient, the clinician and the clinical team.
- Promote interventions of proven benefit.
- Reduce ineffective investigations and treatment.
- Improve the consistency of care.
- Legal protection for the clinician.
- Highlight variations in practice.

MDTs frequently offer guidance to the clinician. This guidance is often based on published guidelines with a locally specific variation. In addition to giving guidance, MDTs may provide additional benefits to patient care by:

- Speeding up inter-disciplinary care provision.
- Coordinating care between specialties.
- Agreeing local policies and pathways.
- Providing a forum for case based or disease discussion.
- Sharing knowledge, learning and experience.
- Collecting data and audit.

Recommendations in guidelines and from an MDT are arrived at by consensus among a group of interested "experts". There are many factors that influence the recommendations including:

- The evidence. Some guidelines and some recommendations within guidelines are based on robust published evidence, such as a meta-analysis or double-blind randomised controlled trial. Unfortunately, frequently, such evidence is limited. In which case the guideline is subjective, reflecting the opinion and experience of a panel. Nonetheless, guidelines are generally perceived to be "best practice", and to be based on the best available evidence. Good guidelines reference the evidence and include an assessment of the quality of the evidence.
- The cost. Frequently, recommendations are influenced by cost in which the cost of an investigation or treatment is balanced against the cost of not intervening or the likely improvement in the quality of life. Quality-adjusted life years (QALY) can be used as a crude measure of benefit to which a value can be ascribed. A QALY is defined as 1 year of life in good health as measured by a patient's ability to carry out normal daily activities. In many guidelines the emphasis given to cost is not apparent. Good guidelines declare the influence of cost.
- Local circumstances. Local guidelines, including the recommendations from an MDT, may also be influenced by local circumstances, such as resource availability, patient demographics, cultural and social differences, previous experience and audit results. Unfortunately, this is not always apparent. Good guidelines declare when other factors influence the recommendations.
- Opinion. When the evidence is limited, there is a tendency to fill the void with opinion. The expectation is that the opinion of an expert panel is of greater value than the opinion of an individual clinician even when it is likely to be based on less information. However, the opinion of a panel may represent the opinion of one or two dominant individuals.

The potential disadvantages of guidelines and recommendations from an MDT include:

- Research evidence is inadequate, incorrect, irrelevant, misleading, equivocal or ambiguous.
- Errors in compilation due to a lack of rigorous assessment of the evidence or lack of representation by all interested parties.
- A marginal gain may be relevant to a large population but is not necessarily relevant to the individual.
- Recommendations tend towards the average rather than excellence.
- There is a potential for bias. For example:
  o Lead-time bias: when the diagnosis is made earlier but there has been no change in the end point.
  o Length-time bias: when the test detects more slowly progressive conditions that have a better prognosis.
  o Selection bias. Trials often exclude some patient groups, such as children, the elderly or pregnant women, or are biased towards some ethnic groups.
  o Financial bias. There may be an emphasis on cost.
  o Personal bias from panel members.
  o Service bias. For example, advocating services that are available or underutilized.

- Guidelines are often based on patients with a single problem and need to be applied with caution when a patient has multi-morbidity.
- Guidelines can be used to restrict clinical choice and autonomy. They are based on what a third-party think is in the best interests of the patient. Recommendations are not tailored to meet the wishes and needs of an individual. A patient may have a different set of values or wishes.
- Guidelines can be used to assess clinical practice rather than provide recommendations.

Guidelines and the recommendations from an MDT should include the opportunity for variations in practice. Good care is dependent on acting in the best interests of the patient and includes shared decision making. Therefore, the HCP should discuss recommendations and options with the patient in the same way they would discuss any management plan. In a minority of patients, the recommendations within a guideline may be inappropriate or unwanted. For example, when the patient has multiple medical conditions or when the patient has firm views on what care they want. Strict adherence to a guideline risk's putting the desire to conform to the guideline before the wishes and needs of the patient. Recommending a guideline should not be at the expense of individualised care. Therefore, before recommending a guideline ask yourself:

Is the guideline relevant to the patient and the problem?
Does the guideline align with what I would recommend?
Is the guideline implementable?
Are the recommendations appropriate to this patient?

If there is a divergence from the guideline, ask yourself:

What is different?
Why is there a difference?
Is the difference appropriate?

It is not uncommon that a deviation from the recommendations in a guideline or from an MDT is considered bad practice with governance, medico-legal and professional implications. Deviation from the recommendations within a guideline or from the consensus view of an MDT should be made only after careful consideration and with the agreement of the patient. The reasons should be documented to avoid future misunderstandings and potential recrimination.

Use the internet, apps or artificial intelligence to help plan management

The increasing number of available tests and treatments means that it is more challenging than ever to know not only what is available but also what is indicated and appropriate. In the past, reference books were used to provide guidance, but increasingly the internet is the library of choice. There are an increasing number of apps and tools available to help the HCP, and anyone else who wants to look something up, and, in the future, access to AI decision making algorithms will be available and used. However, as previously discussed, apps, AI and the internet should be used appropriately because there are many potential pitfalls.

Measures to ensure information from the internet is used appropriately include:

- Accurately learn and understand available information from the patient.
- Remain focused on the person with the problem, and not only on the problem.
- Define the aims of the search.
- Define the information being sought.
- Use trusted sources.
- Critically assess the source.
- Cross reference information.
- Ensure the information is internally consistent.
- Keep it simple.
- Remember, you are responsible for recommending a management option.

Choose the Most Appropriate Management Option

It is important to ensure management not only aligns with the aims of the consultation and is indicated but also that it is appropriate. Appropriateness refers to the patient, whereas the indications refer to the management option. A management option may be indicated but inappropriate. There are many factors that need to be considered when deciding on which management option is appropriate. These include:

- The patient's personal opinion; their wishes, hopes, fears and expectations. Some patients have firmly held opinions on what management they want or don't want. For example:
  - A patient may not feel the benefit outweighs the risk.
  - A patient may refuse to have an investigation, such as a colonoscopy, or a treatment, such as a statin, because they had an unpleasant experience previously.
  - A patient may have a morbid fear. Such as a fear of hospitals, enclosed spaces, crowds or needles.
  - A patient may be very frightened of having a general anaesthetic or of having an operation under local anaesthetic.
  - The patient may be fatalistic or believe in "alternative medicine", such as mind over matter, "holistic treatment" or "natural remedies".
  - A patient may be influenced by "media" reports or the opinion of friends or family. Opinion may be more important to the patient than reality or fact.
- A patient's fitness. Learning about their lifestyle, how they spend their time and the exercise they take may influence management choice. For example, when a patient leads a sedentary life, it may not be possible to assess the risk of an invasive procedure.
- The social support available or concern about the impact on others.
- Finances, such as the cost of travel or of a treatment.
- Timing. An option may not be at a convenient time for the patient.

Occasionally, it may be appropriate to consider life expectancy when planning management. For example:

- Late complications, that become more likely with time, are particularly significant in younger patients with a long life expectancy. For example:
  - Radiation related complications.
  - Intra-abdominal adhesions following an operation.
  - Late complications are unlikely to occur in a patient with a relatively short life expectancy.
- When the patient is near the end of their life an investigation or treatment, such as a screening test or prophylactic treatment is unlikely to be of benefit.

Learning about the person ensures a management option is not only indicated but also appropriate before it is recommended. For other patients, a recommended management option may turn out to be inappropriate. An assessment of benefit and risk, whether it be by the patient or the HCP, is an important determinant of appropriateness.

Assess the benefits and risks of the management options

Usually, when a management option is indicated it is also appropriate. However, for some patients, the management dilemma is to agree which option is likely to be most beneficial to the patient with least risk. For some patients the decision is clear, for others there is uncertainty, particularly when the benefit-risk equation is close to equipoise or the potential consequences serious. Guidelines, risk assessment tools, publications, audits, local information and personal experience can provide a crude estimation of an individual's risk but benefit and risk assessment is personal; different for each patient, in different contexts, at different times and depending on mitigating factors.

The assessment of benefit-risk is personal

When considering the management option to recommend, ask yourself:

What are the expected benefits?
What are the possible risks?
What is the likelihood of a risk occurring?

What are the possible consequences?

How can risk be mitigated?

Ask yourself, what are the expected benefits?

Benefit usually comes from reassurance, changing life choices or treatment. Investigations, a follow up consultation or referral to another HCP provide benefit only when they lead to treatment, advice or provide reassurance. Occasionally, it is important to consider the benefit to other family members, carers or the wider community. For example:

- Vaccinations benefit the individual and the population by contributing to "herd immunity".
- A benefit of treating an infection or giving an infected patient lifestyle advice is to reduce the infection risk to others.
- Placing a urinary catheter or stoma may help carers of an incontinent patient.

When the treatment is to relieve symptoms, such as the pain relief from an analgesic or nausea relief from an anti-emetic or when the treatment is "curative" the benefit is quickly apparent to the patient. However, the benefit of a preventative treatment or changing a life choice is often delayed and is dependent on trust; trust in the HCP or in the evidence. For example:

- Trust that a vaccine will reduce the risk of a future infection.
- Trust that bisphosphonates will reduce the risk of osteoporotic fractures.
- Trust that statins will lower serum cholesterol and reduce the risk of heart disease.
- Trust that stopping smoking or losing weight will reduce the risk of developing cardio-vascular disease or cancer.

Information and reassurance can be very beneficial for some patients. For some patients sharing information, including the results of a test or the opinion of another HCP or of an MDT, relieves anxiety allowing them to get on with their lives. Similarly, for some patients, a further consultation or the opinion of another HCP can be reassuring not only because it is an opportunity to review progress or change but also because it provides a "safety-net".

Ask yourself, what are the possible risks?

All management options, including "doing nothing", are associated with risk. These include:

- Risk of an adverse reaction or side effect.
- The risk of an early complication.
- The risk of a late complication. For example:
  o Osteopaenia following long-term steroid use.
  o Dependence after long-term opiate or benzodiazepine use.
  o Adhesions following an operation.
  o The risk of cancer, osteo-necrosis, ulceration or a small bowel stricture following exposure to ionising radiation.
- The risk of a mis-diagnosis.
  o Over-investigation increases the risk of a false positive result and a misdiagnosis.
  o Over-investigation increases the risk of over-diagnosis or uncertainty. For example:
    • Starting treatment for prostate cancer on the basis of a raised PSA.
    • Performing a thyroidectomy for a well differentiated papillary thyroid cancer.
    • Inappropriately investigating or treating an incidental finding.
  o A false positive diagnosis may lead to unnecessary treatment.
  o A false negative diagnosis may give a false sense of reassurance and delay treatment.
  o Unnecessary anxiety.
- The risk of bias. There is a risk a result will be mis-represented causing stress or anxiety for the patient or false reassurance and loss of trust. For example:

- o Suggesting that a test excludes cancer.
  - o Highlighting relative risk reduction rather than absolute risk reduction.
  - o Emphasising survival rather than mortality.
- The risk of alienating the patient or losing a patient's trust. For example:
  - o Some patients "expect treatment". A management plan that does not have the support of the patient or is not what the patient expected, such as "doing nothing" can undermine trust and adversely affect the working relationship.
  - o Some patients resent being advised to change their life choices.
  - o Some patients feel "rejected" if they are discharged, whereas others get a false sense of safety and delay re-presenting if the problem persists or deteriorates or a new problem arises.
  - o When there is a process error, such as referral to the wrong HCP or organising the wrong test.

In a minority of patients, it is also important to consider the risk to others. These may include:

- Risk of infecting others. This could be by aerosol transmission, such as from a viral infection, TB or MRSA, or contamination with body fluids, such as Hepatitis B, C, HIV, or Ebola virus.
- Risk from radiation exposure. For example, following a radio-isotope scan.
- Risk of physical or verbal assault.
- An unnecessary investigation or treatment for one patient may put another at risk because their care is delayed.

Many risks, such as an early complication following an operation or a side effect from a medication are well known and become apparent quickly. However, some are rarely considered or only become apparent after time.

Ask yourself, what is the likelihood of a risk occurring?

The likelihood of a risk occurring can be derived from published information, audits, personal experience or one of an increasing number of scoring systems.

Examples of scoring systems available to estimate risk

- P-Possum score to assess operative risk
- The "Wells criteria" to assess the risk of a DVT or PE
- APACHE scoring to assess illness severity
- Atlanta criteria to assess the risk of morbidity and mortality in acute pancreatitis
- TNM classification to assess the risk of mortality from cancer
- The WHO FRAX assessment tool to assess the risk of fragility fractures in patients with osteoporosis
- The ABCD2 score (Age, Blood pressure >140/90, Clinical signs, DM and Duration) to assess the risk of a stroke after a TIA
- The CHADS-VASC score (Age, Sex, Heart failure, Previous stroke, Valvular heart disease, DM) to assess the risk of a stroke in a non-anticoagulated patient with AF.

The likelihood of risk can be presented as an absolute risk or a relative risk.

- Absolute risk is the probability the problem will occur if nothing changes. It can be expressed as a percentage or a ratio.
- Relative risk is the difference in probability between different populations or within the same population over time. It can be expressed as a percentage difference or a hazard ratio. There is no difference in risk when the hazard ratio is 1, whereas a hazard ratio of 0.5 means that the risk is halved, and a hazard ratio of 2 means that the risk is doubled.

For example:

- The population lifetime risk of a man developing bowel cancer is 1 in 15 (6.7%) and for a woman 1 in 18 (5.6%). Therefore, men are 17% more likely to develop bowel cancer, HR 1.2, but the difference in absolute risk is only 1.1%.
- The absolute life-time risk of a 50-year-old developing bowel cancer is 1.8%. However, when the patient has a first degree relative with bowel cancer the risk is increased to 3.4%. The increase in absolute risk is only 1.6% but the increased relative risk is 89%, HR=1.9.

It is important to present absolute and relative risk to the patient with care to ensure there is no bias or mis-understanding. For example, saying to a 50-year-old man the risk of cancer is increased by nearly 90% because they have a first degree relative with bowel cancer gives the impression the risk is very high. However, telling them that the excess risk is only 1.6% or that the absolute risk remains very low at less than 1 in 25 is more reassuring.

A risk is often expressed as a percentage for a population but is binary for an individual; it either happens or doesn't happen. Therefore, rather than state the risk for the patient it may be better to state how sure you are of an outcome or use the third person. For example:

- Rather than saying "You have a 98% chance of not getting bowel cancer" you might say
  o "I am 98% sure you will not get bowel cancer", or:
  o "The evidence shows that overall, 98% of men of your age will not get bowel cancer".

Risk is usually presented as a subjective assessment, such as a "likely or unlikely", "high or low" or an "increased" or "decreased" risk. For example:

- Venesection is likely to cause pain and distress, but the chance of thrombophlebitis or septicaemia is very low.
- An upper GI endoscopy is likely to be uncomfortable, causing the patient to gag, but the chance of aspiration or perforation is very low.
- Heartburn when taking an NSAID is possible, whereas it is rare to get a peptic ulcer.
- A headache following nicorandil is likely and occasionally causes skin and mucosal ulcers.
- Itching or constipation usually occurs when taking opiates but may rarely cause respiratory depression.
- Statins are likely to cause loose stools and may cause liver failure.

Risk likelihood is influenced by many variables including:

- The problem. Frequently, the more severe the problem, the more likely the risk. For example:
  o The risks from hypertension increase as the blood pressure increases. For this reason, a blood pressure of 140/90 mmHg to 160/100 mmHg is considered mild (stage 1), 160/100 to <180 systolic or <110 diastolic is moderate (Stage 2), and >180 systolic or >110 diastolic severe hypertension (stage 3).
  o The risk an abdominal aortic aneurysm (AAA) will rupture increases as the diameter increases. The annual risk is 9% when the diameter is 5.5-5.9 cm, 10% at 6.0-6.9 cm, 32.5% when the AAA >7.0 cm.
  o In a patient with UC, the risk of developing bowel cancer increases with the severity, extent and duration of inflammatory bowel disease.
  For some patients the relationship between exposure and the development of a problem is non-linear. For example:
  o There is a J-shaped association between mortality and BMI or alcohol consumption.
- The patient. When not all the important variables are factored in.
- Time. Point risk refers to the risk at a specified point in time, period risk is the proportion who will get the risk during a given time period, lifetime risk is the proportion who will get the risk at some time in their lives. For example: The lifetime risk that bowel cancer will develop in a patient with ulcerative colitis is about 5%. However, the absolute risk of cancer developing is <2% within the first 10 years, increasing to 8% after 20 years, and to 18% after 30 years.
- The evidence. For the individual it can be difficult to estimate risk because published data can be misleading or may not be relevant to a specific patient. The reasons for this include:
  o The data may be based on a sample population with different characteristics. This is particularly relevant to minority groups.

o The published risk may be less when the trials are conducted in an optimal environment which does not reflect general practice (efficacy vs effectiveness). In a research setting, many clinical variables are controlled. Published data is old data.
o The sensitivity of risk assessments derived from a population with a high disease prevalence will typically be reduced and the specificity increased when applied to a population with a low prevalence.
o The data may be misrepresented or mis-interpreted.
o The likelihood a risk factor will lead to a problem is published as a percentage derived from population studies whereas the outcome for an individual is binary. For example, a patient who smokes may have a 10% risk of developing lung cancer but for the patient it either occurs or doesn't. Patients always remember the smokers who remain well.

Ask yourself, what are the possible consequences?

Most HCPs and patients agree what constitutes a significant risk, i.e., what is "consequential", but fundamentally it is for the patient to decide what is consequential. Examples of risks that are widely recognised to be serious include:

- Death, debility or lasting morbidity.
- Anaphylactic reaction to a medication.
- Septicaemia following an invasive procedure.
- Perforation during an endoscopy.
- Torrential haemorrhage following an invasive procedure.
- Cancer.

Well known, reversible or treatable risks are usually considered less serious. For example:

- A post-operative wound infection may be common but, for most healthy patients, is a relatively minor complication that can be treated successfully and is therefore generally considered to be of limited consequence. Wound dehiscence or necrotizing fasciitis are uncommon, but are serious complications.
- Diarrhoea is a frequent side-effect of antibiotic treatment which for most patients is a mild self-limiting "inconvenience". Pseudomembranous colitis is an uncommon but serious complication.

In general, patients, HCPs and the healthcare community are willing to accept a "minor" and easily treated complication that is more frequent than a serious complication or side effect even when it is uncommon. However, some risks are consequential for some patients but not to the majority. For example:

- Peripheral neuropathy following cisplatin or vincristine treatment for cancer is a serious adverse outcome for a professional pianist or surgeon.
- An ischaemic leg following an abdominal aortic aneurysm repair is a serious adverse outcome for a rambler.
- A late complication, such as cancer following radiation exposure from radiological investigations is a serious adverse outcome.

Some patients want or refuse a treatment, or prefer one treatment over another, despite the likelihood of a serious risk. For example:

- When a patient needs a bowel resection for cancer, they may refuse a stoma despite the increased risk of an anastomotic leak.
- A patient may refuse to have an ERCP for obstructive jaundice because of the risk of acute pancreatitis.
- A patient taking oral anticoagulants for AF and recurrent TIA's may prefer to continue taking anticoagulation medication during an invasive procedure and accept the risk of bleeding rather than the risk of a stroke.

On the other hand, some clinicians may not offer an investigation or treatment, such as an operation, because of the perceived risk to the patient. This is particularly the case when there may be professional consequences from an adverse outcome.

It is not uncommon for patients to be on several different care pathways. If each pathway is managed in isolation there may be unintended risks. For example:

- A patient may be obese and being treated for COPD, asthma, DM and hypertension. Treatment of their osteoarthritis with non-steroidal anti-inflammatory medications (NSAIDs) will help their joint pain and movement but may aggravate their bronchospasm and renal failure.
- A patient with widespread peripheral vascular disease may be receiving treatment for hypertension, heart failure and platelet emboli. Treatment of a DVT with an anticoagulant will increase their risk of a serious haemorrhage.

Ask yourself, how can risk be mitigated?

Risks should always be discussed with the patient in advance and mitigated if possible. If a permanent adverse outcome, such as a stroke, occurs, it is not possible to "turn the clock back".

Hindsight informs learning, foresight implements learning

Many risks can be reduced either by the patient changing a life choice or with medical intervention. For example:

- Stopping smoking to reduce a risk of cancer or heart disease.
- Undertaking a more active lifestyle to reduce peri-operative risk or to increase the tolerance to a peri-operative complication.
- Reducing weight and blood pressure, stopping smoking and exercise to reduce the risk of rupture in a patient with an AAA.
- Optimal management of DM to delay the onset of complications.
- Optimising blood pressure prior to a general anaesthetic.
- Endovascular ablation to treat AF to reduce the risk of a stroke.
- Vaccination to reduce the infection risk.
- Anti-retroviral treatment prior to sexual intercourse with an HIV infected person reduces the risk of infection.
- Stress ulcer prophylaxis in critically ill patients to reduce the risk of bleeding.
- Operating on a hernia to prevent a complication.
- Pre-hydration in a patient with renal failure needing intravenous contrast.
- Lead shielding in children or pregnant females requiring an Xray.
- Pre-operative counselling or sedation to reduce anxiety for a claustrophobic patient requiring an MRI scan.

Some risks cannot be reduced. For example:

- Risks associated with an individual's gene profile.
- Risks associated with age and height.
- Risks associated with past medical conditions.
- Financial or social deprivation.

For some patients, and for some conditions, management to reduce risk intuitively seems to be worthwhile. However, it may expose a patient to other risks, i.e., one risk is exchanged for another. For example:

- Undertaking an investigation to "exclude" an unlikely problem may reveal an incidental finding leading to more investigations or treatment and risk additional complications.
- The risk of dehydration from bowel preparation prior to a colonoscopy.
- The risk of a TIA or PE from stopping or changing an anticoagulant prior to an invasive procedure.
- The risk of transplant rejection from stopping an immuno-suppression treatment.
- Endovascular pulmonary vein ablation to treat AF to reduce the risk of a stroke may lead to cardiac tamponade and the need for an emergency thoracotomy.
- Anti-retroviral treatment prior to sexual intercourse may lead to increased sexual activity and increased risk of other infections.
- Stress ulcer prophylaxis in critically ill patients may reduce the risk of bleeding, but PPI's and H_2RA's are associated with an increased risk of pneumonia.
- Operating on an asymptomatic hernia to prevent a complication, risks a postoperative complication, such as chronic pain.

- Following up a patient to identify a deterioration rather than discharging a patient may delay a consultation with another patient and delay their care.

Consider adherence and compliance

There is always a risk that a patient will not adhere or comply with a management plan.

Adherence is the extent to which a patient follows a recommendation.

There is little point recommending a management plan that will not be adhered to. For example:

- Whether or not the patient takes the prescribed medication.
- Whether the patient follows advice given.
- Whether the patient attends an appointment.

Compliance is the extent or degree to which a patient follows instructions.

Treatment effectiveness is dependent on a patient complying with important instructions. For example:

- When to start or stop a medication, or the dose or frequency.
- Preparation prior to a procedure. For example:
    o Not eating when taking medication to clean the bowel prior to a colonoscopy.
    o Fasting before an operation.

There is little point recommending a management plan that cannot or won't be complied with.

Adherence or compliance errors are a frequent cause of treatment failure. For most treatments, non-adherence only impacts on the patient. However, for some treatments, non-adherence can affect others, such as if the patient is being treated for an infectious disease.

Non-adherence or non-compliance can be unintentional or intentional. The causes of unintentional non-adherence or non-compliance include:

- Administrative errors. For example, not being sent an appointment.
- Delivery errors. For example, not receiving an appointment.
- Forgetfulness. For example, dementia.
- Carelessness. For example, being distracted.
- Ignorance. For example, lack of training, lack of awareness of the importance/significance.
- Confusion. For example, polypharmacy, complex administration patterns.

The causes of intentional non-adherence or non-compliance include:

- Apathy.
- Logistic. For example, unavailability of transport, taking a lot of medications at once.
- Inconvenient, deliberately not attending/taking medication.
- Financial.
- Lack of understanding.
- Lack of trust or confidence in the HCP or health care.
- Choice, personal, social and cultural attitude.

The reasons for and extent to which a patient adheres or complies with a management plan can vary at different stages in the pathway of care or for different management options.

A successful consultation, a good working relationship and the agreement of the patient make adherence and compliance more likely. In general, the more serious the problem or the prognosis the more likely the patient will adhere to the management plan, and the less onerous, inconvenient or difficult the management option the more likely they are to comply. If there is a risk of non-adherence or non-compliance it is necessary to learn and understand the patients' concerns. This will inform management of their concern. Failure to manage their concerns is likely to affect the outcome.

Consider the timing

When considering management, it is also necessary to consider timing. Timing is influenced by many factors including:

- The availability of an investigation or treatment.
- The preparation required. For example:
  o Bowel preparation prior to a colonoscopy delaying when a colonoscopy can be done.
  o Stopping an anticoagulant prior to an invasive procedure.
- The clinical priority.
- The natural history of the condition and prognosis.

Timing influences both the choice of management and when a management is indicated. For example:

- In a seriously ill patient, management is focused on providing immediate organ support, usually oxygen and fluid replacement therapy, to reduce the risk of irreversible damage and restore homeostasis.
- When a patient has a serious infection, treatment may be indicated before a definitive diagnosis is made.
- When a patient is likely to have cancer, investigations and treatment should be undertaken urgently to reduce the risk of the cancer becoming untreatable.
- A patient with severe pain from an impacted ureteric stone may need urgent pain relief before tests are performed to confirm the diagnosis.
- In a patient who is unfit, a hernia may be amenable to a local anaesthetic repair with few risks while it is small, but not when treatment is delayed and it becomes large or develops a complication.
- Delaying an operation may give an opportunity for the patient to get fitter reducing the risks from an anaesthetic but the delay may increase the likelihood of disease progression, a deterioration in the patient's physical condition or a complication and irreversible harm.

For some patients, it may be preferable to delay management. For example:

- When there is diagnostic uncertainty, a period of watchful waiting and timely review is likely to increase confidence in a diagnosis. For example, the investigation of a small pulmonary or liver nodule may be repeated after a period of time to help distinguish between a benign incidentaloma and a cancer.
- To allow risk to be reduced. For example, giving the patient an opportunity to lose weight or stop smoking prior to joint replacement surgery.
- When the risk from delay is minimal. For example, a long wait to treat a small asymptomatic paraumbilical hernia is unlikely to cause harm.

Agreement and consent

Part of ensuring a management option is appropriate is to ensure the patient agrees with the management option recommended and, when indicated, formally consents to it. Planning management should be a collaborative process. It should involve all relevant parties and an agreement reached before the end of the consultation as to what will be done next. Ensuring agreement not only respects autonomy but also increases the likelihood of compliance and adherence: after all, there is little point recommending a management plan that will *not* be complied with or adhered to. Learning about the patient as a person ensures the patient's views inform management and the discussion about management. If it becomes apparent that there is a difference between what a patient wants or expects and what is recommended, available or likely, this should be discussed and managed to avoid future psychological or emotional consequences, such as disappointment, stress, anxiety, anger or hostility, or a loss of trust and confidence in the HCP and a breakdown in the working relationship.

For many management options, such as whether to review the patient or to perform a "routine" blood investigation, only the agreement of the patient is needed. Some management plans, such as those with risks, should only be organised with the informed consent of the patient. When planning management:

Ask yourself, is consent indicated?

For some simple interventions, such as to take blood or insert a urinary catheter, a verbal consent is all that is required. However, when there is a risk of a complication a written consent is indicated. If there is uncertainty written consent is indicated.

In the UK, for consent to be valid the individual should be an adult who has the mental capacity to make a voluntary and informed decision to consent to or refuse an investigation or treatment, even if refusing treatment could result in harm or death. Therefore, before discussing consent with a patient:

Ask yourself, does the patient have the mental capacity for informed consent?

As part of the consent process the patient needs to understand the rationale for the test or treatment and the expected benefits, the options or alternatives, the risks and to know what is involved. Discussing consent is a process which should include:

- A discussion of the problem being managed, the aims and indications, likely benefits and potential risks. All investigations and treatments are associated with risk, which should be explained to the patient. When a particular risk is increased, such as when there is a known safety concern, or is consequential this should be highlighted in the discussion.
- When there is choice, the options should be discussed.
- Highlighting any deviation from the recommendations within a guideline or from the consensus view of an MDT. Any deviation should only be undertaken with the agreement of the patient. The reasons should be documented to avoid future misunderstandings and potential recrimination.
- An explanation of what the investigation or treatment involves for the patient. The details of many investigations or treatments are highly specialised and only known to experts in the field. Nevertheless, when an HCP is recommending an investigation or treatment, they should not only know the indications and contraindications but also should have working knowledge of what is involved, including the benefits and risks. This information should be shared with the patient when consenting a patient.
- Ethically, placebo treatments should only be used within the context of a clinical trial with appropriate fully informed consent.

In the UK, when the patient lacks the capacity to consent to a management option, such as when they have a significant mental health condition, a guardian or independent advocate can be appointed to act in the patient's best interests (Mental Health Act 1983). In an emergency, investigations or treatment may be undertaken in the best interests of the patient, preferably with the agreement of more than one suitably experienced clinician.

The Management Options Available

The management options available include:

- Discharge.
- Recommending changing a life choice.
- Recommending an investigation.
- Recommending a treatment.
- Recommending referral to another HCP.
- Recommending another consultation.

The aims, indications and possible consequences are different for each. Therefore, before recommending a management option, ask yourself,

What are the aims?
Is it indicated?
Is it appropriate?
How should it be managed?

Discharge

There is frequently a desire to "do something" even when the evidence suggests reassurance and discharge is the most appropriate option. Doing something just for the sake of it reflects indecision, whereas discharge indicates self-assurance. Discharge should be a positive decision, made carefully and deliberately based on information available, although occasionally, discharge is indicated when other management options are not indicated. Before discharging a patient:

Ask yourself, what are the aims of discharge?

The usual aim of discharging a patient is to avoid an unnecessary consultation. Most patients prefer not to attend consultations or to have investigations or treatments for many reasons, including because they are an imposition, inconvenience or are unpleasant. For some patients, the aim of discharge is to reassure the patient other management options are unnecessary, such as when a course of treatment is complete, inappropriate or contra-indicated, or when the risks outweigh the benefits.

Occasionally, the aim is to conclude the relationship with the patient because they do not accept the opinion of the HCP or no longer want to see the HCP, such as when there has been an irretrievable breakdown in the HCP-patient relationship.

Ask yourself, is discharge indicated?

Discharging a patient is indicated:

- When the patient can be reassured that the presenting problem does not need further medical care. For example:
  o A minor viral illness.
  o A short period of diarrhoea and vomiting.
  o A strained muscle.
  o Anal pain from a thrombosed external pile.
  o A broken toe.
  o After a small superficial abscess has discharged.
- When a treatment is started with a high likelihood of success and a follow up consultation or further investigations are not indicated. For example:
  o When a minor bacterial infection is treated with antibiotics.
  o When skin inflammation is treated with cream.
  o When a minor operation is performed, such as an operation to repair a hernia.
- When the problem has been successfully treated.
- When management of the problem is the responsibility of the patient.
- When other management options are not indicated or the risks outweigh the benefits.
- When the patient does not want investigations or treatment.
- When the patient no longer wants to see the HCP.
- When there has been an irretrievable breakdown in the HCP-patient relationship.

A secondary consequence of discharge is that it increases the availability of health care resources for other patients. However, this should rarely be an indication to discharge the patient.

Ask yourself, is discharge appropriate?

Medically, discharge is appropriate when it is indicated and meets the management aims. However, for some patients it may be inappropriate for various reasons, including:

- When the patient is likely to be very upset or dissatisfied if they are discharged, such as if they feel they are not being taken seriously.
- Discharge may undermine trust in the HCP and health care system.
- Discharge may alienate the patient.

It may be inappropriate to discharge a patient if there is a chance of a false negative test result. False reassurance may lead to a delay before the patient re-presents, particularly among patients who don't like to "trouble the HCP" or "talk about their health".

Ask yourself, how should discharge be managed?

Discharge should be managed to ensure it is accepted as appropriate by the patient and is safe. Providing a detailed explanation of the problem, reassuring the patient about their problem and starting a treatment, giving lifestyle advice or explaining why other management options are not indicated can introduce the idea that discharge is indicated and appropriate. In summary, the process leading to discharge may include:

- Sharing information about the problem and checking understanding.
- Starting treatment likely to be successful, reassuring the patient or providing lifestyle advice or following a successful treatment.
- Explaining possible warning symptoms, what to be aware of or to look out for.
- Reassuring the patient that they can return should their symptoms recur, deteriorate or a new problem arise.
- Describing future options, such as what they should do if the problem changes, recurs, persists or deteriorates. When discharge is a "wait and see" or a "watchful waiting" option, the patient should know they can return at a later date should the problem persist, recur or deteriorate. "Watchful waiting" can be more useful than doing something prematurely or inappropriately.
- Ensuring they agree to the management plan.

Discharge may conclude the pathway of care but it should not conclude the availability of care.

Recommend changing a life choice

Traditionally, health care has focused on managing a problem for the patient: usually prescribing a medication or recommending an operation. However, the successful management of an increasing number of health problems is dependent on the patient changing a life choice, such as their behaviour or lifestyle. Life choices with medical consequences include exercise, diet and avoiding smoking, stress or excessive alcohol. The consequences of changing a life choice may not only be transformational for the patient but also have profound consequences for future demand on the health service. These are frequently under-estimated and under-appreciated by the patient.

Ask yourself, what is the aim?

Changing a life choice is usually with the aim of reducing a risk in the hope of improving health, quality of life or longevity. For some patients, it is with the aim of treating, preventing or delaying the onset of a problem or alleviating symptoms, help function or increase productivity. Nationally, the aim may be to reduce demands on health and social care.

Ask yourself, is a life choice change indicated?

Changing a life choice is indicated when it is likely to benefit the patient and is amenable to change.
Changing a life choice is indicated before problems develop. For example:

- Reduce weight before developing DM or metabolic syndrome.
- Reducing or stopping alcohol consumption before problems, such as liver cirrhosis or chronic pancreatitis develop.
- Reducing or stopping drug taking or gambling before becoming addicted.

For some patients, changing a life choice is indicated to treat a problem. For example:

- Reduce weight to reduce the strain on a joint.
- Stopping smoking and increasing the walking distance to treat claudication or prevent deterioration.
- When a patient presents with a repetitive strain injury it may be appropriate to give advice on how to avoid overuse or repetitive actions.

Some changes are specific to the patient and their problem. For example:

- Patients prone to renal stones should keep hydrated, eat calcium rich foods and avoid a protein rich diet. Vitamin C supplements, sodium and oxalate may reduce the risk of developing recurrent stones.
- Patients with an increased risk of developing colon cancer may reduce their risk if they eat a diet high in fibre and low in processed food or fatty meat.
- Some medications have adverse effects that can be reduced or avoided with lifestyle change. For example, reducing sun exposure when taking a sensitizer such as amiodarone or avoiding grapefruit and citrus fruits when taking statins or calcium channel blockers.

It is important to distinguish between a life choice that is correctable, such as to stop smoking and one that is essentially fixed or irreversible, such as physical, medical, psychological, financial and some domestic or social circumstances. Recommending changing a life choice that cannot or will not be changed is not indicated. When irreversible harm has occurred, changing a life choice may no longer be indicated. For example, when a patient has metastatic lung cancer from smoking, recommending they stop smoking is no longer indicated.

When the patient is adamant that they do not want to change or do not want to discuss change, a discussion is contra-indicated.

Ask yourself, is it appropriate to discuss changing a life choice?

Discussing changing a life choice is appropriate when it is likely to benefit the patient and the relationship with the patient is good enough, because a discussion can be challenging. The HCP needs to have the self-confidence to challenge the patient's current lifestyle or behaviour and the patient needs to be receptive to change. Discussing changing a life choice may be indicated but inappropriate if it is likely to have adverse consequences which may include:

- A loss of trust.
- A loss of confidence.
- Disagreement.
- A breakdown in the working relationship.
- Undermine self-belief.
- A feeling of being blamed.
- Psychological consequences, such as stress, depression or a neurosis.
- The opposite outcome from that intended.

Ask yourself, how should change be managed?

Changing a life choice is a transformation. It does not happen by chance; it needs to be managed. Implementing change is the responsibility of the patient but the HCP has a responsibility to raise the topic and help the patient if it is relevant to patient care.

Choosing the right time to discuss changing a life choice is important. Ideally, it should be relevant to the context. The development of a medical condition is often a good opportunity to discuss changing a life choice, as long as the problem is reversible. If discussing change is mis-timed it is likely to be counterproductive.

Before starting the conversation, ask permission. Asking permission empowers the patient, because they can say "no": the patient may not agree or want to discuss change or it may not be appropriate or indicated at that time. Asking permission also ensures the patient is in a listening frame of mind; receptive and attentive, focusing on the topic rather than thinking about other matters.

There are many different ways change can be managed. Traditional directive methods include:

- Reasoning, using statistics.
- Begging and imploring patients.
- Scaring patients with warnings or threats about what might happen if they don't change.
- Emotional blackmail, such as making reference to the impact on other family members.
- Hoping.

However, these are rarely successful for many reasons:

- They may appear to lack empathy and understanding: "He/she [the HCP] doesn't understand!"
- They may be considered disrespectful: "It's none of your business."
- They may be interpreted as being confrontational, because they are being imposed on the patient: "Are you telling me what to do!"

A non-directive approach using questions to raise awareness of the problem, to help the patient take responsibility and to own the problem, to identify barriers and to decide on their own solutions is more likely to be successful because the patient owns both the problem and the solution.

Whichever method is used preparation is important. Before discussing change, learn about the person and the person as a patient to understand the patient's background and gain an insight into their pressures, challenges and constraints and to establish a good working relationship. Change is more likely to be achieved if there is a good working relationship and the patient trusts and respects the HCP, their opinion and recommendations, and believes the science. Knowing the patient will help set the right tone, indicate the language to use and how much challenge is indicated. Too much challenge, or not a good enough rapport and the patient may feel resentful, anxious, or bullied, too little and meaningful change is unlikely. If the working relationship is not good enough, then discussing changing a life choice may not be appropriate. (Figure 27).

Figure 27: Illustrating the balance between rapport and challenge needed to bring about change

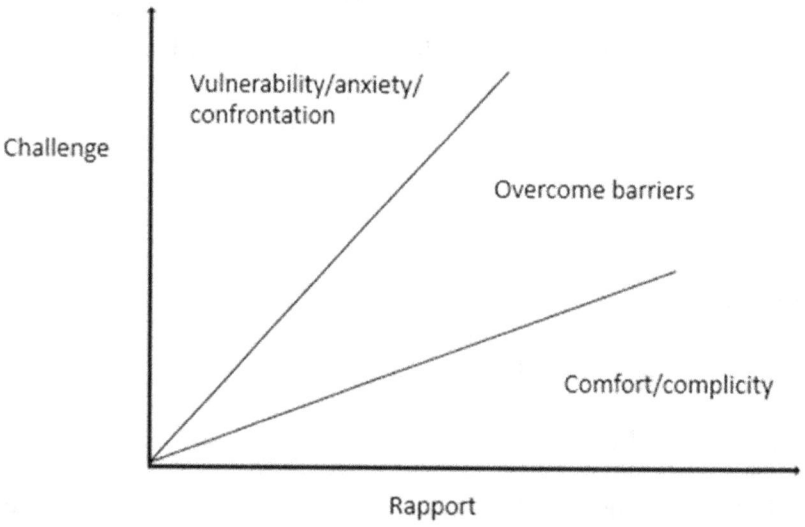

Through asking questions patients are helped to identify their own barriers (Figure 28). For example,

Is awareness or knowledge a barrier?
Is responsibility a barrier?
Do they lack motivation?
Is self-belief a barrier?

Discussing the problem raises awareness and helps the patient accept responsibility. This is the first step in finding a solution. The patient may have been unaware their life choices are causing medical problems or may not have considered that they are responsible for their problems. In which case, accepting responsibility for a problem is a barrier.

It may become apparent while discussing the problem that the patient lacks knowledge. For example, they may be unaware of the risk and the consequences of their lifestyle choice. When taking responsibility or a lack of knowledge are barriers, sharing information to increase their knowledge and understanding may be helpful. This may include handouts, on-line resources or seeing a specialist, such as a dietician. However, it should be remembered that frequently, for the patient, their opinion or the opinion of key influencers within their social group may be more important than reality or fact from an HCP.

Figure 28: A figure illustrating how ranking the size of each barrier can help identify the priority for managing barriers to change

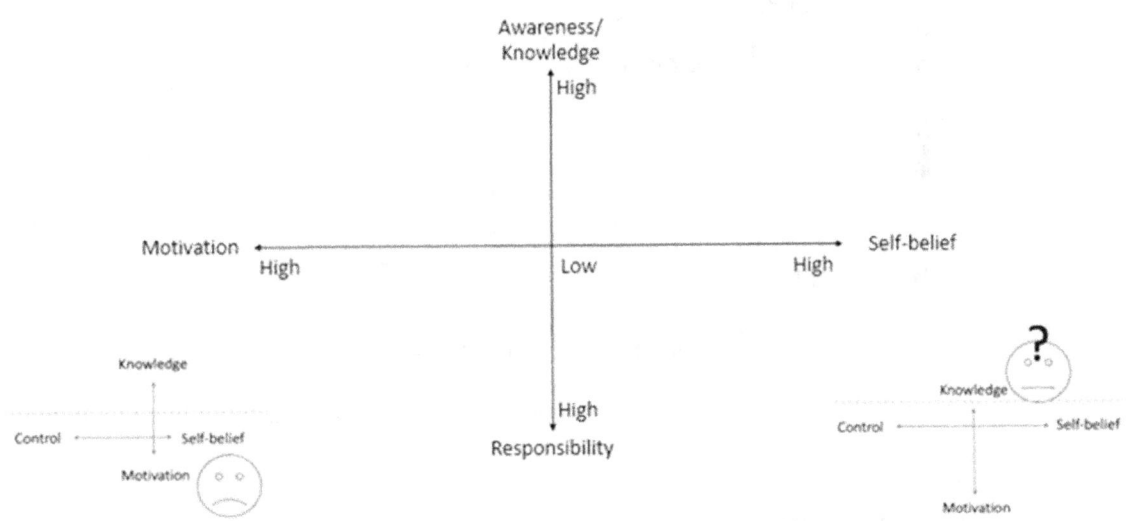

Patients frequently lack the desire to change, such as when their life choice is an enjoyable habit. Some patients lack motivation because there is peer or family pressure. Patients will only change if they want to. When motivation is a barrier, the focus of the conversation should change from discussing the problem, which may seem too big to resolve, to discussing solutions that are achievable. Small, incremental changes, "baby steps", are often more achievable than a "giant leap". For example, keeping cigarettes in a cupboard or using a smaller wine glass rather than going "cold turkey". For some problems it is important to distinguish between motivation and addiction. Some problems, such as smoking, drinking alcohol, excessive eating or taking drugs are an addiction. The patient may want to stop but are unable without specialist help.

Patients often lack the self-belief because previous attempts to change have failed. If the patient lacks self-belief, the inner negative thoughts, feelings and the pressures that prevent change should be recognised and, if indicated, discussed from a medical perspective without attributing blame, finding fault or being judgemental. The aim is to move from negative thoughts, such as guilt, inadequacy or failure, to positive problem-solving thoughts. The emphasis should be on doing what is right, playing to your strengths, focus on the inner positive thoughts, past successes and the benefits of a positive outcome. Not everything is easy and not everything works first time. Previous mistakes or failures can be a platform for future success. Sometimes, when a patient is fixated on negative thoughts, asking a set of questions they will say "yes" to will change their mindset and open the door to being able to ask a question they would normally say "no" to. You may get a different answer if they have a "yes" mindset. Make making the change easy and keeping the status quo more difficult and reward success.

Changing life choices is the responsibility of the patient and it is more likely to be successful when the patient identifies and wants to implement their own solutions. However, the patient may need help. This could include help from family, friends, a support service or from the health service. For example:

- Dietary advice in DM, to reduce weight or to avoid lipids.
- Physiotherapy to alleviate back pain and increase exercise tolerance.
- Bio-feedback to help faecal incontinence.
- Mind-body treatment, such as, mindfulness, hypnosis, cognitive and behavioural therapy, music or art "therapy".
- Prescribing medication. For example, nicotine to help the patient stop smoking.
- Treating an underlying medical condition may help the patient. For example:
  o A joint operation or treating coronary heart disease may improve mobility enabling a patient to increase activity and lose weight.
  o Treating depression may increase motivation and self-belief.

Figure 29: A figure summarizing the method to manage change

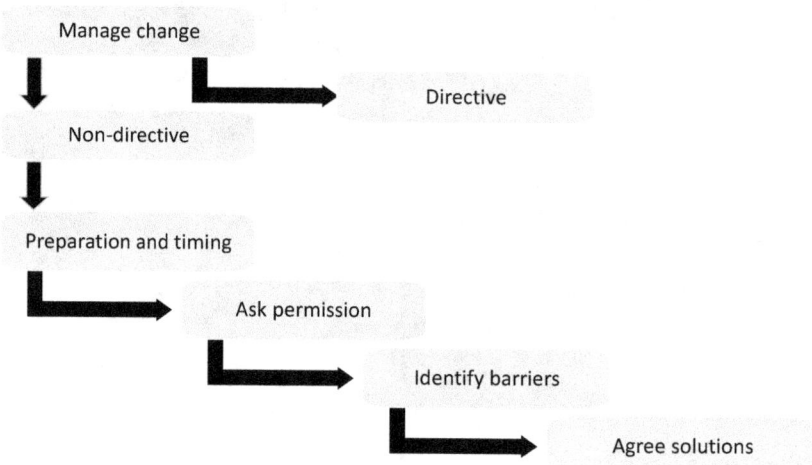

Recommend an investigation

Investigations are an increasingly important part of patient care and are increasingly being performed. Indeed, most consultations lead to an investigation. Not only do patients expect them but also HCPs frequently rely on them. Before organising an investigation ask yourself:

What is the aim?
Is an investigation indicated?

Frequently, tests are requested to screen for an asymptomatic problem, in which case the indications are different. Therefore, before organising a screening investigation, ask yourself:

Is a screening investigation indicated?

An investigation may be indicated and meet the management aims but before it is recommended it is also important to consider the patient. For some patients, there are personal issues that may affect whether or not an investigation is appropriate. Therefore, always ask yourself:

Is the test appropriate for the patient?

An investigation is undertaken to provide more information so it is the result that is important.

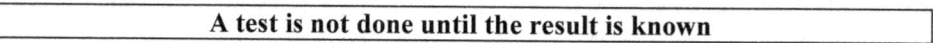

A test is not done until the result is known

The result should answer the question and be followed by action, such as a treatment, another investigation or to share information.

Investigations are a means to an end, not an end in themselves

Therefore, just as it is important to ensure the test is appropriate so it is also important to ensure the result is likely to be meaningful. Therefore, before requesting an investigation ask yourself, What will the result mean?

There are many factors that influence when a test should be undertaken. Therefore, before requesting a test, ask yourself:

When should a test be requested?

Ask yourself, what is the aim of the investigation?

Investigations are undertaken for a variety of different reasons and some investigations are undertaken for several different reasons. In summary, the aims of an investigation include:

- To formulate a diagnosis
    - To confirm a diagnosis. For example:
        - The measurement of serum bilirubin is indicated to confirm a diagnosis of jaundice in any patient clinically suspected of being jaundiced, and to assess the severity of the jaundice.
        - A CXR with the aim of confirming a diagnosis of pneumonia.
    - To make a diagnosis. For example:
        - An electrocardiogram (ECG) to diagnose abnormalities in the electrical activity of the heart. Serum troponin measurement is indicated with the aim of diagnosing an AMI if the ECG suggests acute cardiac ischaemia.
        - Sending a sputum for MC&S to identify the likely pathogen causing a chest infection.
    - To exclude a diagnosis. For example:
        - Measuring beta hCG with the aim of excluding pregnancy.
        - A colonoscopy to exclude bowel cancer.
        - A Doppler USS to exclude a DVT.
    - To screen for asymptomatic problems. For example:
        - A CT chest and abdomen with the aim of screening for asymptomatic metastatic disease or recurrent cancer in a patient treated for cancer.
        - An FBC, urea, creatinine and electrolytes to screen for haematological and biochemical abnormalities.
    - To determine the location of the abnormality causing the problem. For example:
        - A CT angiogram to determine the location of occlusive vascular disease.
        - A carotid Doppler USS and an echocardiogram to determine the source of an embolus.
    - To determine the type of problem.
        - Measuring the WBC count or the CRP to determine if there is an inflammatory response.
        - An abdominal CT scan to distinguish between a structural problem, such as adhesions, cancer and an inflammatory problem, such as a Crohn's stricture.
- For assessment of:
    - Severity. For example:
        - Measuring the WBC count or the CRP or performing a colonoscopy in a patient with ulcerative colitis to assess the severity and extent of the inflammatory response.
        - Early on, patients with an infection may seem relatively well. However, if not treated early they can develop septic shock and death. Measuring the WBC count or the CRP will not only be diagnostic but can also assess the severity of the problem.
        - In some patients, chest pain caused by angina is severe, whereas in others a life-threatening AMI causes only mild chest discomfort or tightness. An ECG, serial troponins and an angiogram will not only be diagnostic but can also assess severity.
        - Assessment of severity of acute pancreatitis using APACHE scoring or the Atlanta criteria.
        - Cancer often presents as a localized problem, such as a change in bowel habit, haemoptysis or haematuria. However, the severity can only be assessed with staging investigations, such as a CT scan.
        - Referral to a psychiatrist may be indicated to assess the severity of a mental health condition.
    - A physical abnormality. For example:
        - An USS to assess the diameter and length of a AAA.
        - An Xray to measure the extent of a deformity, such as a scoliosis.
        - An Echo cardiogram to measure the degree of stenosis and the pressure gradient, across a stenosed aortic valve.
    - Function. For example:
        - Spirometry and arterial blood gas measurement to assess respiratory function.
        - Serum creatinine to assess renal function.
    - Change, including to provide a baseline. For example:
        - Serial creatinine levels to assess a change in renal function.

- Serial CEA or CT scans to assess change in metastatic bowel cancer.
- Serial USS to measure the change in size of AAA.
- Repeat HbA1c to monitor DM.
- Repeat INR to monitor the dose of warfarin.
- Repeat bone density measurement to assess change in a patient on long-term steroids.
- Serial checks of an implant, such as a pacemaker.
  - Future risk or prognosis. The results of investigations are included with clinical assessments as part of many risk assessment tools. For example:
    - P-Possum to assess operative risk.
    - Assessment of prognosis of acute pancreatitis using the Atlanta criteria.
    - Assessment of risk of cancer recurrence with the TNM classification.
    - Using the WHO FRAX assessment tool or the measurement of bone mineral density to assess the risk of a fragility fracture.
- To provide reassurance.

Individual tests can be performed for multiple aims. For example:

- The aims of measuring an FBC may include:
  - To confirm a diagnosis. For example, in anaemia.
  - To make a diagnosis. For example, neutropaenia.
  - To screen for an abnormality. For example, thrombocytopaenia.
  - To understand the type of problem. For example, inflammation.
  - To provide additional information, such as the haematinic profile.
  - To assess severity. For example, the severity of the inflammation.
  - To provide a baseline to monitor change. For example, the response to oral iron treatment of anaemia.
  - For reassurance.
- The aims of measuring serum bilirubin may include:
  - To confirm a diagnosis of jaundice.
  - To exclude jaundice.
  - To understand the location of the abnormality causing the jaundice by measuring conjugated and unconjugated bilirubin.
  - To assess the severity of the jaundice.
  - For assessment of future risk in children.

The aims should be understood and accepted by the patient, the HCP and, for subjective tests, the person undertaking or reporting the test.

Ask yourself, is an investigation indicated?

A test should only be requested if it is indicated. Many factors determine whether or not an investigation is indicated. These include:

- The test meets the management aims.
- The information from the consultation matches the published indications or complies with published guidelines.
- The test is not contra-indicated.
- The test is available. Some tests are undertaken more often because they are available, easy to do and can be done quickly. However, just because a test is available does not mean it should be done: another test may be more appropriate. For example:
  - An abdominal X-ray is often requested to investigate abdominal pain when a CT scan is more accurate.
  - A CXR is often requested to investigate breathlessness and pleuritic chest pain but if a PE is suspected a CT pulmonary angiogram or a ventilation perfusion scan are more accurate.
- The benefit outweighs the risk.
- The patient has given permission for the test.
- The test result will be available in the right time frame. A test may be indicated but if the result is not going to be available in the right time frame it is not indicated.

- The timing is right. This includes:
  - The test is undertaken at the right time during the course of the illness. Undertaking a test too early risks a false negative result or too late and an opportunity for treatment missed. To ensure the timing is right the natural history of the condition should be understood.
  - The timing may need to accommodate investigation or treatment of other medical conditions.
  - The timing may need to suit the patient. Some patients choose to delay or defer having an investigation for various personal reasons.
  - For many "benign" problems, delay is unlikely to irreversibly harm the patient.
- The test is appropriate for the patient.
- The test is likely to give a meaningful result which may change management. For example, when the test is being undertaken to formulate a diagnosis, it should be accurate enough to reliably make the diagnosis.

Test accuracy describes how true, valid or exact the test is. Sensitivity and specificity are measures of accuracy:

- Sensitivity refers to how good the test is at correctly identifying a patient with the abnormality. It is the true positive rate. Mathematically, sensitivity is the number of patients with the abnormality (true positive) divided by the sum of the number with the abnormality and the number falsely negative for the abnormality. In other words, a test with 95% sensitivity will correctly diagnose 19/20 patients with that condition, and 1/20 will be falsely negative. If you want a test to confirm a diagnosis it should have a low false negative rate, i.e., a high sensitivity.
- Specificity refers to how good the test is at diagnosing the abnormality in a sample. It is the true negative rate. Mathematically, specificity is the number of patients without the condition (true negatives) divided by the sum of the number without the condition and the number falsely positive for the condition. A specificity of 95% means a negative test is true in 19/20 patients, and it is falsely positive, in 1/20 patients. If you want a test to exclude a diagnosis it should have a low false positive rate, i.e., a high specificity.

The higher the sensitivity and specificity the more accurate the test.

A table illustrating the accuracy of a CT scan for diagnosing early cancer.

	Sensitivity	Specificity
Small liver cancers	60-70%	70-80%
Early colon cancer	70-90%	>90%
Small lung cancers	90%	90%
Early pleural malignancy	50-70%	70-80%

The "likelihood ratio" (LR) assesses how likely a test will be at giving the expected result (LR+) or how likely a test is at excluding a result (LR-). They are calculated using the formulae:

[LR+] = sensitivity/ (100-specificity).
[LR-] = (100-sensitivity)/specificity.

When LR+ >10 the diagnosis is likely to be true. When LR- <0.1, the test is likely to exclude the diagnosis. For example:

- The sensitivity and specificity of an ECG for the diagnosis of AF is >90%, therefore an ECG is a useful test to both diagnose and exclude AF, LR+ >9, LR- <0.1.
- The sensitivity and specificity of 1mm of ST depression, or T wave inversion on an ECG for the diagnosis of coronary artery ischaemia is little more than 50%, i.e., little better than tossing a coin.
- The sensitivity and specificity of the ECG for the diagnosis of left ventricular hypertrophy is dependent on the size of the R and S waves. If the R wave on an ECG is >12mm in amplitude or the sum of the S wave in V1

and R wave in V5 >35mm the sensitivity for diagnosing left ventricular hypertrophy (LVH) is very low at about 7%, i.e., there are many more false negative diagnoses than true positive diagnoses, whereas the specificity is high 99%, i.e., false positive diagnoses are rare. Therefore, the likelihood of LVH is high: LR+ >7.

- In an anaemic patient, a ferritin of 100 μg/L (reference range 15-300 μg/L) is 60% sensitive and specific for the diagnosis of iron deficiency anaemia. In other words, it is not diagnostic. On the other hand, if the ferritin level is 30 μg/L, the sensitivity and specificity for iron deficiency anaemia is >90%: LR+ >9 and LR- <0.1.
- At a threshold level of 5 μg/L CEA has a sensitivity and specificity for cancer of about 70% and is unlikely to diagnose or exclude cancer: LR+ >2, LR- <0.5. However, at a value of >10 μg/L it is rarely associated with benign disease: LR+ >9, LR- <0.1.

Frequently the results of one test become the indications for another test. For example:

- When an FBC confirms a patient is anaemic, additional tests are indicated to distinguish between anaemia caused by excessive blood loss, chronic disease, haemolysis, a deficiency or a production abnormality and then to determine the cause.
- When a serum bilirubin confirms a patient is jaundiced, additional tests are indicated to distinguish between hyper-bilirubinaemia caused by parenchymal liver disease, biliary obstruction, Gilberts syndrome, haemolysis, ineffective erythropoiesis, resorption of a haematoma, hepatocellular disease, and medications, such as chlorpromazine, carbamazepine, erythromycin, or rifampicin.
- When a WBC, CRP or ESR indicate an inflammatory response, additional tests are often indicated to determine the location of the abnormality causing the inflammation, the type of inflammation and the cause.

Serial tests are frequently indicated to monitor progress or change. For example:

- Repeating the measurement of CRP or a WBC count to monitor the inflammatory response.
- Repeating a troponin to diagnose an AMI.
- Repeating an USS or CT scan to assess the change in the size or appearance of a mass.
- Repeating the measurement of serum cholesterol or HbA1c to assess the response to treatment.
- Repeating a test may be indicated when the result is uncertain or ambiguous.

A test is not indicated:

- When a patient does not want to be investigated. In which case, it is important to ensure the patient knows why the test is indicated and the possible consequences of not performing the test, and this information is documented.
- When treatment is not indicated or is inappropriate, investigating the patient to formulate a diagnosis is also unlikely to be appropriate. For example, when a patient is terminally ill, an investigation is not indicated if subsequent treatment would be inappropriate.
- When a patient is very ill and treatment is indicated before an investigation. For example, a patient with life threatening bleeding may need an emergency intervention rather than a diagnostic investigation.

Unfortunately, it is not uncommon for a test to be requested even though it is not indicated. This may occur when:

- The information learnt is incorrect, misunderstood or misinterpreted.
- The aims are unclear.
- Lack of knowledge of the test indications.
- Over estimation of the accuracy of the test.
- A desire to do something: it may be "easier" to perform a test than to "do nothing".
- Fear of missing something. This may be because of professional insecurity, inexperience or "defensive medicine".

The potential disadvantages of performing a test when it is not indicated include:

- Unnecessary risk to the patient. All investigations are associated with risk, such as a complication, and this should be considered when deciding whether or not an investigation is indicated. Most risks are short term or time-limited with an expectation for a full recovery. Some are uncommon but serious, such as anaphylaxis to iodinated contrast media or cancer from exposure to ionising radiation.
- Unnecessary anxiety, distress and inconvenience for the patient.
- A risk of a mis-diagnosis: either a false positive leading to a mis-diagnosis, or a false negative and false reassurance and delayed treatment.

> **The greater the number of tests requested the greater the chance one of the tests will be falsely abnormal.**

- Performing an inappropriate test on one patient risks delay and possible harm to others who have to wait longer for the test.
- Waste of money. All tests take time and resources. Tests frequently done may be relatively cheap but the overall cost to the healthcare community of performing many such tests can be high.

During the consultation knowledge of the investigation may be used to inform the questions to ask or signs to look for to ensure an investigation is indicated.

Ask yourself, is a screening investigation indicated?

The indications for organising a test to screen for an asymptomatic problem include:

- The patient fulfils the criteria for entry into a National Screening programme. For example:
  o Neonatal screening for a genetic abnormality.
  o Breast cancer screening.
  o Cervical cancer screening.
  o Bowel cancer screening.
- An "extra", "out of program", screening test may be indicated for a patient already within a screening program to provide additional information or to assess change when it is relevant to the diagnosis or planning management. For example:
  o A CT scan may be indicated to exclude cancer recurrence in a patient who presents with a new problem but is already on a screening program to detect cancer recurrence.
  o An AFP blood test may be indicated to exclude hepatocellular cancer in a patient with liver cirrhosis who is already on a screening program.
  o An abdominal USS may be indicated to reassess the diameter of a AAA.
  o An oesophagoscopy may be indicated to re-assess dysplasia in Barrett's oesophagus.
  o Blood tests and eye tests may be indicated to monitor renal function and retinopathy in a diabetic patient.
  o In patients with chronic UC a colonoscopy may be indicated to reassess disease severity or detect dysplasia or cancer.
- Screening for an asymptomatic problem secondary to the presenting problem. For example:
  o Measuring serum electrolytes, urea and creatinine to screen for deranged homeostasis.
  o Serum bilirubin is frequently measured together with a transaminase such alanine transaminase, and alkaline phosphatase, to screen for an abnormality in a patient with biliary colic.
  o A serum troponin, ECG and an echocardiogram to screen for a cardiac abnormality in a patient with peripheral vascular disease.
  o A CXR and urine samples to screen for a source of infection in a patient with a fever.
  o An abdominal USS to screen for a AAA in a hypertensive patient with widespread peripheral vascular disease.
  o Requesting bone densitometry to screen for osteopaenia in a patient presenting with back pain from a vertebral crush fracture.
  o In patients presenting with alcoholic liver cirrhosis measuring AFP to screen for liver cancer.
- Screening for an asymptomatic problem secondary to a risk factor. For example:

- o In a morbidly obese patient measuring serum transaminases and performing a liver USS to screen for NASH.
- o In patients with chronic GORD an endoscopy to screen for Barrett's oesophagus.
- o A mammogram to screen for breast cancer or a colonoscopy to screen for bowel cancer when a first degree relative has cancer.

Variables that influence the indications for a screening test include:

- Demographic information. For example:
  - o Age. For example:
    - The risk of cancer developing increases in older age.
    - When life expectancy is short, a screening test may not be indicated.
  - o Ethnicity may influence risk. For example:
    - The risk of Sickle cell disease.
- Exposure. In general, the likelihood of harm is increased when exposure is more frequent, more severe or more prolonged. For example:
  - o The risk of developing lung disease due to exposure to air pollution.
  - o The larger the wound the more likely a wound infection will occur.
- The number of risk factors. In general, multiple risk factors compound risk. For example:
  - o A post-menopausal spinster with a low BMI who smokes and drinks alcohol has five different risk factors for osteoporosis.
  - o A female on the oral contraceptive pill having a pelvic operation for cancer has 3 risk factors for a DVT.
  - o A 70-year-old female taking steroids and immune-suppression for temporal arteritis who drinks alcohol and smokes has at least 5 risk factors for osteonecrosis.
  - o A 55-year-old centrally obese male smoker and alcohol drinker with a hiatus hernia and gastro-oesophageal reflux has at least 7 different risk factors for Barrett's oesophagus.
  - o A 50-year-old hypertensive, obese (BMI>30) Chinese mother on statins who had gestational DM has at least 5 risk factors for DM.
- Mitigating factors. Measures that reduce risk, such as a lifestyle change or a treatment, may change the indications for a screening test.

Ask yourself, is the test appropriate for the patient?

A test may be clinically indicated but inappropriate. Learning about the person and the person as a patient and having a working knowledge of what the test involves can help determine whether or not the test is appropriate and what test is most appropriate for the patient and the problem. For some people a risk is a safety concern affecting whether or not a test is appropriate. For example:

- Age is usually only a safety concern when tests are performed on children or the elderly.
- Gender is usually only a safety concern when a woman may be pregnant. For example, the risk of exposing the foetus to ionising radiation.
- A previous allergic reaction may be a safety concern. The risk of anaphylaxis is increased among patients who have previously had an anaphylactic reaction.
- A previous non-allergic reaction may be a safety concern.
- Infection risk to the patient. For example, immunocompromised patients.
- Infection risk to others. For example, patients colonised by MRSA, ESBL or C. difficile.
- Bleeding risk may be a safety concern. For example, patients taking anticoagulant medications, hemophiliacs or patients with Von Willebrand's disease.
- Thrombosis risk may be a safety concern. For example, patients with protein C deficiency or who have had recurrent thromboses.
- Other relevant information may be a safety concern. For example, performing an invasive investigation when the patient is a Jehovah Witness.

When there is a safety concern there is a need to balance risk and benefit. The impact of safety concerns on management and the options available should be discussed with the patient because their opinion may influence management. For example:

- Delaying a radiological investigation until a baby is delivered.
- Delaying an invasive investigation until anti-coagulants can be stopped.
- Treating MRSA colonisation before performing an invasive investigation.

An increasing number of tests are available, so there is often a choice. For example:

- A pelvic problem could be investigated by a trans abdominal USS, a trans-vaginal USS, a CT scan, an MRI scan, a laparoscopy or an endoscopy.
- The heart could be investigated by an ECG, an exercise ECG, a 24-hour ECG or BP, a trans-oesophageal echo, a trans-thoracic echo, a CT angiogram, an MRI scan or an angiogram.
- The colon could be investigated by a flexible sigmoidoscopy, a colonoscopy, a barium enema, a CT scan, a CT pneumocolon or an MRI scan.
- Investigating an intra-abdominal mass with an USS, a CT scan, an MRI scan or a laparoscopy.
- Investigating a painful knee joint with an X-ray, an arthroscopy, an MRI scan or a CT scan.

When discussing a test with a patient, it is not necessary to know in detail how the test is done, the technology behind the test, nor to be able to do it but it is necessary to have a working knowledge of the test not only to determine if the test is appropriate for the patient but also to explain what is involved. There are many factors to consider before making a recommendation. For example:

- Position. Some tests require the patient to be able to adopt certain positions or stay for prolonged periods of time in a particular position. This may be difficult for some patients. For example, patients with COPD or orthopnoea or with a fixed deformity, such as ankylosing spondylitis or kypho-scoliosis, may not be able to lie flat.
- Size. Severely morbidly obese patients may be too large to fit into an MRI scanner or may be too heavy for an investigation table.
- Disability. Usually, it is possible to accommodate a disability but additional time and resources may be needed. For example, helping a patient with a disability lie on their side for a colonoscopy.
- Fear and anxiety. Patients worry about many things including what the test involves or what the test will show, but some patients are so frightened or have a phobia that they will not tolerate the test. For example, a claustrophobic patient is unlikely to tolerate an MRI or a needle-phobic patient an injection.
- What the test involves. Some tests can be so embarrassing or distressing for a patient that they are unable to tolerate the test. For example, a mammogram, a trans-vaginal or scrotal USS, a cystoscopy, a defaecating proctogram, a gastroscopy, a liver biopsy or trans-rectal biopsy. Some tests can be socially difficult and unacceptable to the patient. For example, 24-hour pH/oesophageal manometry.
- The preparation. Some patients cannot tolerate the preparation required. For example, drinking the bowel preparation prior to a colonoscopy.
- Financial and logistic difficulties. For some patients travel, taking time off work, or being away from a dependent precludes having the test.

Ask yourself, what will the result mean?

An investigation is indicated only if the result is likely to meet the aims. Therefore, before recommending a test it is important to know what the result will mean. For example:

- A blood CRP is a non-specific marker for inflammation. Although inflammation is frequently caused by an infection, a raised CRP is not diagnostic for an infection but it may be an indication for further investigation.
- "Cancer markers", such as CEA or PSA are frequently considered to be tests for cancer. However, a raised cancer marker does not mean the patient has cancer. The result is likely to be an indication for further investigation.

Some tests are reported in a binary way; the result either shows an abnormality or is negative. For example, genetic, antibody or microbiological tests. Some results describe the appearance and often include an opinion as to the likely diagnosis. For example, histo- or cyto-pathological tests, imaging or endoscopic tests. Although, the results of such tests are usually reported in a binary way, as with numerical tests, there is a range in which the result is more likely to be "normal" or "abnormal", i.e., a reference range. For example:

- Histopathologically, inflammatory bowel disease is characterised by the extent and distribution of the mucosal architectural abnormality, the cellularity of the lamina propria and the cell types present.
- Cytological and architectural abnormalities and immunohistochemistry are used to identify dysplasia.
- The size, shape and attenuation of a lung nodule are used to distinguish between a benign and a malignant lesion on imaging.

The reference range for a test is usually determined from the average or mean value plus or minus 2 standard deviations from the mean of a large number of representative individuals. Therefore, 95% of the results from normal individuals will be within this range and only 5% outside the range.

Agreed adult clinical biochemistry reference intervals (UK Pathology Harmony Group). NB for some tests e.g. serum troponin, the result is dependent on the analysis method.

- Serum Sodium—133-146 mmol/L
- Serum Potassium—3.5-5.3 mmol/L
- Serum Urea—2.5-7.8 mmol/L
- Creatinine—62-115 μmol/L in men, and 53-97 in women
- Serum Chloride—95-108 mmol/L
- Serum Bicarbonate—22-29 mmol/L
- Serum Phosphate—0.8-1.5 mmol/L
- Serum Magnesium—0.7-1.0 mmol/L
- Serum Albumin—35-50 g/L
- Serum Total Protein—60-80 g/L
- Serum Osmolality—275-295 mmol/kg
- Serum Alkaline Phosphatase—30-130 μ/L
- Serum Bilirubin (total) <21μmol/L
- Serum Adjusted Calcium—2.2-2.6 mmol/L
- Serum Urate—200-430 μmol/L in men, and 140-360 in women
- 24 h Urine Calcium—2.5-7.5 mmol/24h
- 24 h Urine Urate—1.5-4.5 mmol/24h 24 h
- Urine Phosphate—15-50 mmol/24h
- 24 h Urine Magnesium—2.4-6.5 mmol/24h

Biological variables that influence the reference range include:

- Demographic information.
  - o Age. For example:
    - In a child or adolescent with healthy growing bones a serum alkaline phosphatase is normally higher than in adults.
  - o Gender. For example:
    - Men with a larger muscle mass than women tend to have higher creatine kinase (CK) concentration in their bloodstream.
    - Pregnancy may affect many biochemical or haematological variable.
  - o Ethnic group. For example:

- The creatine kinase reference range usually refers to white Caucasians. Other ethnic groups may have higher values.
- African Americans have higher HbA1c than both Mexican Americans and non-Hispanic Whites.
- Lifestyle. For example:
  o Vigorous exercise can affect blood concentrations of creatine kinase, cholesterol, aspartate aminotransferase, and lactate dehydrogenase.
  o Some blood tests can be affected by caffeine, tobacco, alcohol, and Vitamin C or by stress or anxiety.
- Previous or ongoing disease or treatment.

In general, the greater the result deviates outside the reference range, the more likely the result is abnormal. Some tests raise the diagnostic threshold to 99% to increase the specificity, or use a change over time rather than the reference range. For example:

- In patients with liver disease such as hepatitis, haemochromatosis or cirrhosis an AFP of 10 ug/L has a 70% sensitivity and specificity for liver cancer. At 40 ug/L the sensitivity increases to 90%. However, the specificity remains 70%, i.e., the AFP remains normal in 30% of patients who have liver cancer.
- A serum ferritin of 100 ug/L is 60% sensitive and specific for the diagnosis of iron deficiency anaemia. If the ferritin is 30 μg/L the sensitivity and specificity for iron deficiency anaemia increases to >90%.
- The upper limit of the reference range for HbA1c is 42 mmol/L. However, the threshold for diagnosing DM is often set at >48 mmol/L (6.5%). The range 42-48 mmol/L may be considered "pre-diabetes".
- The upper limit of the reference range for CEA is 5 ug/L. At a level of 5 ug/L, a CEA has a sensitivity and specificity for cancer of about 70%. When the value is >10 ug/L, the sensitivity and specificity increase to >90%. An increasing level in a patient previously treated for bowel cancer indicates recurrence. A threshold value of CEA>20 ug/L indicates metastatic bowel cancer.
- The threshold for diagnosing an AMI is often dependent on serial serum troponin levels. A level of 0.1ug/L measured using a highly sensitive assay is likely, >99%, to be abnormal particularly if confirmed when repeated several hours later.

For many tests, increasing specificity is at the cost of reduced sensitivity and vice versa. If the sensitivity and specificity are each 50% the test is no better than tossing a coin.

The wider the reference range the less likely a test will demonstrate an early abnormality. For example:

- If a patient's creatinine in health is close to the lower limit of the creatinine reference range, say 65 μmol/L, their renal function can nearly halve before the serum creatinine exceeds the upper limit of the reference range (115 μmol/L).

The accuracy of a test is influenced by analytical and biological variables.

Analytical variables that may affect the accuracy of a test include:

- General errors. For example:
  o Poor communication, fatigue, distractions, and complacency.
  o Staff shortages and excess workload.
  o Misleading or incorrect clinical information, errors of omission or transcription.
  o Data entry errors, mislabelling of request forms or of results.
  o Equipment errors.
  o Lack of knowledge, training or inexperience.
- Process or pre-test variables. For example:
  o Sampling errors, such as in histopathology.
  o Preparation errors.
  o Stability in transit and the effect of delays/temperature.
  o Confounding factors. For example, hypocapnia on an ABG may be caused by an anxious hyperventilating patient.
- Test variables. For example:

- o Test limitations. For example, If a patient has pulmonary fibrosis, it may be difficult to detect a new nodule within widespread pulmonary scaring on a CXR.
- o Expertise and frequency or the technician performing the test. For example, an expert colonoscopist may notice a subtle change in mucosal architecture and distinguish between an early sessile cancer, a sessile villous adenoma or inflammation.
- o Technical errors. For example, contamination, malfunction, reagent/enzyme quality, calibration errors and poor standardization.
- o Inter-assay or inter-observer variability.
- o Intra-assay or intra-observer variability.
- o Confounding factors. For example, a high platelet causing a falsely elevated serum potassium concentration.
- Post-test variables. For example:
- o Variable selection criteria for "healthy reference" population.
- o Diagnostic threshold: 95 or 99th percentile of healthy reference population.
- o Inconsistent or changing the unit or measurement or the reference range.
- o Mis-interpreting the units: for example, a change of 200ng/L "sounds" a higher value than 2ng/mL.

Biological variables that may affect the accuracy of a test include:

- The bodies compensatory mechanisms, including buffering, sequestering and re-distribution. For example:
- o Intravascular potassium is buffered by intra-cellular potassium and influenced by acid-base metabolism. Therefore, a large change in total body potassium is needed before there is a small change in serum potassium.
- o Intravascular calcium and magnesium are buffered by the intracellular compartment and the bones and influenced by potassium and acid base metabolism. Low serum calcium or magnesium indicates a deficiency but, because most is in bones, normal serum calcium does not exclude a negative total body calcium.
- o The albumin concentration is affected by many factors including hydration, capillary permeability in addition to synthesis and loss.
- o Blood acid-base is both buffered and changes are compensated for through changes in breathing and renal function.
- o The liver metabolism can compensate for increased portal venous blood lactate so that serum pH or lactate levels may not reflect the severity or extent of bowel ischaemia.
- Functional reserve. For many organs, such as the liver or kidneys, the functional reserve far exceeds the everyday demands and they are able to tolerate significant injury before resting function is affected and investigations show an abnormality.
- Regenerative capacity. Some tissues and organs are able to regenerate, such as liver, endometrium, intestinal mucosa, blood cells, blood and lymphatic vessels, so that the initial damage is temporary. Other tissues and organs are able to regenerate following minor injury, such as the kidney, bone, or a peripheral nerve. Tissues with minimal regenerative potential, such as muscle or ligaments, repair with scar tissue.
- Timing. If the time course of the development of the abnormality being measured, and the timing of the test do not align the test result may be misleading. For example:
- o In a patient with inflammation, there is a lag of up to 12 hours before the CRP rises. Conversely, there is a lag of up to 24 hours before a high CRP starts to fall. Therefore, using CRP as marker of inflammation may be falsely negative if measured too early, or falsely positive if measured late, following treatment.
- o When a patient has ingested a large dose of a hepatotoxin, such as paracetamol, there is a lag of up to 24 hours before blood transaminase levels rise.
- o A patient may have overwhelming sepsis yet the blood cultures only show an infection after 5 days of incubation.
- o The serum amylase level may return to normal within a couple of days of an episode of acute pancreatitis. Therefore, a result within the reference range does not exclude pancreatitis when symptoms started several days or more previously.
- Variables related to the investigation. For example:
- o When the patient is very lean, it can be difficult to distinguish tissue planes on a CT scan.

o   In an obese patient or when there are a lot of gas filled bowel loops it can be difficult to visualise intra-abdominal structures using an USS.

The probability that a patient with a positive test result truly has the condition is called the positive predictive value (PPV) of a test. It is calculated using the formula:

PPV = [sensitivity x prevalence]/ [sensitivity x prevalence] + [(1-specificity) x (1-prevalence)]

The probability that a patient with a negative result truly does not have the condition is called the negative predictive value (NPV). It is calculated using the formula:

NPV = [specificity x (1-prevalence)]/ [(1-sensitivity) x prevalence + specificity x (1-prevalence)]

Measures that can increase the predictive value of a test include:

- Choosing the right test for the right reasons. The more closely the clinical features match the indications for a test, the higher the likelihood the test result will be abnormal. In other words, the higher the prevalence of the abnormality, the more likely the test result will be truly abnormal, i.e., accurate. This is the "pre-test probability" of the test.

> **Performing the right test for the right reasons increases the likelihood the result is true**

This is best illustrated with reference to an example:
When a patient is reported to have breast cancer on a mammogram, what is the chance/probability that she actually has breast cancer?

The prevalence of cancer in a 40-year-old woman is one in a 100 or 1%. Conversely, 99/100 women of that age do not have breast cancer. If the specificity is 90%, the report is falsely positive in 1/10 women. Therefore, although 99 of the 100 women do not have breast cancer, 9 (10%) of them will have a false positive mammogram. Therefore, if the test is positive, the probability the woman has breast cancer is 10%.
The predictive value of the test can be increased by increasing the prevalence of breast cancer in the sample being investigated, i.e., increasing the pre-test probability. For example:
If the test is performed in an elderly woman from a sample with a 10% prevalence of breast cancer, the probability a positive mammogram is true increases to almost 50%.
- The predictive value of a test can also be increased by increasing the accuracy of the test. Using the previous example:
If the specificity of the mammogram is increased to 99% only 1/100 will be a false positive and the probability the 40-year-old woman has a true positive mammogram is increased to 50%.
- Reduce the likelihood of analytic error with training, familiarity, procedures, protocols, standardisation and quality control. When the test is a descriptive test, reduce subjective variation by using standardised reporting, double checking, multidisciplinary teamworking, audits or a "second" opinion.
- Interpret the results together with the clinical information. For example:
  o   The likelihood of a liver or bone lesion being a metastatic deposit is increased if the patient has pre-existing cancer and the cancer has a high likelihood of spreading.
  o   The sensitivity and specificity of a CXR for the diagnosis of clinically suspected pneumonia ranges from 70-90%. The more classical the radiological signs, the greater the likelihood.
  o   The likelihood of ECG changes being caused by an AMI is increased if the symptoms and troponin changes are typical.
  o   The likelihood elevated transaminase levels diagnose NASH is increased if the patient is morbidly obese.

> **Learn about the person, the patient and the problem to ensure the test result is correctly interpreted.**

- Perform a different sort of test. For example:

- o Investigating a liver lesion with an USS, a CT scan and an MRI scan.
- o Investigating a radiolucent bone deposit seen on an X-ray, with a bone scan and a CT scan.
- o Using different stains or immuno-histochemistry in histopathology.
- o Investigating a patient suspected of having an AMI with an ECG and blood troponin.
- o Investigating a patient suspected of having NASH with serum aminotransaminases, HbA1c, triglycerides and cholesterol and a liver USS.

The accuracy of a test is increased when the results from different tests are concordant.

However, tests that use different methods may not give the same result. This is between-test analytic variation. The extent of the variation depends on the precision of the method. For example, the size of a liver lesion may vary between an USS, a CT scan or an MRI scan.

- Repeat a test after an interval or perform serial tests.

When a test is repeated it is important to correctly interpret the significance of change. A meaningful change is often referred to as the "critical difference" or the "reference change value". It is defined as the smallest difference between sequential results likely to indicate a true change. It is usually expressed as a percent or as an absolute value. Critical difference is influenced by within individual and between individual variables:

- Intra-individual or within-individual variation is the variation that occurs when a test is repeated using a series of samples from the same patient. Within individual variation can be caused by biological, diurnal or seasonal cycles, the effect of diet, exercise, stress, artifact, distortion or sampling error.
- Inter-individual variation or intra-sample variation refers to the variation that occurs when a test is repeated using the same sample. Reproducibility describes how much variation there is between repeated tests when all the variables remain the same. Reproducibility is important for ensuring accuracy when measuring change both for subjective and objective tests, including laboratory tests. Ideally, the test will give the same result regardless of the number of times the sample was analysed. For example:
  - o The intra- and inter-individual variation of serum electrolytes is approximately 5%, so that the critical difference is >10%. In other words, a change of >10% in the serum concentration is likely to be significant. For example, a fall in the serum potassium concentration from 3.5 mmol/L to <3.0 mmol/L, a fall in the calcium from 2.3 mmol/L to <2.0 mmol/L or in the magnesium from 0.7 mmol/L to <0.6 mmol/L are likely to be significant.
  - o The inter-individual variation for albumin is 9% and the intra-individual variation 3%, so the critical difference is >15%. In other words, a fall in the albumin from 40 g/L to 35 g/L is unlikely to reflect a real difference in the albumin concentration.
  - o The within individual variation for blood glucose level (BGL) is approximately 6% and the inter-individual variation 2-4% so that the critical difference is >10%. In other words, a rise in the blood glucose level from 5 mmol/L to 5.5 mmol/L may not be significant.
  - o The within individual variation for RBC parameters is approximately 5%, and the inter-individual variation 3-5% so that the critical difference is >15%. In other words, a fall in the haemoglobin concentration from 140 g/L to 125 g/L may not be significant.

When a test is to be repeated, it is important also to consider timing. Some changes are not linear, they may plateau, change exponentially or have a tipping point. For example:

- Serum lactate levels only increase when production exceeds the capacity of the liver and other tissues to metabolise lactate.

Ask yourself, when should a test be requested?

For some problems and some patients, the timing of the test may be important. Most tests are requested following the consultation or when the result of another test is known. For some patients, other factors influence when a test should be requested. These include:

- Some tests only become abnormal after an interval. For example:
  - There is a lag of up to 12 hours before a CRP rises.
  - A troponin rise can be detected 2-4 hours after transmural myocardial necrosis to reach a maximum after 6-9 hours.
- Some tests or test results are not available in the required time frame. For example, in an emergency, a VQ scan is likely to take too long to perform or report when a PE is suspected.
- Some tests are requested because the results are available quickly. However, just because a test is available does not mean it should be done: another test may be more appropriate.
- The patient's availability may affect when a test can be performed. Some patients choose to delay or defer having a test for various reasons.
- An increasing number of patients have complex medical conditions and are on a number of different care pathways. Occasionally, this may affect the timing of a test.
- Natural history of the problem. The result may depend on the timing of a repeated test. For example:
  - A serum amylase may return to normal several days after the onset of acute pancreatitis.
  - CRP remains elevated for up to 24 hours before starting to fall.
  - A troponin remains elevated for at least 7 days.
- Change over time or response to treatment. Some patients with some problems are only investigated when the problem persists, deteriorates or does not respond to treatment.

Recommend a treatment

Most clinical problems eventually lead to a treatment. Some patients want and expect treatment, even if it is unlikely to help them. After all, many people self-medicate with "remedies" bought from chemists or "health" shops in the hope that they will be helped or to reassure themselves that they are doing everything they can to help themselves. If a patient is helped, even if this is likely to be a placebo effect, this can be reassuring to them.

Historically few effective treatments were available and many treatments were little better than a placebo. Increased medical knowledge has led to many more treatments being available. Nevertheless, few treatments are definitive treatments, treating the cause of the problem. Most treat symptoms or manage the problem. Before starting treatment ask yourself:

What is the aim?
Is treatment is indicated?

A treatment may be indicated and meet the management aims, but before it is recommended it is important to consider the patient. For some patients, there are factors that may affect whether or not a treatment is appropriate. Therefore, always ask yourself:

Is the treatment appropriate?

There are many factors that influence when a treatment should be started. Therefore, before starting a treatment ask yourself:

When should treatment be started?

A treatment is successful when it meets the aims. Because there are many different aims, it is also important that both the patient and the HCP are clear what would constitute a successful outcome. Therefore, before starting a treatment ask yourself:

What would be a successful outcome?

Ask yourself, what is the aim of treatment?

When considering starting a treatment it is important to be clear on the aims and to discuss these with the patient. There are many treatments, each with different indications, but there are few aims. Ideally, a treatment is with the aim of curing the patient, i.e., treatment is definitive. For example:

- Changing life choices can occasionally be a definitive treatment. For example, stopping drinking alcohol to treat alcohol addiction or losing weight to treat type II DM.
- Antimicrobial, anti-viral or anti-fungal medication for a microbiologically proven infection.
- Avoiding gluten in coeliac disease.
- Repair of a hernia.
- An appendicectomy for appendicitis.
- Thrombolysis of thrombo-embolic disease, such as a stroke, a PE or peripheral ischaemia is definitive treatment for the complication, but not for the cause.

Occasionally, a trial of treatment is started and the successful response to treatment is taken as confirmatory evidence for the diagnosis. For example:

- Taking a lactose free diet in suspected lactose intolerance.
- Taking antimicrobial medications to treat a suspected bacterial infection.

For many problems a definitive treatment is unavailable and the aim of treatment is to alleviate symptoms. Treatment to alleviate symptoms can refer to:

- Non-specific symptomatic treatment, such as rest, analgesics for pain relief, antiemetics for nausea, laxatives for constipation or an anti-spasmodic for colic or muscle spasm.
- Specific treatment, such as splinting a fracture, lancing an abscess, providing oxygen to treat breathlessness or nitrates to relieve angina.

For many problems changing life choices may also provide symptomatic treatment. For example, losing weight to reduce the pain form arthritis. For some patients and some problems, symptomatic treatment is indicated as an interim treatment while awaiting the results of investigations or while waiting for more specific treatment to take effect or for improvement to occur naturally: after all, time can be a great healer.

Treatments are often recommended with the aim of helping function. This can include the function of an organ, a system or of a body part. Treatment to help function is usually a temporary measure to correct or reverse an abnormality, for symptom relief or to prevent additional harm while, for example, healing occurs, investigations are undertaken or other treatments work. For example:

- Oxygen supplementation to minimise hypoxic organ damage.
- Intra-venous fluid supplements to restore or maintain circulating volume, cardiac output and perfusion of vital organs, such as the kidneys.
- Diuretics to reduce circulating volume, improve cardiac function and alleviate breathlessness in heart failure.
- Anti-inflammatory medication to reduce the inflammatory response, improve joint function and reduce pain.
- A cast, internal or external fixation to immobilise a long bone fracture to allow function while the fracture heals.
- Loperamide to treat diarrhoea, improve lifestyle or reduce the risk of hypovolaemia.
- Colonic stenting to relieve large bowel obstruction, reduce the risk of perforation and enable an elective operation.

Some treatments are aimed at slowing the rate of disease progression. For example:

- Steroids or immune-suppressant medications reduce inflammation and the rate of consequential damage.
- Anti-hypertensive medications reduce the blood pressure slowing the rate of damage to the heart.
- Chemotherapy to slow the rate of growth of cancer.

Treatment is increasingly undertaken with the aim of reducing the risk of future problems. This could include reducing the risk of an illness or a complication that may otherwise have arisen. For example:

- Giving intra-venous fluids to prevent renal failure in a fasted patient.
- Treating an asymptomatic inguinal hernia to prevent bowel obstruction.
- Performing a sub-total colectomy or bilateral mastectomy to prevent cancer in a genetically high-risk patient.

- Pre-operative antibiotics to reduce the risk of a wound infection.
- Starting antibiotics early in a patient suspected of sepsis to reduce the systemic inflammatory response and reduce the risk of overwhelming sepsis.
- Prescribing statins to reduce the risk of heart disease.
- Prescribing anti-platelet medication to reduce the risk of a stroke in a patient with AF.
- Starting low-molecular weight heparin to reduce the risk of venous thrombosis.
- Starting furosemide to reduce the risk of an arrhythmia in a patient with hypercalcaemia while waiting for calcium chelating treatments to work.

Frequently a treatment is started for multiple aims. For example:

- Immuno-suppression treatment of colitis will not only reduce the risk of a future problem or disease progression but also improve the symptoms of diarrhoea.
- Treatment of hypertension will provide symptom relief, improve cardiac function, reduce progression of atherosclerosis and also reduce the risk of a complication, such as a heart attack or stroke.

Ask yourself, is a treatment indicated?

A treatment should only be started if it is indicated. The indications for most treatments are published. Ideally, a treatment should only be started if it has a proven effectiveness for treating the problem based on the results from a meta-analysis or double-blind randomized controlled clinical trial. Unfortunately, such evidence is not always available.

The treatment indicated will vary between patients, to meet different aims and depending on the context and the information available. It is important to consider whether a preventative treatment is also indicated. For example:

- In a breathless patient with heart failure treatment with diuretics is indicated to increase diuresis to improve cardiac function and give symptom relief by reducing breathlessness. If the symptoms of angina and the changes on an ECG and a coronary artery angiogram demonstrate stenotic coronary artery disease an angioplasty or coronary artery stenting may be indicated with the aim of improving myocardial perfusion. Changing life choices, such as to stop smoking, reduce weight, and undertake more exercise, and preventative treatments such as statins to reduce lipid concentrations are indicated with the aim of reducing the risk of recurrence or progression.
- A femoral shaft fracture is very painful. Splint immobilization of the fracture and analgesics are indicated with the aim of relieving symptoms and preventing further harm by reducing the risk of additional tissue damage and further bleeding. If haemorrhage is sufficient to cause hypovolaemia a blood transfusion may be indicated with the aim of restoring circulating blood volume and preventing a secondary problem such as shock. If the fracture is compound, then wound toilet and antibiotics are indicated with the aim of reducing the risk of a wound or bone infection. Treatment with an intra-medullary nail may be indicated to immobilise the fracture, to relieve symptoms and improve function by allowing early mobilization and reduce the risk of a future complication, such as mal-union. If the patient has osteoporosis, a bisphosphate medication may be indicated to reduce the risk of a future fracture.

Many factors should be considered when determining whether or not a treatment is indicated. These include:

- The information from the consultation matches the published indications or complies with published guidelines.
- The treatment is not contra-indicated.
- The treatment is available.
- The treatment will be available in the right time frame.
- The treatment meets the management aims.
- The treatment is appropriate for the patient.
- The treatment is likely to be effective.
- The timing is right. This includes:
  - The treatment is undertaken at the right time during the course of the illness. For example, a radical cancer operation should be undertaken before the cancer has spread.

- The timing may need to accommodate investigation or treatment of other medical conditions. For example, delaying starting anti-coagulants until an invasive procedure has been performed.
- The timing suits the patient. Some patients choose to delay or defer starting a treatment for various reasons.
- The benefit outweighs the risk.
- The patient consents to the treatment.

> **Starting the right treatment for the right reasons increases the likelihood the treatment will be successful**

For some patients, treatments are not indicated and for others they are contraindicated. For example:

- A treatment is not indicated if it is unlikely to benefit the patient. For example:
  - Preventative treatments such as antihypertensive medications or statins are not indicated for patients nearing the end of life.
  - Ethically, placebo treatments are not indicated. Placebo treatments should only be used within the context of a clinical trial with informed consent.
- Contraindications can be absolute or relative. For example:
  - In patients with an iodine allergy, intravenous contrast for a radiological treatment, such as a stenting, is absolutely contra-indicated.
  - Poor renal function is a relative contraindication to the use of intravenous contrast during a radiological treatment, because the contrast may cause further deterioration in renal function.
  - Ionizing radiation is a relative contraindicated in children and fertile females who may be pregnant.

Unfortunately, some treatments are recommended for the wrong reasons. For example:

- The information learnt is incorrect, mis-understood or mis-interpreted.
- Mis-diagnosis.
- Overdiagnosis.
- The treatment is contraindicated.
- Ignorance of other options.
- Over estimation of the effectiveness of the treatment.
- Lack of guidelines, restrictions or limitations.
- Treatment is wanted by the patient even though it is not indicated.
- Lack of confidence, inexperience or insecurity. It is easier to treat a patient, to be "doing something", rather than to observe a patient over time or review a patient.

The potential disadvantages of excessive, incorrect or inappropriate treatment include:

- Unnecessary risk to the patient.
- False hope or expectations.
- Distress and inconvenience for the patient.
- Waste of money.

During the consultation the information learnt should indicate whether or not a treatment is indicated and knowledge of the treatment may be used to inform the questions to ask or signs to look for.

Ask yourself, is a treatment appropriate?

It is important to consider whether and what treatment is appropriate for the patient. The treatment may be considered the best treatment but if the patient cannot undertake or tolerate the treatment or does not want it, it cannot be started.

> **Learn about the person, the patient and the problem to ensure the treatment is appropriate**

All treatments are associated with risk but some risks are increased when there is a known safety concern. Safety concerns to consider include:

- Age: particularly regarding treatments in children and the elderly.
- Pregnancy: many treatments are contra-indicated in pregnant females or their safety and effectiveness are uncertain.
- Previous adverse reaction. The risk of anaphylaxis is increased among patients who have previous other anaphylactic reactions.
- An interaction between medications. An increasing number of patients, particularly the elderly, are taking more than one medication to manage comorbidity or to prevent future illness. There is a risk of an adverse interaction when a new treatment is added. It may be necessary to review whether all of them are appropriate. Some medications can be stopped or the dose reduced ("deprescribing"). Deprescribing should be planned and supervised, following a careful discussion with the patient.
- Increased infection risk. For example, immunosuppression treatment.
- Increased bleeding risk. For example, anticoagulant medications.
- Increased thrombotic risk. For example, taking the oral contraceptive pill.

When there is a safety concern, the risk and benefit balance is individual. Some safety concerns, such as anaphylaxis, are an absolute contraindication whereas others are a relative contraindication and for some it may be possible to make a change that mitigates the risk. The impact of safety concerns on management and the consequent potential risks to the patient should be discussed with the patient when planning an investigation as part of consent.

There are many other patient related variables that may influence whether a treatment is appropriate. These include:

- Co-morbidity.
- Other medications.
- Physical factors, such as:
  o Performance status. This is particularly relevant for a general anaesthetic or invasive treatments.
  o Disability. For example, some treatments need the patient to be dextrous and coordinated, so are unsuitable for patients with a severe tremor or some disabilities. Some treatments require the patient to be able to adopt certain positions or stay for prolonged periods of time in a potentially uncomfortable position. This may be difficult for some patients. For example, patients with COPD, orthopnoea, ankylosing spondylitis or kypho-scoliosis may not be able to lie flat. Usually, it is possible to accommodate a physical disability but additional time and resources may be needed.
  o Size. Some treatments can be particularly challenging in morbidly obese patients.
  o Access. For example:
    - Swallowing disorders. Some patients are unable to swallow tablets.
    - Vascular access can be very difficult in some patients. For example, intravenous drug takers or obese patients.
    - Anal stenosis may prevent a colonoscopy.
- Psychological factors, such as:
  o Fear, anxiety and phobias. Patients worry both about what the treatment involves and the risks. For example:
    - Some patients have a fear of needles.
    - Some patients are frightened of what the treatment involves. For example, an invasive procedure or an operation such as a haemorrhoidectomy.
    - Some patients are frightened by the preparation. For example, bowel preparation before a colonoscopy.
  o Resentment. Some patients are already taking a lot of tablets and do not want to take more.
  o Embarrassment. Some treatments can be embarrassing for a patient. For example, inserting suppositories or pessaries or having a circumcision.
- Symptomatic improvement. Adherence tends to be better when the patient notices an immediate improvement.
- Social, financial or cultural factors, such as:

- o The inconvenience and costs of getting prescriptions.
- o Travel to a centre for specialist treatment.
- o Some treatments significantly disrupt everyday life. This is particularly the case if the treatment is dependent on another health care professional. For example, wound management or stoma care.
- The duration of the treatment. What a patient will tolerate may depend on whether a long course of treatment is required or a short course. Patients are more likely to tolerate a treatment that is short term rather than being long term, such as preventative treatment in an asymptomatic patient. For some patients, taking the treatment becomes a habit, part of their everyday life, not necessarily liked but tolerated. For others it is a burden they resent.

An increasing number of treatments are available, so there is often a choice. For example, a choice between different antibiotics, different anti-coagulants or different anti-hypertensive medications. When there is a choice, learning about the person and the person as a patient and having a working knowledge of the treatment, what it involves and how it works can help determine the most appropriate treatment to recommend. There are some general principles that can be used to inform choosing one treatment in preference to another. These include:

- Balance benefit and risk. All treatments are associated with risk, and the safety concerns influence risk. Some risks, such as side effects, are common and unlikely to be serious in most patients. For example:
  - o Anti-histamines causing drowsiness.
  - o Codeine causing constipation.
  In other patients these risks may be more serious. For example:
  - o Drowsiness causing a driver to have a road traffic accident.
  - o Severe constipation causing stercoral perforation.
  Most risks are short term or time-limited, with an expectation for a full recovery, but some are permanent. For example:
  - o Peripheral neuropathy following cisplatin or vincristine treatment for cancer is often permanent.
- If a previous treatment worked it may work again, and vice versa.
- A definitive treatment is preferable.
- Patient choice.
- When available, recommend a lifestyle change rather than a prescription medicine or an intervention. For example:
  - o Increase the walking distance for a patient with intermittent claudication.
  - o Change the diet. For example:
    - Avoid fatty foods in NASH.
    - A low carbohydrate diet in DM.
    - A low residue diet in adhesion SBO.
    - Avoid foods that precipitate an episode of biliary colic.
- Consider whether help from another HCP is indicated. For example:
  - o Physiotherapy to treat back pain.
  - o Bio-feedback to treat faecal incontinence.
  - o Speech therapy following a stroke.
  - o Acupuncture for pain relief.
- For some problems, mind-body treatments, such as psychotherapy, mindfulness, hypnosis, cognitive and behavioural therapy, music or art "therapy" may be helpful.
- In general, low risk or low-cost treatments should be used before high risk or high-cost treatments.
- Consider long-term or preventative benefits of a treatment and late complications or risks.

Treatment should always be discussed with the patient and this should include discussing choices, and the benefit-risk balance, particularly when it is close to equipoise or the risks are consequential.

Ask yourself, when should treatment be started?

Treatment is usually started following the consultation or when a diagnosis has been made. For some patients, other factors influence when a treatment should be started. These include:

- Availability. Some treatments are unavailable in the required time frame. For example, in an emergency there is little benefit in requesting a treatment that will take a long time to start. Some treatments are started because they are available quickly. However, just because a treatment is available does not mean it should be done: another treatment may be more appropriate.
- The risk of irreversible harm from delay. For example:
  o If a PE is suspected, interim parenteral anticoagulation is indicated before the results of investigations are known.
  o If sepsis is suspected antibiotics and organ support are indicated before infection is proven.
- Some patients choose to delay or defer starting treatment for personal reasons.
- Some treatments are not immediately available.
- An increasing number of patients have complex medical conditions and are on a number of different care pathways. Occasionally the provision or timing of one treatment may influence another. For example, treatment may need to be delayed until anticoagulation can be safely stopped or treating an abdominal aortic aneurysm may have to await a carotid endarterectomy.

Ask yourself, what would be a successful outcome?

A successful outcome is when the treatment meets the aims. In other words, the treatment is effective for the individual and helps the patient. For this reason, it is important to determine the aims of the treatment in advance and measure success against these. It is very important that the patient also knows and understands the therapeutic aims and also measures the outcome against these aims. If a patient expects an outcome that is unlikely to be achieved, they are likely to be unhappy. The many different ways the effectiveness of a treatment may be assessed include:

- Cure.
- A change in symptoms. For example, less pain, sickness, itching or relief of constipation.
- A change in signs. For example, reduced cellulitis in response to antibiotics, increased urine output in response to rehydration or reduced blood pressure in response to anti-hypertensive treatment.
- Functional improvement, such as an increased range of joint movement, walking distance, improved peak flow or urinary flow.
- A change in laboratory parameters. For example, rehydration can be measured by reduced haematocrit, reduced serum creatinine and reduced urine osmolality.
- A change in appearance on clinical imaging. This could include a change in the size, shape or attenuation of an abnormality, such as a mass.
- Slow disease progression/deterioration.

The effectiveness of some preventative treatments is only apparent in the long-term by the absence of a problem based on large population samples. For example, pre-exposure HIV treatment or vaccinations to reduce the risk of infection. It is difficult for patients and HCPs to recognise the success of such treatments whereas failure is always highlighted.

It should be noted that therapeutic effectiveness is not the same as efficacy. The results published when treatments are trialled in the "ideal" research environment show the efficacy of a treatment but this does not necessarily reflect their effectiveness in general clinical practice. On the other hand, sometimes treatments benefit a patient despite the absence of published evidence of efficacy or effectiveness. The reasons for this include:

- The research has not been undertaken.
- There is a placebo effect. Treatment success may be influenced by patient expectation.
- A treatment is effective but the measured outcome in research studies may not be statistically significant. This may be for many reasons, such as:
  o The sample population being studied is different.
  o The sample size is too small.
  o The variance in the measured outcome is wide so small changes that may be of benefit to an individual are not statistically significant.
  o The patient may be in a sub-set not included within published studies or a small sub-set of a larger sample.
  o For a population there is no statistical difference on average, but for the individual there is a difference because they are at the tail end of the normal distribution.

- Therapeutic effectiveness is rarely binary, i.e., all-or-none. Usually, a range of therapeutic outcomes can occur.

A treatment is more likely to be effective if:

- It is what the patient wants and expects. If the patient does not want a treatment, or a treatment does not meet a patient's expectations they will be dissatisfied.
- The patient believes it will work. If a patient is pessimistic about a treatment, it is unlikely it will be effective or credited with any improvement.
- It has been effective in the past.
- The patient trusts the HCP and the science.
- There are few side effects or complications.

The HCP and the patient should know what outcomes are possible, what outcomes are to be expected and what to hope for. If there is a difference between a patient's expectations and the likely outcome of treatment it is important to manage the patient's expectations to avoid:

- A loss of trust.
- A loss of confidence.
- Disagreement.
- A breakdown in the working relationship.
- Disappointment.
- Psychological consequences, such as stress, anxiety, anger or hostility.

For some patients, a treatment can be stopped after completing a course but, for many patients, treatment needs to be continued, such as when a treatment is intended to manage a problem rather than cure it. This should be discussed before starting treatment.

Recommend a referral to another HCP

For many patients, management includes referral to another HCP, such as a cardiologist, a rheumatologist, a physiotherapist or a dietician. Before making a referral:

Ask yourself, what is the aim of referral?

A referral should be made with a specific aim. These are "the terms of reference" for the HCP receiving the referral. They should be understood by both the patient and the HCPs involved. The aims of making a referral to another HCP include:

- To formulate a diagnosis or refine a differential diagnosis. For example:
  - A referral to a specialist, such as a neurologist, a cardiologist or a surgeon for their opinion.
  - A referral for a second opinion to confirm or exclude a diagnosis or to resolve uncertainty.
  - Some patients are referred to a specialist to screen for an asymptomatic problem. For example, referral to an ophthalmologist to screen for eye disease in a diabetic patient.
- To manage the problem. Sometimes decisions about management are complex, have significant risk or are too difficult for the patient or the HCP to make on their own. Other opinions may provide additional information about management.
- To provide treatment. For example, referral to a physiotherapist or a surgeon.
- For assessment. For example, referral to an anaesthetist for pre-operative assessment.
- For reassurance. This could be confirmation of a diagnosis or a treatment or to exclude a problem.

Ask yourself, is referral indicated?

There are many different specialist HCPs available and the indications for making a referral are different. Occasionally there are guidelines to inform when a referral is indicated or it may be appropriate to talk to the relevant HCP. Often if a referral is considered it is indicated.

Referral is not indicated when it is made for the wrong reasons, such as a desire to do something, a fear of missing something (which is different from suspecting a problem) or to transfer, divert or deflect a problem. A referral is contra-indicated when the patient refuses.

Ask yourself, is referral appropriate?

Most patients are reassured when they are referred to another HCP. Indeed, in a minority of patients, a referral can restore or revive trust in the HCP and health care system and some patients are upset or dissatisfied if they are not referred. This may be because they feel they are not being taken seriously or are upset that they are not getting a treatment. A referral to another HCP may be inappropriate when:

- It is likely to cause distress or inconvenience for the patient.
- It is likely to undermine trust and confidence.
- It may lead to false hope or expectations.
- It is a waste of resources.

Ask yourself, how should the referral be managed?

Use information about the person, the patient and the problem and from the examination to ensure the referral is to the right team and the aims, indications, timing and the context are appropriate. A referral to another HCP is a request. It should use established procedures and pathways. Organising a referral needs to be managed by the HCP. Pre-requisites to making a referral are:

- The referral should meet the management aims and indications and be appropriate.
- The patient should give consent.
- Relevant information is made available.
- Choose the right time.
- Choose the right context.
- Choose the right person or team to refer to.

Recommend a follow-up consultation

Often the first consultation is one of many in a pathway of care. Any follow up consultation should have a purpose; there is no place for a "routine follow up". Before organising a further consultation:

Ask yourself, what is the aim?

Before recommending a follow up consultation it is important to be clear on the aims of the follow up consultation and to discuss these with the patient. The aims include:

- To formulate a diagnosis, review a list of possible diagnoses or understand the problem following a period of time for change to occur, investigations to be undertaken or a trial of treatment.
- To re-assess severity, to inform management, after a period of time.
- To screen for a secondary problem or complication.
- To share information with the patient, to keep the patient informed. This could include sharing the results of an investigation, the opinions of another HCP or to discuss the pathway of care or management planned.
- To provide treatment.
- To discuss consent.
- For reassurance. Some patients are reassured by the "safety net" of a follow up consultation. When patients are trying to change a life choice, a follow up consultation may be indicated with the aim of providing reassurance.

Ask yourself, what are the indications for a follow up consultation?

If the diagnosis is uncertain and the patient is unlikely to come to harm from a period of "watchful waiting" a follow up consultation may be indicated. For example:

- To review the symptoms and signs in the hope of resolving diagnostic uncertainty. Close monitoring with careful review at an appropriate time interval provides an opportunity for a meaningful review. The problem may resolve, symptoms or signs can be re-considered and new ones may become apparent.
- To assess change. For example:
  o To monitor disease progression.
  o To assess the response to treatment.
  o To check for the development of a complication.
- For information exchange. The importance of information exchange to the care and well-being of the patient and their family should not be under-estimated. Increasingly, patients want more information, not less and the consultation is an opportunity to ensure both parties are fully informed. Patients often have additional questions and concerns that they either do not express during the first consultation or arise subsequently and a further consultation gives them an opportunity to discuss these.
- To make decisions about future management.

A follow up consultation is contra-indicated if the patient refuses.

Ask yourself, is a follow up consultation appropriate?

When there is uncertainty whether a follow up is indicated or not it should be discussed with the patient. This should include a discussion of management choices and the benefit-risk balance. Information about the person may indicate whether a follow up consultation is appropriate.

An unnecessary follow up consultation is inappropriate because it not only causes unnecessary distress and inconvenience for the patient but also is a waste of time and money and may reduce the opportunity for a consultation with another patient.

Applying Method to the Consultation

Information learnt throughout the consultation should inform management and management should inform some of the questions to ask or signs to look for (Figure 30).

Figure 30: Illustrating the information to inform management

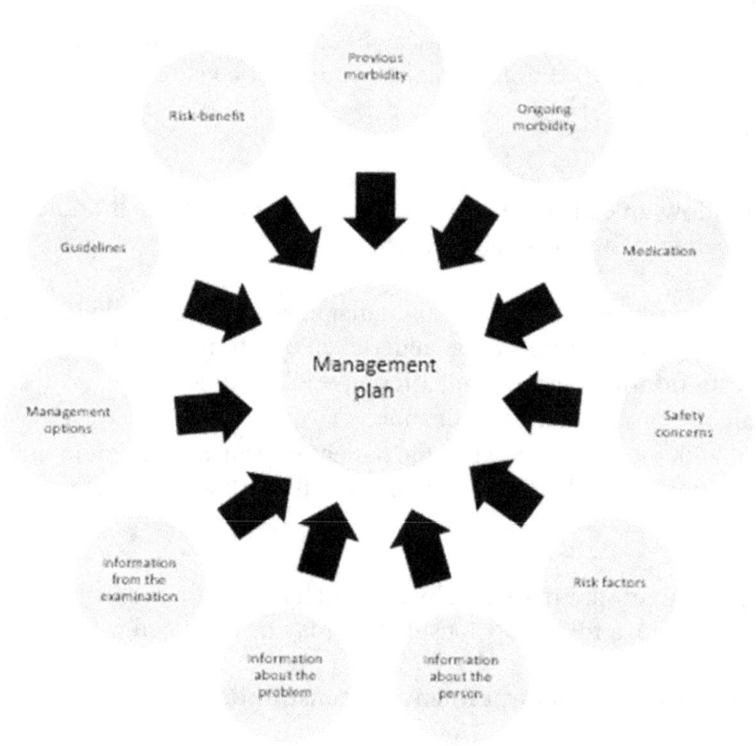

Use headline information and the introductory conversation to inform management

First impressions and the patient's description of their presenting problem will indicate when urgent management is indicated. This may include analgesics to help a patient in severe pain, oxygen to help a very breathless patient or, in the emergency department, following an emergency protocol.

Demographic information and information already known about the patient may influence the management options available and the benefit-risk equation. For example, some management options are indicated only in males or females and some are high risk or contraindicated at extremes of age. The patient's description of their presenting problem together with other headline information is used to determine the aims of the consultation and the initial focus of the consultation. The aims of the consultation together with information about the person, the patient and the problem and from the examination will inform management aims.

While listening to the patient, at the start of the consultation, ask yourself:

> Is emergency management indicated?
> What are the management aims?

Figure 31: Illustrating the questions to ask yourself at the start of the consultation

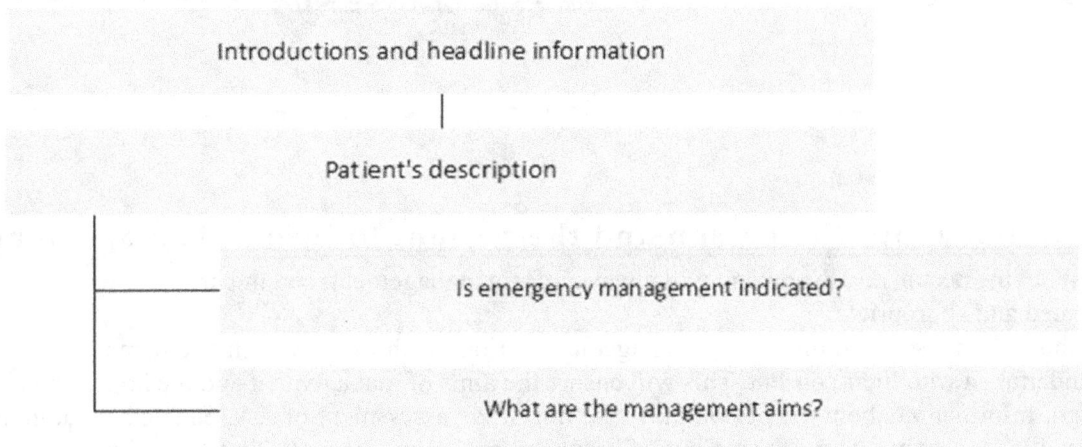

Use information about the problem to decide on management

Learning about the problem is the key to understanding the problem and formulating a diagnosis. This will determine the aims of management, what management is indicated and timing (priority). Learning about the symptoms and signs will inform management to alleviate symptoms. When a diagnosis is made specific treatment may be indicated. When the diagnosis is uncertain or there are a number of possible diagnoses, an investigation or a trial of treatment may be indicated. Questions should be asked to ensure a management option is indicated and, when there is choice, to determine the most appropriate option. Additional questions may be indicated to ensure the benefits and risks are fully understood and the timing is right.

In summary, while learning about the problem, ask yourself:

> What are the management aims?
> What management plan is indicated?
> What is the management priority?
> What are the benefits and risks?
> What additional information is needed?

Figure 32: Illustrating the questions to ask yourself while learning about the problem.

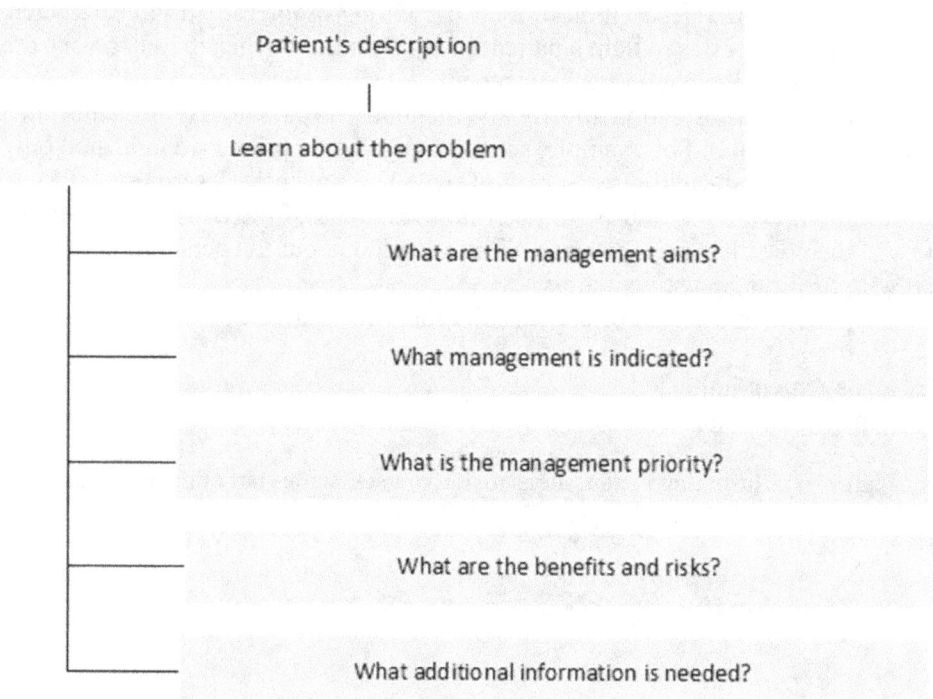

Use information about the person and the patient to inform management

Learning about the person and the patient will always inform management, and in particular whether a management option is indicated and appropriate.

Learning about the person and discussing management options with them will ensure management is appropriate and is being undertaken with their consent. This will ensure the aims of management and the hopes and expectations of the patient align. Information about the person may also inform an assessment of risk, enable a meaningful discussion of risk and benefit, and help ensure the timing of management is appropriate. Together, this is likely to increase compliance and adherence.

Information about the patient should always be considered before recommending a management option. For most patients, there are no concerns but this should not be assumed. In some patients, information may change management, such as when a treatment is contra-indicated, in others information is relevant to the problem. For example:

- When the patient presents with breathlessness, likely to be caused by asthma and information about the person indicates they are exposed to a lot of air pollution, a lifestyle change may be indicated in addition to bronchodilators.
- When the patient presents feeling ill, with a headache likely to be caused by carbon monoxide poisoning from an open fire a change at home, such as avoiding using the fire or improved ventilation, may be indicated and a carbon monoxide detector installed.
- When a patient with DM presents feeling ill, the diagnosis may include a metabolic abnormality, such as ketoacidosis or renal failure or an occult infection, such as a urinary tract infection. The blood glucose should be measured and urgent investigations to check homeostasis are indicated.
- The differential diagnosis of recurrent central abdominal colic, bloating and a feeling of nausea includes intermittent small bowel obstruction. When the patient has had a previous laparotomy, this may be caused by post operative adhesions.

While learning about the person and the patient, ask yourself:

What information is relevant to planning management?
What management is appropriate?

What are the benefits and risks?
Are there any contra-indications?
What additional information is needed?

Figure 33: Illustrating the questions to ask yourself while learning about the person and the patient.

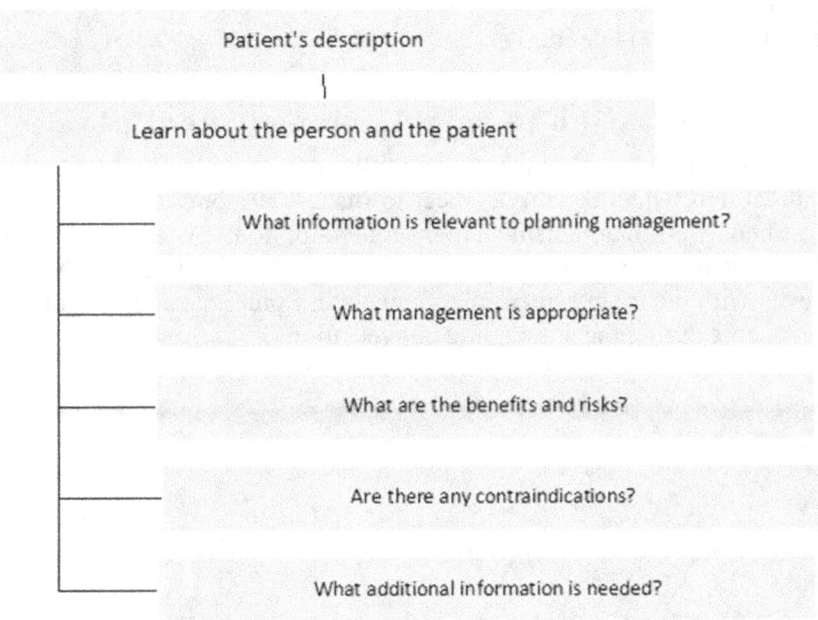

Use the examination to inform management

When the patient presents with a visible or palpable abnormality, the examination is likely to determine management. For other problems, the examination is likely to influence the choice of management and the priority. Frequently, the examination will influence the benefit-risk balance, if only to confirm the safety of a management option (Figure 34).

Figure 34: Illustrating the questions to ask yourself while examining a visible or palpable abnormality.

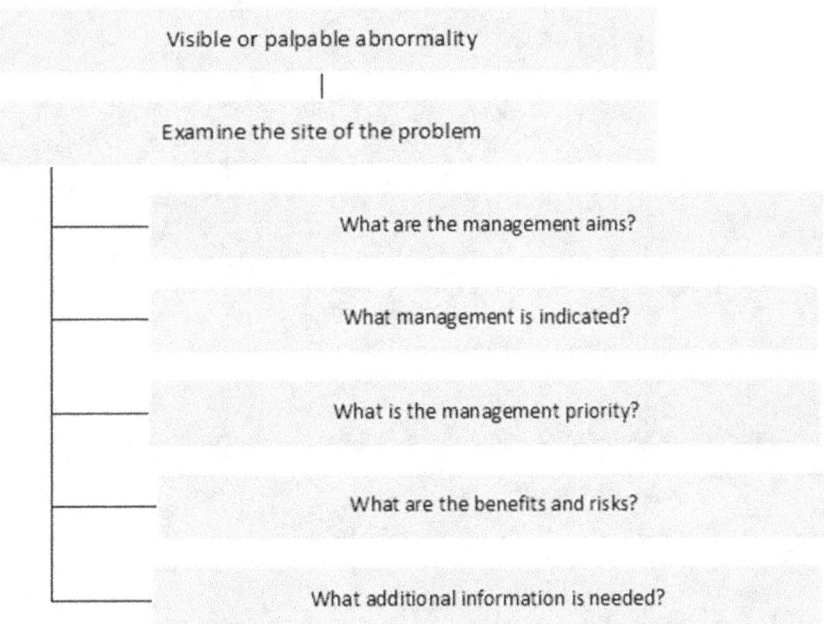

When the patient presents with a visible or palpable abnormality, while examining the site of the abnormality, ask yourself:

What are the management aims?
What management plan is indicated?
What is the management priority?
What are the benefits and risks?
What additional information is needed?

Use the concluding conversation to agree a management plan

Part of the concluding conversation should include a discussion of the management options, a recommendation on the best option for the patient and, when there is choice, to discuss the options. It may be appropriate to review a guideline to inform management. Before organising a management option, it is important to ensure that the patient has a good understanding of what is involved, the likely benefits and risks and checking that these are acceptable to the patient and the patient agrees with the management recommended. Some management options require consent. If so, discussing consent usually occurs during the concluding conversation.

Section 2
Application of a Clinical
Method to the Consultation

Chapter 5
Starting the Consultation

Abstract

Organising the consultation requires a functioning administration team, effective and efficient organisation, good communication and the right staff and facilities. A well-organised consultation lays the foundation for a good working relationship and a meaningful consultation. The pre-consultation preparation, first impressions, the way the patient is welcomed and the introductory conversation set the tone for the rest of the consultation.

The introductory conversation starts every consultation. A good start is likely to lead into a relaxed consultation. A relaxed consultation is more likely to be a meaningful consultation. A meaningful consultation is more likely to be a successful consultation, in which the outcome meets the aims and the patient is happy. This is likely to give the patient confidence, establish a good relationship and ensure a reservoir of goodwill for the rest of the pathway of care. On the other hand, if the pre-consultation preparation is problematic the consultation is likely to have a difficult start. If the start of the consultation is difficult, the rest of the consultation is likely to be difficult and the patient may leave unhappy or dissatisfied. This is likely to have repercussions for the rest of the pathway of care.

Introductions should be courteous, respectful and suit local convention. A social introductory conversation will help relax the patient and provide an opportunity to assess the patient, such as their behaviour, how ill they are, their higher brain function and whether or not they have special needs. This information together with previous information known, the context of the consultation, demographic information and the information about the presenting problem makes up the headline information and determines the aims and the initial focus of the consultation.

Most patients with a new problem expect to talk about their problem early in the consultation, after all, that is why they are there. However, this does not mean it should always be the initial focus of the consultation. It may be more appropriate to learn about the person or about the person as a patient before focusing on the problem. This approach may help an anxious patient relax or build a working relationship when the patient is challenging and ensures the focus is on the person with a problem, rather than solely on the problem. Similarly, when the patient is normally "fit and well" or has multiple ongoing medical problems or are taking numerous medications, learning about the person and the patient ensures background information is considered when learning about the problem. A flexibly managed consultation is more likely to be a meaningful consultation undertaken in the best interests of the patient.

In summary, the importance of a well organised consultation and a good start to the consultation is out of proportion to the quality and quantity of information exchanged. The headline information and the introductory conversation at the start also determine the aims and initial focus of the consultation.

Introduction

The pre-consultation organisation, the staff and facilities and the introductory conversation are disproportionately important. They set the tone and agenda for the rest of the consultation and the consultation sets the tone and agenda for the rest of the care pathway.

"You never get a second chance to make a first impression"

Will Rogers

A good start is likely to lead to a good rapport and a relaxed consultation. A relaxed consultation is likely to lead to a meaningful consultation and a meaningful consultation is likely to be successful. Conversely, issues, such as organisation or communication difficulties prior to the consultation or a bad start to the consultation tend to have lasting adverse consequences. The start is also an opportunity to set the agenda for the rest of the consultation. The headline information and the introductory conversation determine the aims and the initial focus and ensure information exchange is in the best interests of the patient.

The aim of this chapter is to describe how the start of the consultation informs the rest of the consultation.

Organizing the Consultation

Organising a consultation starts when a referral is received and accepted (Figure 35).

Figure 35: Illustrating referral pathways

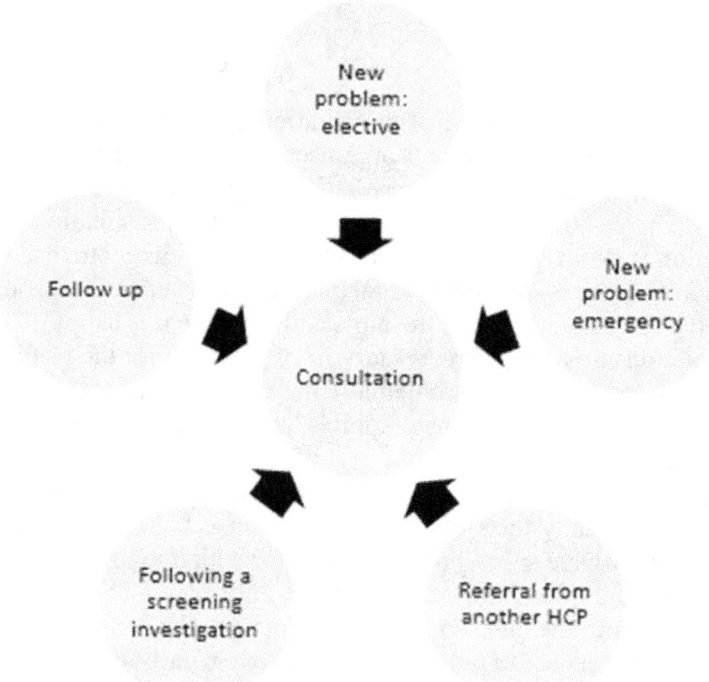

Patients want a consultation with an HCP for different reasons and can be referred via different routes and at different stages in their care pathway. The types of referrals and examples of the reasons for a referral include:

- "Self-referral", in which the consultation is initiated by the patient, the patient's family, carers or the emergency services. The reasons for self-referral include:
  - For help with a new problem.
  - A change in a pre-existing problem.
  - To discuss their risks and plan management when a close relative has been diagnosed with a heritable condition.
  - For reassurance.
  - For treatment, such as a travel vaccination.
  - For a report, such as a disability assessment.
  - To access a service, such as an open access endoscopy service, a "one stop" clinic or to perform a minor surgical procedure.
- Referral from another HCP. Usually, a referral from another HCP occurs after an initial assessment has been made by an HCP. The reasons patients are referred include:
  - For help to formulate a diagnosis.
  - To plan management.
  - When emergency care is needed.
  - To provide treatment.
  - For reassurance.
  - For a second opinion.
- Referral following a screening investigation. Increasingly a new consultation occurs following a screening investigation. For example, following a cervical smear, faecal occult blood test, a mammogram or "well-person screening".
- A further appointment. A further appointment occurs within an ongoing pathway of care. For example:
  - To discuss the results of an investigation and plan management

- ○ When an ongoing problem has changed.
- ○ To check for change.
- ○ To monitor response to treatment.
- ○ For assessment, such as a pacemaker check, to check blood pressure or DM control.

Once a referral has been received it needs to be accepted as being appropriate, prioritised and an appointment made with the relevant HCP in an appropriate facility. Most consultations are for a non-urgent problem but some are time critical. In which case, the consultation needs to be organised either urgently or as an emergency. The type of consultation organised and the duration of the consultation should be appropriate to the patient, the HCP and the problem. Some consultations are with a specialist and require trained staff, specialist equipment and facilities, whereas others can take place in a multi-purpose facility.

Scheduling a consultation, communicating with the patient and ensuring the patient is seen in the right place by the right people at the right time requires competent staff, good cooperation and collaboration (Figure 36).

Figure 36: The organisation required to set up a consultation between the doctor and patient

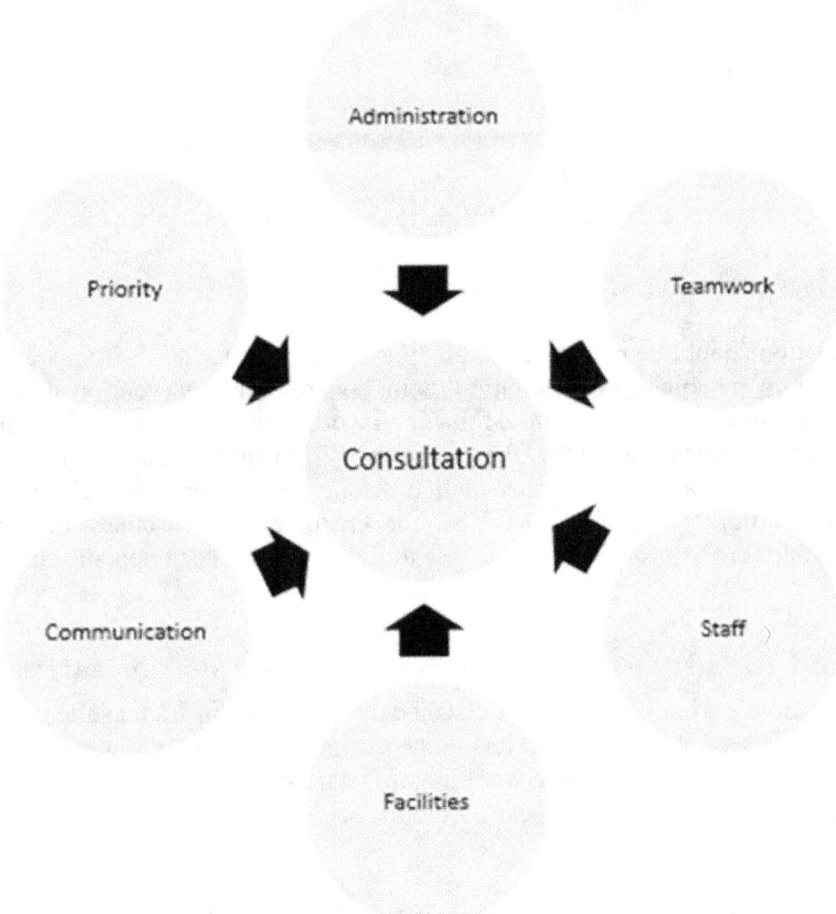

A well-organised consultation lays the foundation for a good working relationship and a meaningful consultation, whereas problems with the pre-consultation organisation are likely to adversely affect the start of the consultation. For example:

- If there are delays, uncertainty or confusion, such as when an appointment is rearranged.
- When the type of consultation is inappropriate to the patient or the problem. For example, organising a telephone consultation when the patient needs to be examined.
- If the patient sees the wrong specialist.
- If the consultation is in the wrong setting or necessary equipment is lacking.
- When the timing is wrong, such as when a consultation to discuss the result of an investigation occurs before the result is known.

Traditionally, a face-to-face consultation has been the default type of consultation but increasingly media-based consultations are being organised using a telephone, a video link, the internet or a radio. Regardless of the type of consultation it is important sufficient time is allocated for a meaningful exchange of information. In general, this is 10-15 minutes but for some specialist consultations up to an hour may be necessary. To ensure this time is efficiently used good preparation is essential.

The advantages and disadvantages of a face-to-face consultation

A face-to-face consultation enables a natural dialogue in which the conversation is dynamic, concordant and spontaneous and is necessary if the patient is to be examined. The conversation together with facial expressions and body language communicate the message. A face-to-face consultation allows interruptions, including affirmations or disagreement and humour. There is an opportunity for empathy and shared emotions, such as happiness, sadness, anxiety or stress, and these are recognised more easily. A face-to-face consultation is more likely to develop a rapport, build confidence and trust, and to show support and understanding than a media-based consultation. It is a social interaction, a shared experience, that counts towards "social capital" and is likely to have long term benefits.

A face-to-face consultation is indicated when:

- There are appropriate facilities and staff.
- The patient is unable to communicate using other media.
- An examination is likely to be required.
- Specialist equipment is needed.
- The consultation is likely to be complex, transformational, rather than simply a transaction in which information is exchanged.
- The consultation may be difficult or challenging.

A face-to-face consultation should be conducted in an appropriate setting that is both safe and private. This could include an office, a clinic room, a cubicle, a resuscitation room, a ward or an intervention suite. A private environment is more confidential and likely to foster trust, essential for a good working relationship. If the consultation occurs behind a curtain or partition, it should be remembered that there is privacy from sight but not sound.

Most consultations need an examination couch and a strong light source for close inspection. Increasingly consultations use specialist equipment such as an USS for the breast or vascular surgeon, a slit lamp for the ophthalmologist, a colposcope for the gynaecologist, access to imaging for an orthopaedic surgeon or a sigmoidoscope for the colo-proctologist.

The advantages and disadvantages of a media-based consultation

A media-based consultation is a conversation at a distance using a medium such as the telephone, a video link, the internet or a radio. A media-based conversation suits some people but is feels unnatural and difficult for others. Communication focuses on the spoken word and recognition of facial expressions and body language are compromised. It is difficult to show empathy and is less likely to contribute to "social capital".

A media-based consultation is indicated when:

- The patient is unable to attend a face-to-face consultation. For example, when:
  o Patients are confined to their home.
  o There are mental health concerns preventing face to face contact, such as agoraphobics.
  o Close proximity is contra-indicated, such as during an epidemic.
  o Health care is needed for remote inaccessible communities or remote areas, such as the Arctic or Antarctic, deserts or mountainous regions or for isolated communities, such as after landslides, floods or earthquakes.
- It is convenient for both the patient and the HCP.
- An examination is unlikely to be required.
- There is a good working relationship.
- The consultation is transactional. For example:
  o To inform the patient the result of an investigation.
  o To check that the patient is responding to a treatment.
  o To exchange information about a procedure, such as an endoscopy or an operation.

The conduct of a media-based consultation is different from a face-to-face consultation. Recommendations to ensure a media-based consultation is likely to be successful include:

- Ensure the patient is happy and able to hold a media-based consultation.
- Ensure it is unlikely to compromise information exchange.
- Use a secure telephone, internet or video-link to connect the HCP and the patient.
- Preferably use a headset to free the arms for taking notes or accessing resources, such as a computer.
- Undertake checks at the start of the conversation, such as:
  - Check that each party can hear and understand each other.
  - Introduce yourself and check the identity of the patient.
  - Check that they agree to talk.
  - Check that it is a good time to talk.
  - Check it is a safe place to talk.
  - If there are several people included, check the patient consents to other people hearing the conversation.
  - Check that they are unlikely to be disturbed.
  - If it is being recorded, check that the patient consents to a recording being made.
- Speak directly to the person.
- Speak in turn and wait for the other person to finish before speaking. Avoid interrupting or talking at the same time.
- The tone and content of the conversation is important. Use empathy and understanding as you would in any conversation.

Potential problems with a media-based conversation include:

- There is an increased risk of a misunderstanding.
- There is an increased risk of appearing uncaring.
- An inability to examine the patient.
- Technical problems. For example:
  - Problems with the sound and vision quality.
  - Transmission delays and a time-lag which can interrupt the flow of the conversation, cause frustration and lead to misunderstanding.
- Communication problems. For example:
  - Some people are unable to communicate using the medium.
  - Lip reading and sign language may be compromised.
  - Non-verbal cues may be missed.

Measures may be available to mitigate these problems, such as a service where speech is transcribed into writing or there is a simultaneous sign language interpreter for deaf people, and some signs can be described or sent as a picture or video. However, for some patients a face-to-face consultation is indicated following the media-based consultation.

Prepare for the Consultation

Each patient is special and should be given your undivided attention. Ensure they become the focus of your attention by completing all the work from the previous consultation and learning available information about the patient before starting the consultation. This should include learning the name of the patient and demographic information, the context of the consultation and reviewing documented medical information before meeting with them. When reading through medical information, it is essential to ensure the information refers to the right patient and not to another patient.

The Introductory Conversation

The aims of the introductory conversation are to check the right patient is being seen, to create a favourable impression, to help the patient relax and to lay the foundation for the rest of the consultation. The introduction is the start of learning about the person and should lead into the consultation. First impressions are very important to establishing a good working relationship. How the patient appears and behaves influences how we talk to the patient, the questions asked, the way they are asked and the answers that are expected. How we appear and behave influences what the patient thinks, the working relationship, trust, respect and the information they feel comfortable sharing.

Establishing a good working relationship is a pre-requisite to a meaningful exchange of information, essential for a successful consultation.

Introductions should be courteous, respectful and suit local convention. It is conventional to welcome a patient by name, to smile and at the same time introduce yourself:

Hello/Good morning/afternoon [name], my name is [name].
Thank you for coming today [name], my name is [name]?

The introductions should confirm the patients name and their age or date of birth.

Can I please check your name and date of birth/age?

All in-patients should have such information attached to them in some way, such as with a wrist band. In the emergency setting the patient details may be unknown and a temporary unique identifier is used. This is then matched to the true identity as soon as this is known.

When a patient is accompanied by a family member, guardian or a friend, or the HCP is accompanied by another person, such as a nurse or student, their presence should be acknowledged and they should be introduced. It may be appropriate to ask:

Who is accompanying you today?
Have you come alone or is someone with you?

When a person has a known disability focus on the person rather than the disability and avoid defining them as a disabled person. When their disability may need to be accommodated ask discretely, without making it seem like an issue. For example:

Do you need assistance?
Can I help?
How can I help?
Would you like help?

When the person has a known disability, such as being deaf, it may be appropriate to ask:

Can you hear and understand me?

When the person is partially sighted, it may be appropriate to ask:

Would you like me to describe your surroundings?

Introductions may include asking the patient what they want to be called. Some people want to be called by their first name, others by their surname. Most people demonstrate the social, behavioural and physical characteristics expected of a male or female within the society they live and are happy to be referred to using a title such as Mr, Mrs or Miss. Occasionally, their gender identity and expression influences what they want to be called and may influence the conduct of the consultation. An incorrect assumption can adversely affect the working relationship. If there is the possibility of doubt, ask:

What would you like me to call you?
How do you like to be addressed?

Gender identity or expression should not influence the working relationship. However, the HCPs gender may concern some patients or their families. If there is a perceived concern it may be appropriate to give the patient an opportunity to express their concern. The questions to ask could include:

Do you feel comfortable talking to me about your problems?
Are you feeling OK talking to me?
Is there something you want to raise?

Most patients are slightly nervous or anxious at the start of the consultation. If so, they are more likely to relax if, following introductions, the conversation is about something neutral and non-clinical, such as their trip, the weather, their journey, their name, where they live, how they spend their time or something about the appointment or about yourself. For example:

How was your trip?
How was the traffic?
Have you come far?

If you know the patient from previously it may be appropriate to talk about a more personalized topic, such as an interest or a holiday.

Last time I saw you, you were about to go on a holiday. How was it?

If there has been an issue prior to the consultation it is often helpful if it is raised early to ensure the matter is dealt with rather than let it fester. This could be done with a question, a statement or an apology. For example:

I understand there were some problems organising this consultation?
It's really busy today, I am sorry you have had to wait.

Giving the patient an opportunity to talk about themselves or holding a social conversation at the start of the consultation may seem "frivolous", "unnecessary", a "waste of time" or a "distraction" but it is likely to help build a rapport, it shows the patient that they are being treated as a person with a problem and not just another complaint and it may help "break the ice" for a nervous patient. A relaxed patient is more likely to feel able to talk freely about more personal matters.

The Headline Information

The headline information includes previous information known about the patient, the context of the consultation, demographic information, first impressions and information about the problem (Figure 37). This information is used both proactively at the start of the consultation to determine the aims and initial focus of the consultation, while learning about the person, the patient, the problem and during the examination to inform formulating a diagnosis and planning management, and retrospectively in a summary of key information about the patient at the end of the consultation or when recording or presenting information to another HCP.

Figure 37: To illustrate the information that makes up the headline information

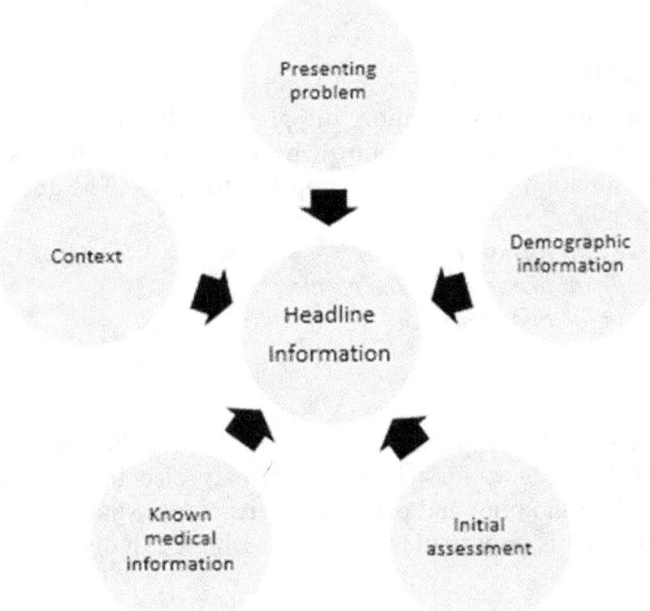

Information known about the patient

Prior to starting the consultation, it is important to have read available background information about the patient. This is likely to include demographic information such as:

- Age.
- Gender.
- Marital status.
- Ethnicity.
- Language.
- Religion.
- Education.
- Occupation.

Most people are or have been patients at some time in their lives and many patients are seen in a consultation following an investigation, including a screening investigation, or as a follow up within a pathway of care or following referral from another HCP. In which case, the records will contain background information. Always familiarise yourself with available information before meeting the patient because it is likely to be relevant to the consultation and their care. Occasionally, when aspects need to be confirmed, explained or clarified it is appropriate to ask relevant questions early in the consultation. Ignorance or misunderstanding of such information is not only potentially dangerous for the patient but, if it is suspected by the patient, may undermine trust and confidence, adversely affecting the working relationship.

When there is no relevant background medical information, it is likely the patient is "fit and well" emphasising the fact that it is unusual they are now presenting with a problem. In which case, learning about the patient can be undertaken early in the consultation to quickly check that they do not have any undocumented relevant past or ongoing morbidity, treatments or safety concerns. The questions to ask could include:

I notice from your medical records that you have not had any previous medical conditions. Is that true?
Normally you seem to be very well. Have you had any previous medical conditions?

An increasing number of patients have conditions that are managed but not cured, such as asthma, DM, COPD, hypertension, cancer, psoriasis, migraine or arthritis, and are taking multiple medications or have been recently investigated. In which case, reviewing this information with the patient early in the consultation may be indicated.

Your records show that you are being treated for [condition]. Is that true?
Can I check what medications you are taking to treat [condition]?
I note that you have been treated for [condition] in the past. Have you had any other medical problems?

The context of the consultation

The context refers to the reason for the consultation, the place of the consultation in the care pathway and the urgency of the consultation. Usually, the context is known by the HCP and the patient prior to the consultation. Nevertheless, at the start of the consultation it is usually appropriate to check. The questions to ask could include:

I understand you want to see me about [new problem]?
You have just had a [test] would you like to know the result?
Can I check you know the reason for this consultation?

First impressions

Potentially a lot of information about the person can be learnt from the way a patient enters the room, their movement and posture and from their voice. First impressions may also be influenced by the patient's physical appearance and facial expression, their clothing and personal hygiene and what they say. However, first impressions should be interpreted with caution and it is important to avoid being biased, judgemental or assigning a stereotype.

Information about the problem

When a patient presents with a new problem, following a screening test or a referral from another HCP the consultation proper starts by asking an open question that gives the patient an opportunity to talk about their problem in their own words. The questions to ask could include:

How can I help?
What is the main problem?
What is wrong?
What is worrying you?
Tell me about [the problem]
Tell me what is wrong

When a patient is seen following an investigation, it may be appropriate to check the patient knows why the consultation is occurring, what the patient knows and the findings of the test. When it follows a screening test, it may also be necessary to explain the reasons for the screening test. It may then be appropriate to ask questions to learn whether or not they have any symptoms or a change in their symptoms. The questions to ask could include:

You have just had [test]. How did you find it?
We are meeting because you have just had [test]. Can I first ask, have you noticed any new symptoms/change?
Before we talk about the results of your test, can I ask, have you noticed anything wrong/any symptoms?
It may be appropriate to ask leading questions or look for specific signs relevant to the test. For example:

- When the patient is seen following a test to screen for faecal occult blood the questions to ask could include:

Have you noticed any blood in your stools?
Have you noticed a change in your bowel habit? Have you had any anal symptoms, such as pain?
Have you had any abdominal pains?

- When the patient is seen following a mammogram it may be appropriate to explain that a breast examination is indicated.

When the patient is being seen as a follow up or following a referral from another HCP, information about the problem is already known. After summarizing known information, such as the problem or the reason for the consultation, it may be appropriate to ask:

What has happened since we last met?
Has anything changed since you saw [HCP]?

Determine the Aims of the Consultation

The core aims of a consultation are to establish a working relationship, exchange relevant information, formulate a diagnosis and plan management (Figure 38).

Establishing a working relationship is a core aim and maintaining it is an ongoing task. A good working relationship has many benefits, it enables a meaningful exchange of information during the consultation and is likely to help ensure adherence and compliance with future care.

For the patient, information exchange is about learning and understanding information about their problem, the opinion and recommendations of the HCP. For the HCP, information exchange is about learning and understanding relevant and appropriate information about the person, the patient and the problem and identifying or excluding relevant signs on examination. For most patients and most consultations, exchanging information is an enabler. It is undertaken with the aims of formulating a diagnosis and planning management. While talking to the patient, it is not only necessary to think about what questions to ask but also what signs should be sought, and while examining the patient, it is not only necessary to think about what signs to look for but also what additional questions to ask.

For most consultations, formulating a diagnosis is a principal aim of the consultation and is the reason for the exchange of information. Ideally, the aim is to formulate a definitive diagnosis in which both the cause and pathogenesis are known. However, when this is not possible, the aim is to use the available information to formulate a descriptive diagnosis or make a list of possible diagnoses and exclude unlikely diagnoses. A working diagnosis or differential diagnosis then informs management. Formulating a diagnosis is dependent on the HCP using their clinical and cognitive skills, their knowledge of medicine and the basic sciences and method to learn, understand and interpret available information. It does not happen be chance.

Figure 38: Illustrating the aims of the consultation.

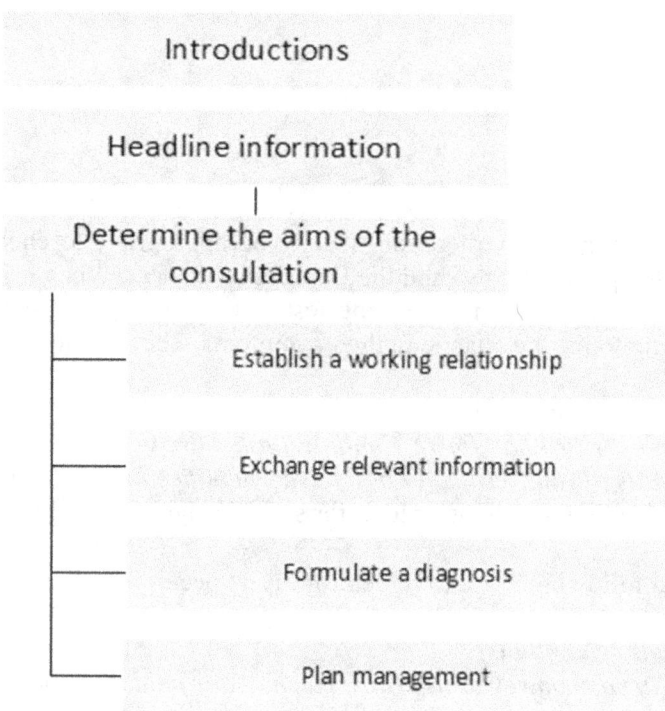

An agreed management plan is the outcome of the consultation. Management options should be considered throughout the consultation and be used to inform the questions to ask or signs to look for. Ideally, management includes definitive treatment. However, this may not be possible for many patients and many problems. In which case, management involves requesting investigations with the aim of formulating a diagnosis or learning more about the problem, discussing changing life choices, starting treatment to alleviate symptoms, help function or reduce the risk of a deterioration or a complication or organising a follow up consultation to assess change, for screening or for reassurance.

The introductions and headline information are used to determine the principal aims of the consultation. The principal aims will vary between patients and between consultations. For example:

- When a new patient is seen by the HCP for the first time, the principal aims are usually to exchange relevant information to learn more about the person and the patient and to establish a working relationship.
- When a patient presents with a new problem, the principal aims of the consultation are to exchange relevant information to formulate a diagnosis and plan management.
- When the consultation follows an investigation or a course of treatment and the diagnosis is known, the aims are usually to exchange information and plan management.
- When the patient is seen for the first time following an investigation, the aims are to establish a working relationship, exchange information and plan management.
- When the consultation is in response to a referral from another HCP the aims are determined by the referring HCP.
- When there are problems with the working relationship, establishing or re-establishing a working relationship is likely to be an initial aim of the consultation.

The principal aims may change during the consultation in response to the patient and the information learnt. For example:

- When learning about the patient reveals they have significant or complex ongoing or past medical conditions, information exchange to learn about the patient may become an important aim of the consultation.
- When a patient becomes very emotional or exhibits challenging behaviour, establishing a working relationship may become the main aim.

Determine the Initial Focus of the Consultation

The introductory conversation and the headline information will determine what to talk about first or what part to examine first (Figure 39). Learning about the problem early on is often what the patient expects: after all that is usually why they are there! However, if it is undertaken early in the consultation there is a tendency for the HCP to focus on the problem rather than on the person with a problem and the relevance of information about person and the patient to the presenting problem may be missed.

Figure 39: Illustrating an overview of the consultation.

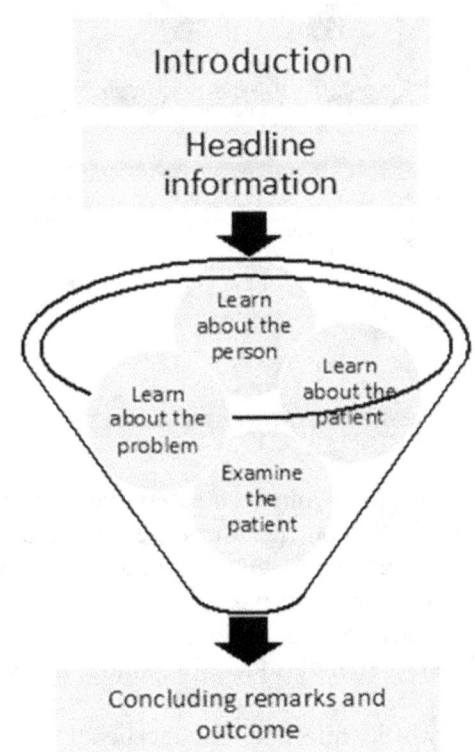

Use first impressions to inform the initial focus of the consultation

Even though the introductory conversation is an informal social conversation, it is important to listen carefully to what the patient says, their choice of words, the tone they use, what they don't say and silences, to be alert to subtle signs, facial expressions and body language. With most patients there is nothing that is unusual or unexpected and the introduction is simply a springboard to a meaningful conversation about their problem. However, occasionally first impressions influence the conduct, the aims and the initial focus of the consultation. For example:

- When a patient's behaviour or special needs are challenging, learning about the person may become the focus for the consultation with the aim of establishing a working relationship.
- When a patient has behavioural or learning difficulties or a mental health condition it may be appropriate to adapt the consultation to meet their needs.
- When a patient is manifestly emotional, managing this may be the initial focus of the consultation.

When talking to the patient during the introductory conversation it is important to ask yourself:

Are you at risk?
Is the patient very ill, in severe pain or very breathless?

Does the patient have special needs?
Is their appearance consistent with what you would expect?
Is their affect and behaviour consistent with what you would expect?
Is their "higher" brain function consistent with what you would expect?

First impressions and the headline information will also determine the aims and initial focus of the consultation.

Figure 40: Illustrating the questions to ask yourself at the start of the consultation.

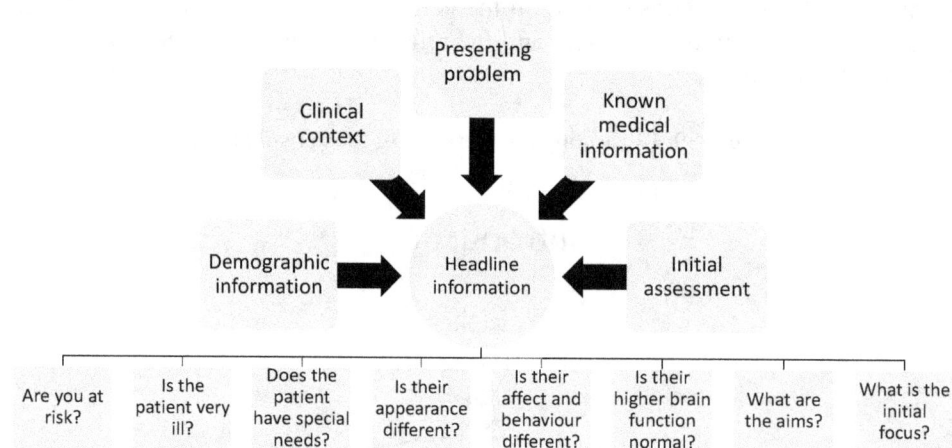

Ask yourself, are you at risk?

When seeing a patient, it is important to ensure your own safety and the safety of other members of staff. If it is necessary to ask the question, "are you at risk?" your health or wellbeing are probably at risk. In which case, take measures to ensure you are safe. On a road, for example, this is obvious; you don't want to become the victim of a road traffic accident while caring for another. In a clinic the risks may not be immediately apparent but can be real. For example, you may be threatened by an aggressive patient or family member or, when alone with a patient, be placed in a compromising position that could be misinterpreted. It is therefore, important, whatever the setting, to ensure measures are in place for your own safety.

In almost all contexts a chaperone is worthwhile both for the benefit of the patient and yourself. Certainly, a chaperone should be present when examining a patient of the opposite sex, a child or when an intimate examination needs to be performed, such as a rectal, breast or genital examination, or if there is any concern about how the patient may react during the consultation. Similarly, it may be appropriate for a family member, friend or carer to accompany the patient.

Ask yourself, is the patient very ill, in severe pain or very breathless?

Some patients are very ill, very breathless and some are obviously in severe pain when seen. This can be overwhelming, making everything else inconsequential. It is easy to recognise when a person is very breathless or in severe pain but not necessarily when someone is ill. The features characteristic of an ill patient include:

- A "grey" complexion with sunken eyes, dry lips and tongue. The cheeks may be flushed and the breathing rapid and shallow. They may be peripherally cold and slightly sweaty. They may have a hunched appearance with evidence of weight loss and muscle wasting.
- A change in their behaviour or functional performance. When a patient appears listless and lacks energy, is apathetic and disinterested, and work and everyday tasks are difficult.
- A change in their thought processes and conversation. Thinking, decision making and response times become slow, conversation may be confused or mono-syllabic.

- A change in their clothing and appearance. When ill, a patient may appear dishevelled and have "bad breath". Bad breath may indicate pathology, such as intestinal obstruction, liver disease ("hepatic fetor"), uraemia or diabetic ketosis.

Most patients with a perceived emergency call a help line (111 in the UK), an emergency number (999 in the UK, 911 in USA) or self-refer directly to an emergency department where they are managed by a specialist team according to predetermined protocols. However, occasionally a very ill patient is seen in the non-urgent setting. They may be a new referral or a patient with a known previous condition who suffers a relapse or a recurrence or a patient with an ongoing medical condition who suffers a deterioration or a complication. Indeed, it is not unusual for a patient on a pathway of care to wait for a pre-arranged clinic appointment rather than organise an earlier appointment despite becoming very ill.

There are many texts and articles describing the management of the medical emergency. In general, when the patient appears ill the pace, aims, focus and format of the consultation change (Figure 41).

Figure 41: A figure to illustrate the focus of the consultation in an emergency consultation.

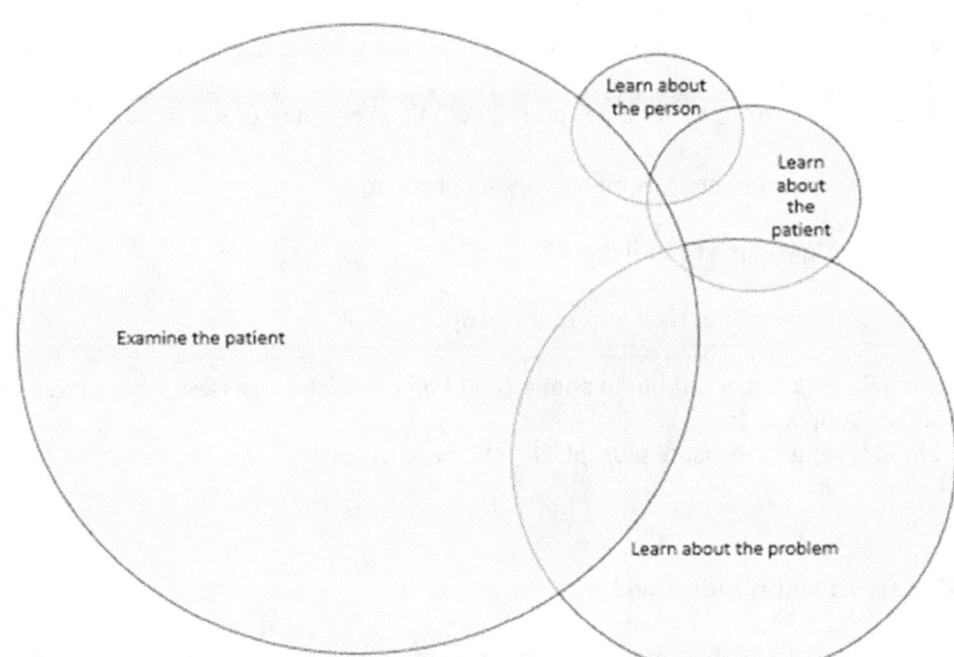

The initial aims are to rapidly assess the systemic impact of the problem on the patient, start urgent treatment to prevent irreversible harm and alleviate symptoms, to learn about the presenting problem and to examine the patient to identify high priority diagnoses and to assess the systemic impact on the patient.

- First assess the airway.

Ask yourself, could the airway be obstructed?

Relieve, bypass or treat any airway obstruction because significant obstruction can cause hypoxia.

- Assess their breathing while talking to the patient and examining the chest.

Ask yourself, is breathing normal?

If the patient is breathless give them oxygen, if they have a wheeze and are struggling to breathe give a bronchodilator for bronchospasm. If there are signs of a pneumothorax insert a chest drain.

- Assess the peripheries, feel the pulse and measure the blood pressure.

Ask yourself, could they be in shock?

If the patient is peripherally cold, with tachycardia, hypotension and tachypnoea they are likely to be in shock. Diagnose and treat the cause. For example, intravenous fluids for hypovolaemia, antibiotics for sepsis, diuretics or inotropes for heart failure, antihistamines or steroids for anaphylaxis.

- Learn about the patient, including ongoing morbidity and treatments and known allergens.
- Learn about the problem and pro-actively consider common medical emergencies.

Ask yourself, what high priority diagnosis is likely?

Common medical emergencies include:

o Severe infection, such as a chest or urinary tract infection or septicaemia.
o Severe bronchospasm. Usually caused by asthma or a hypersensitivity reaction.
o A pneumothorax.
o Acute cardiac failure caused by an AMI or an arrhythmia.
o Acute "brain failure". Usually caused by a stroke, an intracranial haemorrhage or a seizure.
o Diabetic keto-acidosis.
o Haemorrhage, such as from varices, a ruptured ectopic pregnancy or a ruptured AAA.

- While learning about the problem start managing the problem.

Ask yourself, what investigations are indicated?

Investigations are likely to include as a minimum (Appendix 2):

o Blood testing for glucose, a full blood count, blood biochemistry to assess "liver, renal and bone function", clotting and a group and save.
o Arterial blood testing to measure pO_2, pCO_2, pH, base excess and lactate.
o An ECG
o A CXR

Ask yourself, what treatment is indicated?

Start or plan a treatment to correct abnormalities, help vital organ function and alleviate symptoms. This is likely to include:

o Supplemental oxygen.
o Intravenous fluids.
o Analgesia for pain.
o Antimicrobials if sepsis is suspected.
o Correct a metabolic abnormality. For example, intravenous glucose to reverse hypoglycaemia or insulin to treat diabetic ketoacidosis.

A seriously ill patient should be given urgent supportive treatment, before the results of investigations are known

When the patient is genuinely in severe pain, they need symptomatic treatment with an opiate before they are able to give a reliable account of their illness. When this has taken effect, it is possible to learn about the problem and prescribe appropriate analgesia. Appropriate analgesia may include:

o A GTN spray for angina.
o A triptan medication for migraine.
o A splint for a fracture.

- o Drainage of an abscess.
- o Hyoscine for colic.
- o Diazepam for muscle spasm.

Having made an initial assessment, organised basic investigations and started emergency treatment there is time to learn detailed information about the person, the patient and the problem and examine the patient using standard methodology.

Ask yourself, does the patient have special needs?

Some patients have special needs. This could include "everyday" needs, such as wearing spectacles or a hearing aid, or more complex needs, such as being unable to understand or speak the language, a physical or learning disability, a mental health condition or a phobia. These needs may already be documented in the medical records or may be likely because of a known condition. For example, patients with Parkinson's disease or following a stroke are more likely to have difficulties with communication. When there may be a special need it is appropriate to ask and to find out what help they need. When a special need is likely to influence their care, learning and understanding about the person and their special need may be the initial focus of the consultation.

If a meaningful exchange of information is not possible, learning information from other family members or carers and the examination become the focus of the consultation.

Ask yourself, is their appearance consistent with what you would expect?

Physical appearance changes over time. The appearance of the face, hair and skin change as we get older: there is a tendency for muscle bulk to reduce, obesity to increase and skeletal changes, such as scoliosis, to progress. For many people these are "normal" changes. When the patient's appearance conforms to expectations, it does not influence the consultation. However, occasionally, such as when there is a mismatch between appearance and expectations, it may change the aims, focus and format of the consultation. For example:

- If a patient appears much "younger" or "older" than their chronological age it may be appropriate to learn more about them as a person and as a patient to assess their "biological" age.
- When a patient is unexpectedly dishevelled or dirty it may be appropriate to learn whether they have neglected themselves through choice or because they are very ill or live in difficult home circumstances.
- When a patient's clothes appear too big for them it may be appropriate to ask if they have lost weight.
- Some signs indicate underlying medical conditions. For example:
  - o A hemiplegic gait and facial palsy following a stroke.
  - o A barrel shaped chest and clubbing indicating COPD and emphysema.
  - o Sarcopaenia indicating carcinomatosis.
  - o A "pill-rolling" tremor is characteristic of Parkinson's disease.
  - o Yellow sclera are characteristic of jaundice.
  - o Coarse facial features are characteristic of acromegaly.
  - o Moon face and buffalo hump are characteristic of Cushing's syndrome.

If there is a suspicion, it may be appropriate to ask relevant questions or look for associated signs early on or when learning about the problem or examining the patient.

A patient's appearance should be interpreted with caution because first impressions can be misleading or lead to bias, inappropriately influencing the relationship or the care provided.

Ask yourself, is their affect and behaviour consistent with what you would expect?

It is normal to feel unhappy, anxious, reticent, wary or even slightly frightened when attending a consultation. In which case, learning about the person as part of a social conversation early in the consultation is an opportunity to relax the patient, to show you care and will try to help. When these feelings or emotions are profound, they may prevent a meaningful consultation. In which case, learning about the person may become the initial focus of the consultation (Figure 42).

However, some patients will only talk about personal thoughts and feelings when they trust the HCP and the timing and context are right.

Ask yourself, is their higher brain function consistent with what you would expect?

Higher brain function is the ability to think independently, to problem solve, generate hypotheses, to plan and make decisions, to remember, to reason, to communicate, to remain attentive, respond appropriately and co-operate. Conversation, behaviour, thinking and memory are proxy measures of higher brain function. When a patient manifests a short-term memory deficit, unusual changes in behaviour, such as swings in thoughts, thought processes and mood that are out of context, or the patient appears confused or delirious, having delusions (a certainty in false beliefs) or hallucinations (when sensations seem real but are not) their higher brain function is abnormal. When deranged higher brain function is suspected, learning about it becomes the initial focus of the consultation because it determines the reliability of information exchanged and whether consent can be valid. There are different ways to learn about higher brain function including:

- Learn information about the patient's lifestyle as a proxy measure of higher brain function. For example, are they able to live independently?
- Undertake a formal mental state assessment.

Figure 42: A figure to illustrate the initial focus of the consultation when building a working relationship with the patient is the principal aim of the consultation.

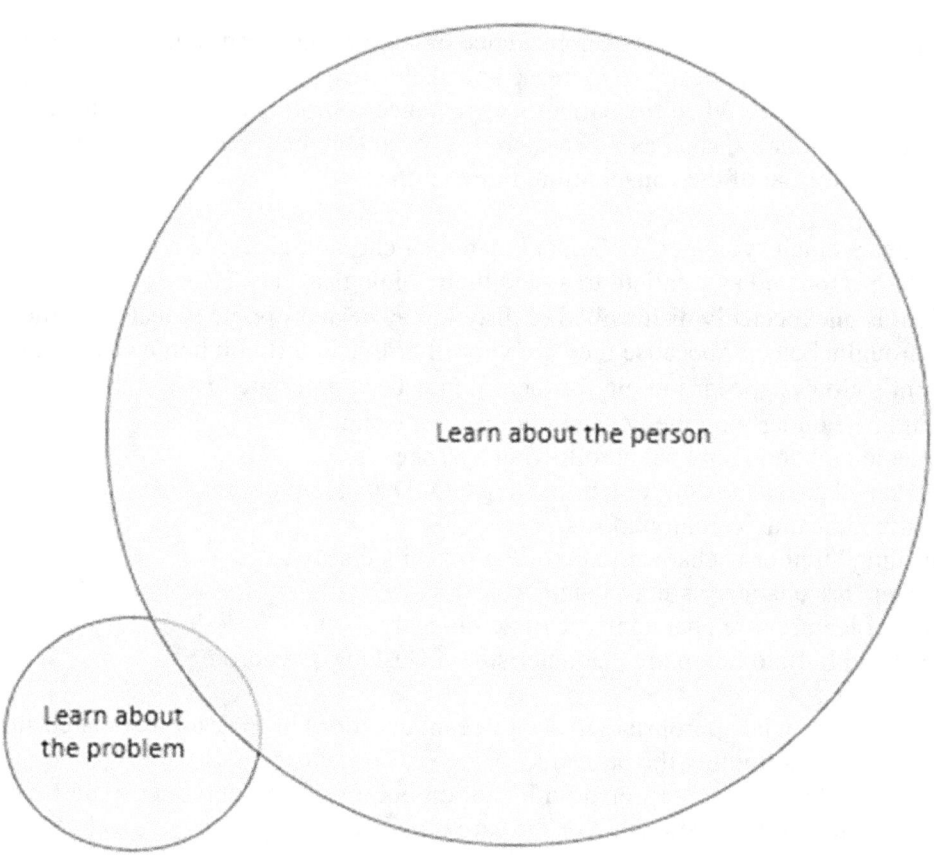

When higher brain function is so abnormal that it undermines the credibility of information from the patient it may be possible to learn information from other family members or carers. The examination may then become the focus of the consultation (Figure 43).

Figure 43: A figure to illustrate the focus of the consultation when higher brain function precludes a meaningful conversation.

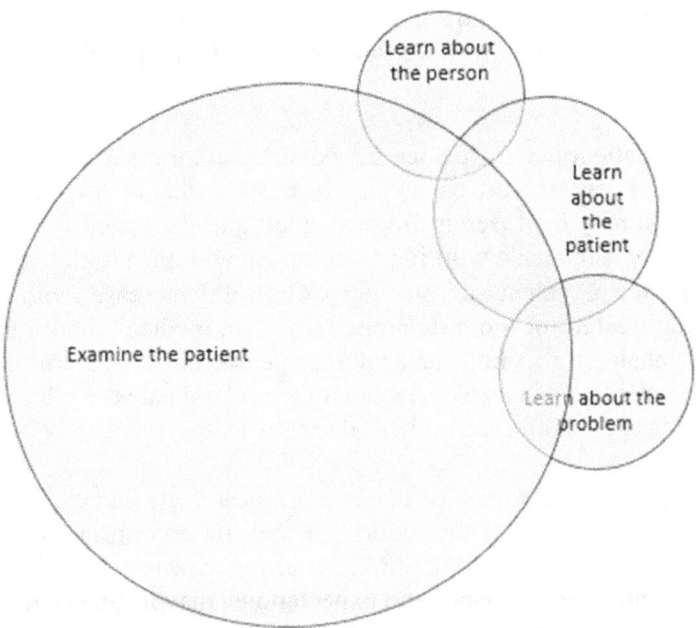

Use Background Medical Information to Determine the Initial Focus of the Consultation

Most patients expect their problem to be discussed first. After all, that is what they want help with. However, when there is limited background information or an extensive medical background, learning about the person and/or the patient may be the initial focus of the consultation both to contextualise the problem and because the information may be relevant to the diagnosis or management of the presenting problem (Figure 44). Frequently, learning about the patient leads to learning about the person and, in particular, learning the impact their medical conditions have on their lifestyle or functional performance.

Figure 44: A figure to illustrate the format of the consultation when a patient has either no co-morbidity or a complex medical background:

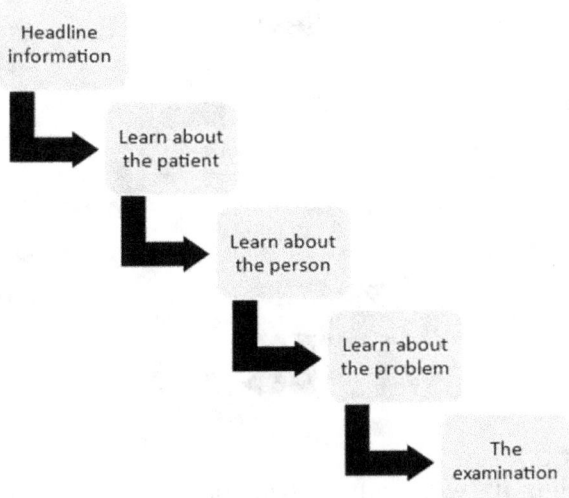

177

Use Demographic Information to Determine the Initial Focus of the Consultation

Demographic information, and age, gender and ethnicity in particular, is not only relevant to formulating a diagnosis and planning management but also influences how we talk, the tone the language used and may determine the initial focus of the consultation. For example:

- The age or gender of the patient may influence the conduct and the pace of the consultation, the initial focus and the questions asked, the way they are asked and the answers that are expected. For example, the conduct of a consultation with a child may be different from an adult and the initial focus in young children may be on learning about the person to establish a working relationship with the child, to gain their confidence.
- Age and gender influence the prevalence of morbidity. Morbidity increases with age so that two thirds of people aged >65 years are being treated for more than one long term medical condition. For example, taking insulin for DM, a salbutamol inhaler for asthma or azathioprine for ulcerative colitis. Conversely, the absence of medical conditions and risk factors in an elderly patient would indicate their "biological" age is likely to be less than their chronological age. Therefore, in older adults the initial focus may be on learning about the patient rather than about the problem.
- Lifestyle, occupation and family relations influence our hopes, fears and expectations and may be risk factors for disease. For some patients, such as the elderly, it may be appropriate to learn about the person before learning about the problem because lifestyle may be a proxy measure of their functional performance which, together with information about their wishes and expectations, may influence management options. For others, it can usually be assumed that any concerns will arise when discussing management.

Use the context to inform the initial focus of the consultation

The context is an important determinant of the aims, focus and format of the consultation.

When a patient presents with a new problem the principal aims are to exchange relevant information to formulate a diagnosis and plan management. The nature of the problem determines the initial focus of the consultation.

Figure 45: A figure to illustrate the focus and format when the patient presents with a new problem.

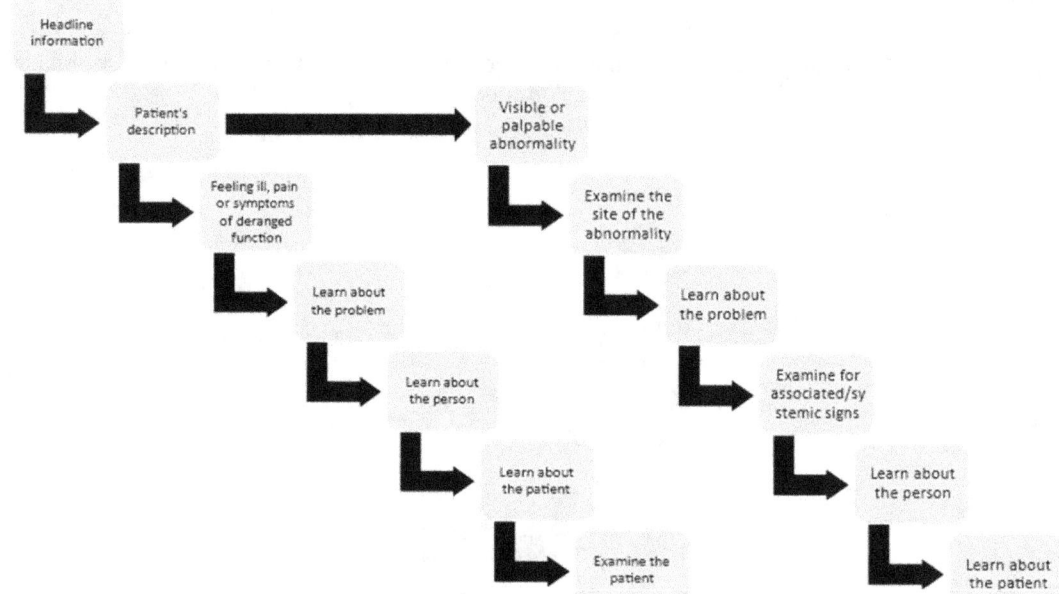

When the patient presents feeling ill, with pain or symptoms of a functional problem, the initial focus of the consultation is on learning about the problem and then, when indicated, on the examination.

When the patient presents with a visible or palpable abnormality, the initial focus is on examining the site of the abnormality and then on asking questions to learn about the problem. Usually, learning about the person and the person as a patient is undertaken later in the consultation when it is appropriate, such as to inform management planning (Figure 45).

When the consultation follows an investigation, a course of treatment or a previous consultation within a pathway of care, it is usual to start the consultation by checking the patient knows the reason for the consultation and to share information, such as the results of a test or to learn about any change.

When the consultation follows a screening investigation and the diagnosis is known, it is usual to start the consultation by ensuring the patient knows why the consultation is occurring and to share information about the screening test. This usually leads onto checking the patient is asymptomatic or examining the patient to look for relevant signs.

When the consultation is in response to a referral from another HCP the aims determine the initial focus of the consultation. For example:

- When a patient is referred to a cardiologist to formulate a diagnosis and plan management of a suspected cardiac abnormality, the initial focus is on learning about the problem to formulate a diagnosis, to plan management and inform the signs to look for.
- When a patient is referred to a surgeon and the diagnosis is known the initial focus is on learning about the person and the patient to plan management.
- When a patient is referred to an anaesthetist, the diagnosis and management plan are known, so the focus is on assessing their fitness for an operation and planning the anaesthetic.

Use the patient's description of their problem to inform the initial focus of the consultation

When the patient is being seen for a new problem or a change in a pre-existing problem, the patient's initial description of the presenting problem signposts the initial questions to ask or the site of the body to be examined (Figure 46).

When the main problem is a visible or palpable abnormality, such as a skin lesion, a deformity or a mass, an examination of the site of the problem is usually the initial focus of the consultation.

When a patient presents feeling ill, with a pain or symptoms of a functional problem, the patient's description will indicate the questions to ask to learn more about the problem. The patient will usually include a lot of information in their description. For example:

- A 65-year-old man may say "I suddenly developed severe chest tightness this morning".
- A 25-year-old patient may say "I have had a really uncomfortable headache for several days".
- An 80-year-old female may say "The ache in my knee when I walk has now become so bad that I cannot leave the house and spend most of my time sitting in a chair".
- A 50-year-old female may say "My abdominal cramps have got so bad over the last few months that I often have to lie down in bed".

Figure 46: Illustrating the pathway to learning the details of the problem.

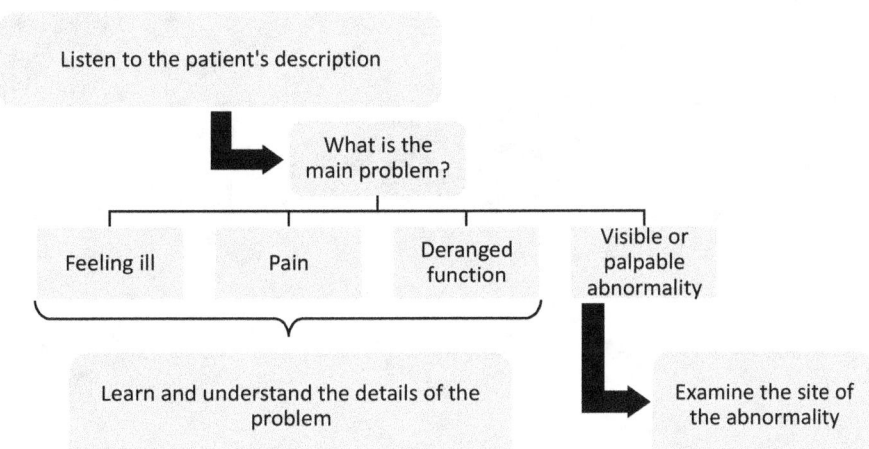

While listening to the patient's description ask yourself:

Are there any trigger symptoms, such as a pathognomonic symptom or a "red flag" symptom, such as unexplained weight loss?
Do the symptoms match a diagnostic pattern?
What is the differential diagnosis?

Trigger symptoms or a pattern signpost the questions to ask or signs to look for to confirm or exclude a likely diagnosis. For other patients the description, together with other headline information may indicate a differential diagnosis (Figure 47).

When the differential diagnosis is short, questions can be asked and signs sought to confirm or exclude individual diagnoses. When the differential diagnosis is long or uncertain, questions need to be asked and signs sought to learn and understand the details of the problem, to determine the location of the abnormality causing the problem, the type of problem and the likely cause to formulate a diagnosis or a list of possible diagnoses. While talking to the patient and examining the patient consider management options.

Figure 47: Illustrating how the patient's description can be used to formulate a diagnosis when a patient presents feeling ill, with a pain or with symptoms of deranged function.

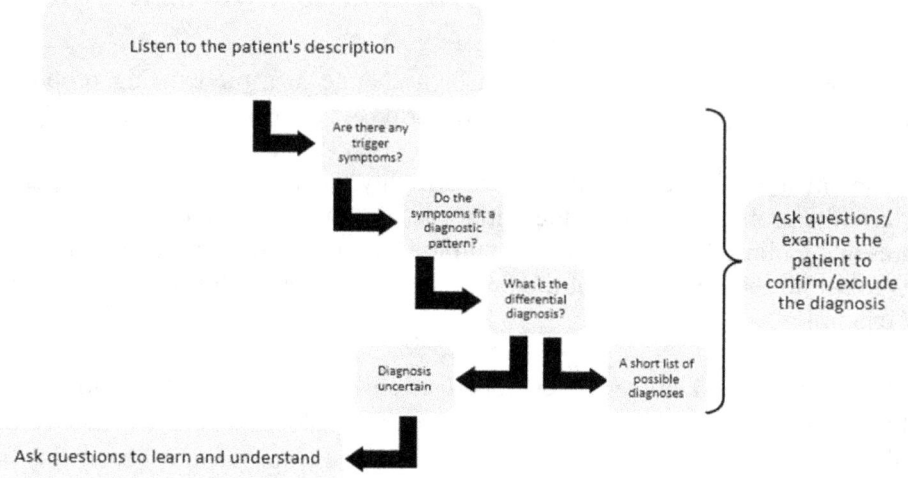

Chapter 6
Learn and Understand Information about the Person

Abstract

The consultation is an important opportunity to learn about the person. Indeed, it may be the only opportunity in a pathway of care that involves many investigations or different treatments. For most patients, learning about the person is undertaken as part of a "cosmetic" introductory conversation to give the problem an identity, to aid recall and to demonstrate an interest in the patient as a person with a problem and not just as a "complaint". Occasionally, there is an indication to learn more information about the person, which could include learning about their home, lifestyle and social circumstances, how they spend their time, their functional performance and capability, their quality of life, personal wishes, views and beliefs, hopes, fears and expectations.

Learning about the person is, by definition, personal to the patient and potentially intrusive. Therefore, relevant information should be learnt in context and when indicated to meet the aims of the consultation. The aims may include, to establish a working relationship, to assess the patient, to contextualise the problem, or to ensure management is appropriate and consistent with their wishes, views, needs, hopes and expectations.

Learning about the person starts with learning demographic information and background medical information before meeting the patient. Talking with the patient at the start of the consultation as part of an "everyday" social conversation, is not only a good way to introduce the consultation, helping the patient relax but also is an important part of learning about the person. First impressions are an opportunity to assess their appearance, behaviour and higher brain function in the context of known demographic and medical information. Most patients appear "normal" and appear to fit an expected socio-behavioural-psychological stereotype and it is unnecessary to learn detailed information about them as a person. However, learning more detailed information is indicated when their behaviour or appearance are different from expected, such as when their behaviour is challenging or there is concern about self-neglect or their diet, with the aims of establishing a working relationship, contextualizing the problem and informing management. Learning relevant details about the person may be indicated later, during the consultation, when learning about the problem, the patient or examining the patient to help formulate a diagnosis or to inform management.

In conclusion, learning about the person is an important part of the consultation which should not be undervalued or taken for granted.

Introduction

The good physician treats the disease; the great physician treats the patient who has the disease.

Sir William Osler

Learning about the person is an important and often undervalued part of the consultation. It is important, because patients are people with problems and not just a "complaint". Each person is unique and should be treated as such and should feel as though they are treated as such. It is undervalued because, traditionally, the emphasis has been on learning about the problem and examining the patient.

Learning about the person not only helps establish a working relationship but also is part of information exchange and may inform the diagnosis and management. For many people, this can be achieved with a short conversation, through verbal and non-verbal clues at the start of the consultation. For others, it is apparent, either at the start or during the consultation that there is a need to learn relevant additional information about the person.

The aim of this chapter is to discuss how learning about the person can inform the consultation.

Determine the Aims of Learning about the Person

The usual aims of learning about the person at the start of the consultation are to help the patient relax and to give the problem an identity, to aid recall. This also shows you respect them as a person with a problem and not just a complaint, which will help build trust and a working relationship. Later in the consultation, the aim of learning about the person may be to assess the impact the problem is having on the patient or to identify risk factors to help plan management. Occasionally, the aim is to inform the diagnosis or to help prioritise a list of possible diagnoses. In summary, the aims of learning and understanding information about the person include:

- Establish a working relationship:
  o To help the patient relax.
  o To give the problem an identity.
  o To reassure the patient that they will be treated as a person with a problem and not just as a "complaint".
- Information exchange:
  o To learn and understand relevant information.
  o As a baseline or background assessment.
  o To inform learning about the problem and the patient.
  o To inform the examination.
  o To inform sharing information with the patient.
  o To document relevant information.
- To inform management planning:
  o To ensure management is appropriate.
  o To ensure management is in context.
  o To assess:
    ▪ The impact on the patient.
    ▪ Future risk.
  o To help prioritise management.
  o To learn what the patient understands about their problem.
  o To increase the likelihood of adherence and compliance with future care.
- To contribute to formulating a diagnosis:
  o To inform the diagnosis.
  o To determine or exclude a cause.

Frequently, information about the person is a risk factor. In which case, relevant information should be documented with other risk factors.

Decide whether Learning about the Person is Indicated

Most patients fit an expected socio-behavioural-psychological stereotype and there is no indication to learn detailed personal information. In other words, their personal life is private and should remain private. Learning about an aspect of a person's personal life is indicated when it is relevant and likely to contribute to meeting the aims of the consultation or the pathway of care. For example:

- Learning about a person's occupational and domestic circumstances may be indicated to identify a cause for a problem, such as pollution as a cause for asthma.
- Learning about a person's occupational and domestic circumstances may be indicated to prioritise care.
- Learning about the impact a problem has on their lifestyle or quality of life may be indicated to help plan management.
- Learning about their functional performance or quality of life may inform decisions about management.
- Learning about their sex life is indicated in patients presenting with a sexually transmitted disease.
- Finding out a person's hopes, fears and expectations, such as their life expectation, may be indicated to inform management.
- Learning about their wishes, views and beliefs may be important when they may have firm religious, ethnic or cultural beliefs that may influence management.
- Learning about their hopes, fears and expectations may be important when considering benefit and risk.

Learning personal details is contraindicated if the patient does not want to talk about them or it is irrelevant to meeting the aims of the consultation.

Decide when to learn Information about the Person

There is no pre-determined time when the focus of the consultation should be on learning information about the person. First impressions and the introductory conversation may indicate it should be the initial focus of the consultation. For example:

- When there is a concern about a patient's higher brain function, such as their memory or recall, asking questions about their lifestyle early on may be used as a proxy measure and inform the reliability of the rest of the conversation.
- When there is concern the patient may live in a challenging environment, it may be appropriate to discuss this further when learning about the problem as it may be relevant to formulating a diagnosis or planning management.

For most patients, learning about the person is undertaken when the information may be relevant to the diagnosis or to planning management. In which case, relevant questions are asked in context. For example:

- When a risk factor for the problem includes lifestyle, it would be appropriate to learn about the person when learning about the problem.
- When the differential diagnosis includes causes associated with a patient's lifestyle, it would be appropriate to learn about the person when learning about the problem.
- When the patient is away a lot with their job, it may be appropriate to discuss this with the patient when planning management.
- When considering a challenging or risky management option or a choice between different management options, it may be appropriate to learn more about the person before making a recommendation.

Often, while listening to the patient it is also important to "listen to your own thoughts and feelings". It is not always clear why such thoughts or feelings occur. They may be hunch, a response to something the patient says, the way they say it, what they don't say or it could be their facial expressions or body language. Nevertheless, such thoughts and feelings should not be ignored because the patient may be signalling that they are thinking about an important relevant personal matter, such as a sensitive or embarrassing topic, a distressing experience or situation, such as domestic violence or sexual or physical abuse. Exploring such feelings by asking questions sensitively is usually indicated and should become the focus of the conversation at that time, because it is likely the patient is ready to talk and the opportunity may not arise again or be appropriate at another time.

Use Demographic Information to Inform the Consultation

Demographic information is part of our identity. Demographic information recorded in the medical record usually includes, age, gender, marital status, occupation, ethnicity, language and religion. It may influence the conduct of the consultation, such as the pace, language used, tone and content and may occasionally be relevant to the diagnosis and management options. Occasionally, learning more about an aspect of their demographic information is indicated. For example:

- To understand more about the impact of aging.
- To estimate biological age and life expectancy.
- To learn relevant information about their sex, gender identity or gender expression.
- To learn about their occupation or hobbies.
- To learn about help or support at home.
- To learn about their relationships.

Age

Age, is not just a number, it is a clinically relevant item of information that should be considered when learning about the person, the patient and the problem and when examining the patient. It impacts on the differential diagnosis, because the probability of a diagnosis is different in different age groups, and on management, because age effects many aspects of our life and attitude to life.

Chronological age is measured from birth whereas biological age is a measure of the accumulated impact life has had on the mind and body. As we go through life, our genes and metabolism change and physical, psychological and medical morbidities accumulate. Different parts of the body and different organs and systems age differently. This is generally known for cognitive function, power and mobility but also applies to organs and systems. For example, a patient's "immunological age" may be different from their "cardio-vascular age".

When learning about the problem:

Ask yourself, how does age inform the diagnosis?

Age is always relevant to the diagnosis because for many problems there is a tendency for some diagnoses to occur in some age groups and the probability of a diagnosis is different in different age groups. For example:

- A 16-year-old man with persistent severe bloody diarrhoea is likely to have colitis whereas an older patient could have cancer.
- A 22-year-old man with abdominal pain for 24 hours may have acute appendicitis whereas in an elderly patient acute cholecystitis or diverticulitis are more likely.
- A 25-year-old man presenting with a mass on his back is likely to have a sebaceous cyst or lipoma. In an older man the differential diagnosis includes seborrheic keratosis and cancer.
- Unilateral hip pain in a young adult may be caused by femoro-acetabular impingement syndrome, hip dysplasia or rheumatoid arthritis. As adults become more elderly the likelihood of a patient developing osteoarthritis increases and the likelihood of a new onset of rheumatoid arthritis reduces.
- A child presenting with a reducible groin swelling is likely to have a patent processus vaginalis, whereas in an adult it is likely to be an acquired inguinal hernia.
- An 80-year-old female feeling unwell with anorexia and weight loss increasing over the last few months is likely to have cancer, whereas a young person may have DM.
- The incidence of cancer increases exponentially after middle age.
- The incidence of some conditions, such as inflammatory bowel disease, breast cancer and Hodgkin's lymphoma are bimodal with a first peak among young adults and a second peak in the elderly.

When a patient's age is a risk factor, it should be linked with information about the patient.
When learning about the patient and the problem:

Ask yourself, how does age inform management?

Chronological age, biological age, life expectancy and life expectation all influence management. Biological age is a subjective estimate or a probability based on the influence of a number of variables on life expectancy. These variables include demographic information, wealth, address, environment, such as exposure to pollution, sanitation and clean water, lifestyle, occupation, hobbies, exercise, stress, sleep, diet, smoking, alcohol consumption, drug taking, and past and ongoing morbidities and treatments, such as DM or atherosclerosis. Chronological age is frequently used as a benchmark against which biological age is compared because estimating biological age is so subjective. When a patient's "biological" age appears to be less than their chronological age it may be said that "you look young for your age" or "you are fit for your age". Other patients, who are in a relatively poor physical or mental condition with significant or multi-morbidity, frequently look older than their chronological age.

In general, chronological age is used to estimate life expectancy and is a strong determinant of a person's life expectation, both of which will influence management. Life expectancy is the amount of time a patient may expect to live. In the UK, at birth, men can expect to live an average of 79 years and women an average of 82 years. The median life expectancy for males is about 82 years and for females about 85 years and the age at which most males die (the mode) is 86 years and for females 88 years (Figure 48). Statistically, the "predicted" life expectancy increases as we get older because some people in the population die at every age. However, for an individual, life expectancy is a probability rather than a true prediction.

Figure 48: Frequency of deaths for different age groups in a typical cohort of 100,000 in England and Wales (Derived from Office for National Statistics 2024). Age at death for the younger group has been excluded.

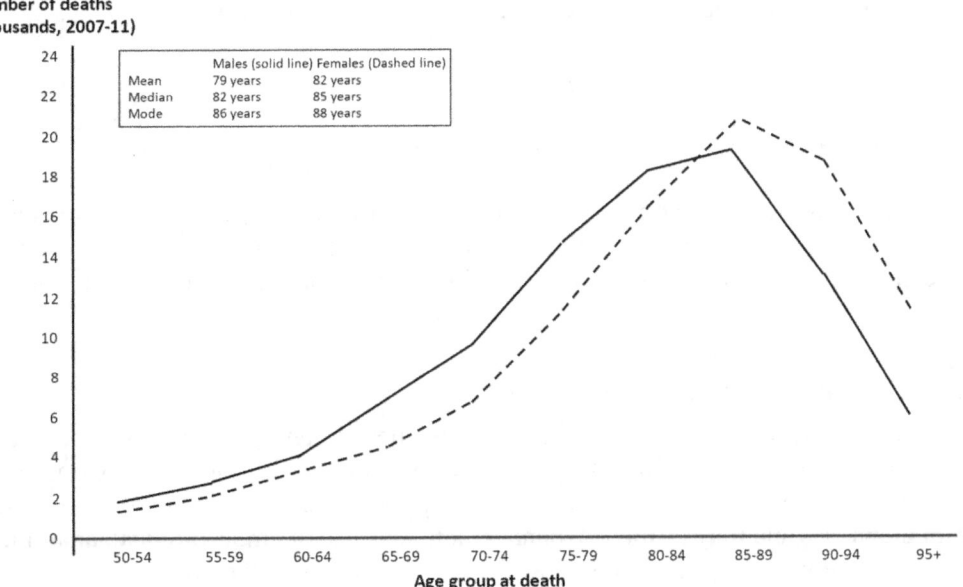

Both chronological and biological age are used to determine life expectancy and management.

Chronological age, biological age, life expectancy and life expectation all influence management in different ways, although biological age and life expectancy are more important than chronological age or life expectation. For example:

- Screening for cervical cancer is indicated in young women because the prevalence is high in this age group.
- In older woman the probability of a positive mammogram is increased because the prevalence of breast cancer increases with age.
- In a patient with a short life expectancy, such as an elderly patient, screening tests or prophylactic treatments are not usually indicated.
- A change in bowel habit is usually investigated with a colonoscopy, whereas a CT scan is indicated in an elderly patient who is unlikely to tolerate the preparation and the procedure.
- An operation on a child is likely to need a general anaesthetic whereas an adult may tolerate a local anaesthetic procedure.
- The choice of treatment may be influenced by age. For example:
  - A herniotomy is sufficient to repair a hernia in a child whereas a prosthetic mesh is indicated in an adult.
  - A young patient with cancer will often want aggressive chemotherapy in the hope of cure, whereas a patient who is elderly may prefer palliative treatment to alleviate symptoms rather than treatment aimed at cure.
  - In a young patient, with a long-life expectancy, radiotherapy may be contraindicated because of the risk of late complications.
  - The risk of an operation may be acceptable in a young patient but not in the elderly.
  - A risk from a treatment and the consequences of a complication are likely to be increased at the extremes of age when physiological resilience and tolerance are reduced.

When learning about the person, it may be appropriate to ask about life expectation. It may be appropriate to ask:

How long do you think you will live?
Have you ever considered how long you will live?
*Most people of your age, live till they are ** years old. Do you think you will live that long?*
*Most people with your condition live another ** years. Do you think you will live that long?*

Should they have an unrealistic expectation or are very pessimistic about their life expectancy this can be discussed. However, great care should be taken when discussing life expectancy, because it is a probability not a prediction. It is better to be approximate than to be wrong. For example, it may be appropriate to say:

You may live many [months/years] yet.
It is likely you only have a few [weeks/months] to live.
People of your age/with your condition can expect to live another [months/years]

While examining the patient:

Ask yourself, does age inform the examination or the signs?

Age per se does not usually affect the examination except at the extremes of age when the conduct of an examination is likely to be different. Occasionally, the aim of the examination is to assess function to inform an assessment of biological age. Conversely, information from the examination may inform an estimation of biological age or life expectancy.

Sex, gender identity and gender expression

Sex is a biological assessment based on the patient's chromosomes, organs and hormones. People can be born male, female, intersex or have an abnormal sex chromosome. When a person is born intersex; they are genetically male or female but have the reproductive or sexual anatomy of the opposite sex or are "mixed sex". Sex influences the probability of different diagnoses and may influence management because of embryological, anatomical, physiological and pathological differences between males and females. When learning about the problem:

Ask yourself, how does a patient's sex inform the diagnosis?

Differences between males and females may influence the location of the abnormality causing the problem, the type of problem and the diagnoses. Some diagnoses only affect males, such as prostate or testicular cancer and others only females, such as endometriosis, uterine fibroids, polycystic ovary syndrome or ovarian cancer. Sex also influences disease probability. For example:

- Breast cancer is much more common in women.
- In young boys the incidence of asthma is higher than young girls whereas in young adults the incidence is higher in females.
- Women are more prone to renal failure than men.
- Women are four times more likely to develop osteoporosis.
- Auto-immune disease is more likely in women.
- Males are at greater risk of sudden death from IHD than women.
- The incidence of AAA is higher in men.
- On average women live longer than men so many diseases of old age are more prevalent in women.
- The average age of women with IHD is ten years older than males.

When a patient's sex is a risk factor, it should be linked with information about the patient.
When learning about the patient and the problem to plan management:

Ask yourself, how does a patient's sex inform management?

Some investigations are dependent on the patient's anatomy. For example, a transvaginal USS or USS guided prostate biopsy. Some treatments are influenced by a patient's sex. For example, in a male, a breast lump likely to be gynaecomastia can usually be observed without treatment, radiation exposure is contraindicated in females who may be pregnant.
When examining the patient:

Ask yourself, how does a patient's sex inform the examination?

A patient's sex may influence the conduct of an examination not only because of anatomical differences but also because a chaperone is indicated when examining a patient of the opposite sex. Anatomical and diagnostic differences may also influence the focus and format of the examination and the signs to look for. For example:

- When a female presents with nodular hepatomegaly and ascites and cancer is suspected, the breasts should be examined to exclude a primary cancer.
- When a female presents with abdominal pain, a vaginal examination may be indicated to examine for a pelvic abnormality.
- In a male, a rectal examination may be indicated to examine the prostate.
- Excessive hirsutism in a female may indicate hypothyroidism.

When the patients gender identity or expression is different:

Ask yourself, does a patient's gender identity and expression inform the consultation, the diagnosis or management?

Gender identity is how the person thinks of themself, whereas gender expression is how the person expresses their gender through, for example, their behaviour or clothing. Non-binary, bi-gender or agender people don't clearly identify with either a male or female identity or are fluid between genders. A trans-gender person chooses to express themselves with an identity that is different from their sex. A patient may have transitioned from one sex to another at some point in their lives, be in the process of transitioning or planning to transition. They may change their appearance, clothing, name, pronouns or have had gender changing surgery and hormone treatment.

When the patient's gender identity or expression appears to be different from their sex it may be appropriate to ask questions about their gender identity early in the consultation because it may impact on the conduct and language of the consultation, such as what they want to be called, and may impact on the questions asked or signs sought on examination and on management. Incorrect assumptions are likely to adversely affect the working relationship. It may be appropriate to ask:

What would you like to be called?
Do you think of yourself as male or female?
How do you wish to be thought of?

Sexual orientation refers to the persons physical or emotional attraction to others. For example, they may describe themselves as "straight", "lesbian", "gay" or "bisexual". Sexual orientation may influence sexual behaviour and practices which may be relevant to the diagnosis. For example, practicing homosexuals are at increased risk of HIV infection.

A patient's close personal relationships

For most patients there is no indication to talk about their close personal relationships, long-term partners or marital status. However, occasionally it is relevant to planning management or the diagnosis, such as on the rare occasion when they are likely to need help with a management, such as a test or treatment, or when there is a suspicion of a significant interpersonal problem. It may be appropriate to ask:

Do you live alone or with someone?
Who do you live with?
Are you [single/married]?
Do you have a close partner or friend?
Does someone help care for you?
Do you have someone who can help you?

When learning about the problem:

Ask yourself, could the patient's close personal relationships inform the diagnosis?

In general, a happy marriage or long-term partnership and good relationships with friends and family is associated with better health, lower risk of morbidity, such as cancer or cardio-vascular disease and a longer life than being single or lonely. This difference is most marked in middle and old age and when divorced or single men are compared with married men. On the other hand, an unhappy marriage or partnership or being the victim of bullying, controlling or threatening behaviour, emotional, psychological, physical or sexual abuse will have an adverse effect on well-being and may be the cause of the presenting symptoms. Abused patients may present with a variety of symptoms including:

- Headaches.
- A mental health condition, depression, stress or an anxiety disorder.
- Disturbed sleep and fatigue.
- Unusual or a change in behaviour, such as being irritable, anxious, insecure, wary or suspicious.
- Low self-esteem: constantly checking with a partner and appearing to have lost their independence. Become isolated and detached from friends.
- Seizures.
- Atypical or unexplained fractures or bruising.
- Musculo-skeletal pains.
- Anorexia or an abnormal diet.
- Nausea, vomiting, weight loss and a change in bowel habit.

When physical abuse is suspected, asking additional questions away from their partner may be indicated. This should only be undertaken when it is safe to do so and there is sufficient trust. It may be appropriate to refer the patient to the appropriate authority or a specialist.

When learning about the problem to plan management:

Ask yourself, could the patient's close personal relationships affect management?

Discussing close personal relationships may be indicated when discussing management. For example:

- When the patient is likely to need transport to get to and from a hospital.
- When the patient is likely to need care at home following a treatment, such as following an operation.
- When the patient is likely to have difficulty maintaining family and social obligations, such as, providing child-care or caring for a disabled person.
- When the problem is infectious and close relations or contacts may need to be contacted.
- When the relationship or social behaviour risks spreading disease, such as HIV or a sexually transmitted disease.

While examining the patient:

Ask yourself, could the patient's close personal relationships affect the examination?

It is unlikely a patient's close personal relationships will affect the examination but when abuse is suspected an examination away from their partner may be indicated.

Ethnicity and race

Ethnicity refers to a group of people who share national, cultural, linguistic, racial or religious traditions, whereas race refers to people who share distinctive physical traits. Usually, a patient's ethnicity or race does not influence the consultation. However, occasionally ethnicity may be relevant to the diagnosis and management.

It is usually appropriate to ask someone about their ethnicity when it is a risk factor for a possible diagnosis. In which case, when learning about the problem to formulate a diagnosis:

Ask yourself, is a patient's ethnicity or race relevant to the diagnosis?

Race is unlikely to be relevant to the diagnosis, whereas ethnicity may affect the probability of a diagnosis, because some conditions are more prevalent in certain ethnic groups. For example:

- There is an increased likelihood of social deprivation in some racial and ethnic groups and this is likely to increase the risk of some diagnoses, such as DM or COPD.
- People of African and Mediterranean descent have an increased risk of sickle cell disease.
- Europeans have an increased incidence of cystic fibrosis.
- African-Americans have high rates of cardiovascular disease, whereas Asians have relatively low rates.
- African-Americans and Indians have high rates of stroke, whereas Asians have relatively low rates.
- Asian-Americans have higher rates of DM than white Americans.
- In general, ethnic minority patients have a lower prevalence of cancer.
- Crohn's disease and UC are more likely in Jews when compared to non-Jews.
- When gene-based knowledge is applied to an individual. Increasingly, gene-based knowledge is being used to predict the risk of a condition arising. However, a lack of ethnic and racial diversity in current genome association studies means that genetic knowledge is not universally applicable. This may affect the likelihood of diagnosing some conditions in some racial or ethnic groups.

When a patient's ethnicity is a risk factor, it should be linked with information about the patient.
When learning about the patient and the problem to plan management:

Ask yourself, does ethnicity or race inform management?

Ethnicity and race may influence the patient's wishes, views, beliefs, hopes, fears and expectations. In some countries, social inequalities between ethnic and racial groups influence health care use or provision, adherence or compliance with care. In addition, ethnicity may occasionally influence investigations, such as whether a sickle cell test is indicated, or treatment, such as when there are ethnic variations in genes responsible for drug metabolism.
While examining the patient:

Ask yourself, does ethnicity or race inform the examination?

It is unlikely the patient's ethnicity or race will inform the examination.

Occupation

Occupation not only refers to paid employment but also to unpaid employment, such as being a carer, and to hobbies or past-times. Giving the patient an opportunity to talk about how they spend their time following introductions is an informal way to learn about them as a person. Usually, how a patient spends their time does not influence the consultation. However, occasionally their occupation may be relevant to the diagnosis, management or to the examination. It may be appropriate to ask:

What is your job?
Do you have any hobbies or interests?

When learning about the problem to formulate a diagnosis:

Ask yourself, is a patient's occupation relevant to the diagnosis?

A patient's occupation may be the cause of the presenting problem. There are many conditions recognised as being caused by occupation. For example:

- Musculo-skeletal disorders, such as repetitive strain injury or carpal tunnel syndrome.
- Dermatitis.
- Respiratory conditions, such as asthma, COPD and pneumoconiosis, asbestosis and mesothelioma.
- Hearing loss.
- Infectious disease.

Many occupations are a risk factor for a condition. For example:

- Air pollution, such as coal dust or silicon is a risk factor for respiratory diseases, such as asthma, COPD or pneumoconiosis.
- Repetitive, heavy manual work or using vibrating tools is a risk factor for osteo-arthritis.
- Exposure to chemicals, asbestos and heavy metals are risk factors for poisoning or cancer.
- Stress and overwork are risk factors for depression.

When a patient's occupation is a risk factor, it should be linked with the problem and documented with other information about the patient.

When learning about the patient and the problem to plan management:

Ask yourself, is a patient's occupation relevant to management?

For most patients, how the patient spends their time does not influence the diagnosis or management except when their occupation is a risk factor for disease or when the problem impacts on their occupation. For example:

- A seizure or an AMI will affect a patient's ability to drive.
- Claudication will affect how far a patient can walk.
- Arthritis may affect a keyboard operator.
- Peripheral neuropathy or a tremor may affect a surgeon's dexterity or a pianist's performance.

For some patient's their occupation may influence the choice and timing of management, such as when organising an investigation for an off-shore worker or planning an operation for a soldier who may be deployed abroad.

While examining the patient:

Ask yourself, is a patient's occupation relevant to the examination?

A patient's occupation may inform the signs to look for on examination particularly if there is a concern they are at risk of a condition, such as COPD or asthma, or are exposed to a risk factor.

Use First Impressions to Inform Learning about the Person

The way a patient enters the room, moves, sits and talks should be observed from the start of the consultation and throughout the consultation. Potentially, a lot of information about the person can be learnt from their physical appearance, clothing and personal hygiene, their gait, movement, coordination and posture, and their voice. The patient's appearance should be assessed in the context of demographic information and lifestyle and, when possible, compared with how they were previously.

When the patient's appearance conforms to expectations it does not influence the consultation, but when there is a special need or a mismatch between appearance and expectations, it may be appropriate to sensitively ask relevant questions or look for signs relevant to meeting the aims of the consultation. At the start of the consultation:

Ask yourself, has the patient a special need?

When there is the possibility that the patient has a special need, it may be appropriate to learn more from the patient, or, when accompanied, the person they are with, about their needs early in the consultation. It may be appropriate to ask:

Do you have any special needs?
What help do you get?
What can you do yourself?
How can we help you?

This is likely to reassure the patient that their needs will be considered, inform information exchange, help establish a working relationship and inform management. Occasionally, it is relevant to the diagnosis.

Ask yourself, does the patient look their age?

Some patients appear to be younger than their chronological age whereas other patients appear older. In which case, learning more to estimate their biological age may be indicated.

Ask yourself, does the patient's appearance conform to expectations?

The clothes people wear and their personal hygiene is a personal matter and unlikely to be clinically relevant. However, occasionally it is relevant to the diagnosis or management and further enquiry is indicated. For example:

- Most patients ensure they appear respectable when attending a consultation, so, if they are dishevelled, they may be very ill. On the other hand, a proud elderly patient may dress smartly for the consultation despite personal difficulties or being very ill.
- If the patient appears to have neglected themselves it may be appropriate to ask questions to learn more about the person and in particular their home and domestic circumstances, because this may influence management. For example:
  o When a wound will need to be cared for.
  o When their appearance suggests there may be a problem, such as caring for a stoma, it may be appropriate to ask about arrangements at home, such as about their bathroom facilities.
  o When their appearance suggests social or financial difficulties that may affect compliance or adherence with management it may be appropriate to check when discussing management.
  Any questions should be asked sensitively, with empathy and understanding. It may be appropriate to ask:

Do you have any difficulties at home?
It must be difficult at home. Do you want to tell me about it?
Can you tell me about where you live?
Have you been finding it difficult to care for yourself?

- When a patient's clothes appear too big for them, they may have lost weight or vice versa. Weight loss may be intentional due to dieting but it may be unintentional and relevant to the diagnosis and management. It may be appropriate to ask questions to determine why they have lost weight.

Have you lost/gained weight recently?
Is your weight the same as it normally is?

- When a patient covers themselves inappropriately, they may be hiding a problem, such as bruises from domestic violence. It may be appropriate to examine them away from other family members.

Ask yourself, is the patient obese or anorexic?

When the patient's weight is outside the reference range and is likely to be relevant to the diagnosis or management it should be discussed. Sometimes it is appropriate to discuss their weight as an introduction to changing a life choice to prevent a future problem. Obesity or anorexia are associated with many different health problems. For example:

- Obesity may pre-dispose to DM, hypertension or NASH.
- Anorexia may be associated with deficiency of vitamins or trace elements.
- Rapid and significant weight loss may indicate an underlying problem, such as cancer or chronic inflammation.

Ask yourself, does the patient's physical appearance indicate a diagnosis, inform management or the signs to look for?

There are many aspects of a patient's physical appearance that may signpost the need to ask specific questions or look for signs. These include the way the patient walks and moves as they enter the room, their posture both standing and sitting, their movements and coordination, their skin, face and facial expressions, and their hands and hand movements. For example:

- Unilateral facial drooping may be caused by a stroke or Bell's palsy.
- Hair loss may be caused by hypothyroidism.
- Some patients in distress or pain move more carefully and adopt a posture that protects or reduces the use of the part affected. For example, an antalgic gait caused by an arthritic hip.
- Patients who are listless and their movements slow and laboured, as if everything is a great effort, may be feeling very unwell.
- How the patient walks and moves may give an initial impression of their overall fitness, highlight a deformity, an abnormal gait, movement or coordination.
- Involuntary movements may be caused by anxiety or old age but can also signify disease.
- A significant loss in height or skeletal deformity could be caused by osteoporosis.
- Restlessness may be caused by thyrotoxicosis.
- Involuntary twitching may be caused by hypercalcaemia.
- A fine tremor may be caused by anxiety, old age or chronic alcohol consumption and a "pill-rolling" tremor is characteristic of Parkinson's disease.

Similarly, the patient's skin and the appearance of the face and hands may be obviously abnormal. This may be relevant to the presenting problem or indicate the need to ask additional questions or look for additional signs as part of learning about the problem. For example:

- Skin turgor may reflect hydration.
- Skin colour may reflect:
  o The peripheral circulation, such as appearing flushed and sweaty from a fever,
  o A metabolic problem, such as appearing yellow in jaundice or sallow due to renal failure.
  o A malar flush due to mitral valve stenosis.
  o Petechial haemorrhage in thrombocytopaenia.
  o Cyanosis indicating a respiratory or circulatory problem.
  o Nicotine staining of the fingers from smoking tobacco.
- Deformity may indicate:
  o Arthritis from manual work.
  o Ulnar deviation of the fingers is characteristic of rheumatoid arthritis.
  o Permanently flexed fingers may indicate a Dupuytren's contracture.
  o Very long digits may suggest Marfan's syndrome.
- The hair and nails may indicate chronic ill health or a nutritional deficiency. For example, koilonychia may indicate iron deficiency anaemia and clubbing chronic illness.

When a patient's appearance is a risk factor, it should be documented with information about the patient.

Ask yourself, does the patient's voice indicate a possible diagnosis, inform management or the signs to look for?

When the patient talks, the sound of their voice should be assessed in the context of their demographic information and, when possible, compared with previously. The sound of the voice or a change in the voice may be relevant to the diagnosis. In which case it becomes part of learning about the problem. For example:

- A rasping gravelly voice may be caused by chronic smoking.
- Slurred speech may be due to a stroke.
- Loss of speech may be due to laryngitis.
- A hoarse voice may be caused by vocal cord paralysis, vocal cord polyps or cancer.
- A change in the pitch to a rough low-pitched voice may be caused by hypothyroidism.

Assess the Patient's Higher Brain Function

Normal conversation requires appropriate behaviour and cognitive function, including their attention and co-operation, appropriate response times, adequate short-term memory, the ability to problem solve, generate hypotheses and make plans and decisions. Anything that disturbs the central neuro-environment, such as a mental health condition, a brain injury, dementia or feeling ill may affect higher brain function and compromise the patient's ability to give a reliable account of their problem, to answer questions properly or to give informed consent. Early in the consultation it is important to assess the patient's higher brain function.

Ask yourself, is the patient's higher brain function sufficient for a meaningful exchange of information?

Lifestyle, occupation and social interactions supplemented with information from the medical records and the introductory conversation are proxy measures of higher brain function. In addition, there may be overt symptoms indicating a problem with higher brain function. For example:

- The patient may appear abnormally agitated. Agitation is abnormal when it is extreme, recurrent or persistent or associated with confusion and disorientation, disordered thinking and talking, irritability, restlessness, abnormal movements and sensations and unproductive activity.
- The patient may appear depressed. They may manifest an overwhelming feeling of sadness. This could include expressing suicidal thoughts or when learning about the person reveal withdrawal from social interaction or impaired performance at work.
- The patient may appear to have a depressed level of consciousness, impaired short-term memory, a reduced ability to concentrate, make decisions or think logically. They may feel less alert and have a reduced environmental awareness.
- The patient may appear confused or disinhibited. What they say may be disorganised, their thought processes, memory and decision making slow and illogical. They may be disorientated, finding it difficult to relate to people, places, objects or time. They may be unable to think ahead or to plan or to think of others.
- They may have abnormal thoughts, or describe beliefs and sensations that are dissociated from reality, including paranoia, delusions (a certainty in false beliefs) and auditory, visual or sensory hallucinations.
- They may have changed their behaviour. This may include:
  o Fatigue, lethargy and apathy.
  o Changed and changeable sleep patterns and daily routines.
  o Changed and changeable appetite and eating.
  o Taking risky substances.

A normal assessment indicates the conversation is likely to be meaningful, the information exchanged reliable and consent can be given. However, there is a lot of inter-personal variability in higher brain function, which can make assessment difficult. Minor changes may be caused by an illness, grief, overwork, stress or fatigue. Minor changes are understandable and likely to be temporary. However, changes are abnormal when they are disproportionate or extreme, out of context, unexplained or persistent. They can be unpleasant and distressing for both the patient and family.

When there are symptoms suggesting a problem with higher brain function then the focus of the consultation should be on learning more detail because an abnormal higher brain function may compromise the reliability of any information learnt. The questions to ask could include:

Do you feel you behave differently?
Has anyone commented on your behaviour or personality?
Has anyone noticed that your behaviour or personality has changed?
It may be appropriate to ask specific questions, such as:

Do you quickly forget things?
Do you have to write everything down because otherwise you will forget it?
Do you get lost?
Are there times when you feel confused?
Do you feel very sad?
Do you feel depressed/agitated/restless?
Does your mood swing from elation to depression?
Do you see or hear unusual things?

A formal assessment of higher brain function may be indicated.

The abbreviated mental test assessment.

- Orientation in time (1-5 points)
- Orientation in place (1-5 points)
- Repeat some key words (3 points). For example, "apple", "penny" and "table"
- Attention and calculation (1-5 points). For example, 7+7+7+7 etc, spell WORLD forwards and backwards
- Name some common items (2 points). For example, pencil, watch
- Speak back a phrase (1 point)
- Copy a shape (6 points)

A score greater than 24/30 is normal

Significantly abnormal higher brain function may undermine the reliability of the conversation and information from other family members or carers and the examination become important.

When learning about the abnormal higher brain function:

Ask yourself, does the patient's higher brain function inform the diagnosis?

When abnormal higher brain function is suspected, additional questions are indicated to identify a diagnostic pattern. For example:

- Depression is characterised by persistent or overwhelming unhappiness or sadness and fatigue and lethargy affecting everyday functions including work and social activity.
- Mania is characterised by extreme activity or agitation.
- Bipolar disorders are characterised by profound and sudden mood swings between depression and mania.
- Dementia is characterised by a progressive loss of cognitive function.
- Schizophrenia is characterised by dissociated thoughts and sensations.
- A personality disorder is characterised by extreme or atypical behaviour. For example, obsessive-compulsive disorder, exhibitionism, kleptomania or pyromania.
- A conversion disorder is characterised by altered or abnormal sensory or motor function in the absence of an organic cause. It may be manifest as abnormal movements, posture or gait or abnormal skin, visual or auditory sensations and, in the extreme, paralysis or coma.

For patients with swings or changes in mental health or a sudden onset it is appropriate to ask about precipitating or triggering factors, such as:

- An acute illness.
- Grief – for example, the death of a family member.
- Hormones – for example, menstrual cycle, post-partum.
- Stress and anxiety – for example, post-traumatic stress disorder, forthcoming exams.
- A serious illness – for example, viral infection or trauma.
- Medications.
- Risky substance use.
- Physical, psychological, domestic, financial, behavioural or sexual abuse.

Ask yourself, does the patient's higher brain function inform management?

A patient's higher brain function may influence management when:

- It is the presenting problem.
- It affects informed consent.
- It may affect adherence or compliance.

Ask yourself, does their higher brain function inform the examination?

When an abnormal higher brain function makes the information learnt during the consultation unreliable then a systematic examination may be indicated. A new onset of an abnormal higher brain function is likely to be an indication for a full neurological examination. However, except in an emergency, an examination should only be undertaken when the patient or a legal guardian is able to give informed consent.

Use Information about the Patient's Lifestyle to Inform the Consultation

Lifestyle refers to:

- How the patient spends their time. This could include their occupation, caring responsibilities or hobbies.
- Their home and social circumstances. This could include exposure to air or water pollution, access to sanitation and home facilities.
- Their diet.
- Their financial circumstances when it is likely to affect adherence or compliance, such as with treatment or travel to and from an investigation.

When learning about a patient's lifestyle is part of the introductory conversation the aims are to build rapport and to give the problem an identity. The questions to ask could include:

How do you spend your time?
What do you spend most of your time doing?
What do you do during the day?
Are you employed, retired or do you have other responsibilities?
Do you have any hobbies or interests?

It is preferable to ask how a patient spends their time rather than to assume they are employed because some are unemployed, retired or have domestic or social responsibilities that occupy their time. Usually, there is no need to learn additional information. However, occasionally when their lifestyle may influence the diagnosis or management learning more detail is indicated. For example:

- Learning about a patient's diet may be indicated when there is concern it is a possible cause for the presenting problem or when it may be a risk factor for future problems. A patient's appearance may be the trigger to discuss diet. For example, when a patient is obviously under- or over-weight it may be appropriate to ask questions about what they eat or to discuss referral to a dietician.

What sort of food do you eat?
Do you eat a wide range of foods?
Are there any foods you don't eat?
Do you take any food supplements, such as vitamins?

- When there is a concern air pollution may be causing their breathlessness, it may be appropriate to ask:

Where do you live?
Do you have an open fire at home?
Do you live near a busy road or regularly walk along a busy road?

- When there is a concern that the problem is caused by lead or arsenic poisoning it may be appropriate to ask:

How old is your house?
Do you have lead pipes?
Do you work a lot with lead?
Do you work with arsenic?
Do you have very old paint on the walls of your house?

Ask yourself, does the patient's lifestyle inform the diagnosis?

Occasionally a patient will mention something about their lifestyle that may be diagnostically relevant. Usually, learning about their lifestyle is indicated only when the differential diagnosis of the presenting problem includes a diagnosis that may be caused by their lifestyle. Examples when a patient's lifestyle may be risk factor include:

- When their problem may be caused by their diet, such as type II DM.
- When their problem may be caused by their occupation.
- When the problem may be caused by polluted water or poor sanitation, such as gastroenteritis or cholera.
- When the problem may be caused by air pollution. Pollution from NO_2 and PM2.5 particles is linked to many medical conditions, including respiratory, cardio-vascular and inflammatory diseases and to mortality.
- When the patient may have been poisoned by chemicals or metals, such as arsenic, lead, thallium, cadmium, mercury or copper.

When a patient's lifestyle is a risk factor, it should be included with information about the patient.

Ask yourself, does the patient's lifestyle inform management?

A patient's lifestyle may affect management in a number of ways.

- It may expose them to risk. For example:
  o Exposure to ionizing radiation, such as radon in the home.
  o When their diet may put them at risk of a deficiencies such as pellagra (niacin deficiency) or beriberi (thiamine deficiency).
- A patient's lifestyle may also be used as a proxy measure of performance status and influence the choice of management. For example, a patient is likely to be fit:
  o When the patient works in a physically demanding occupation.
  o When the patient has a physically active hobby or plays sport regularly.
  o When the patient is a full-time carer.
- A patient's lifestyle may influence their health awareness and engagement with health care. A positive attitude is not only associated with better health and longevity but also a better outcome following treatment.
- A patient's occupation may affect the timing of management, such as when it takes them away for long periods.
- Some patients live in difficult circumstances that may affect management, such as managing a stoma or a wound.
- Some patients need help with their daily life, such as getting dressed or undressed, cooking or having a wash. Many patients living with chronic health problems, disability or a mental health condition manage remarkably well in their own environment with their normal support. However, this may be upset by management planned.
- A patient's financial circumstances may interfere with management. For example, being unable to afford treatment or transport.

Ask yourself, does the patient's lifestyle inform the examination?

The patient's lifestyle is unlikely to inform the examination unless it is relevant to the diagnosis. The signs to look for will be determined by the nature of the problem.

Use Information about the Patient's Quality of Life to Inform the Consultation

In general, quality of life is a measure of wellness. Feeling well and thriving, with a good quality of life is important to all of us. The individual is the judge of their quality of life, not the HCP or an external standard.

The introductory conversation and first impressions not only demonstrate an interest in the patient as a person but may also give an insight into their quality of life. For most patients this is sufficient. However, occasionally learning more detail is indicated with the aim of assessing the impact of the problem on the patient. This not only show's empathy and helps build a working relationship but also may be a measure of severity and may influence management. It is unlikely to help formulate a diagnosis or the examination. When learning about a problem, it may be appropriate to ask:

How are you affected?
How does the [problem] affect you?
This must be very difficult for you?
This is a lot for you to cope with?

Sometimes it is appropriate to compare the present with the past. The questions to ask could include:

How has your life changed?
What were you like before?
What could you do before?
What do you miss most?

It may be appropriate to ask specific questions in context about the impact on their relationships, home or work circumstances, personal development, mental health, independence, hobbies and spare time activities, physical, psychological or financial wellbeing. For example:

How does [the problem] make you feel?
You are probably finding this very stressful?
I expect this has meant you have had to change a lot of things?
I expect you are finding it very difficult not being able to [walk/drive/work]?

There are many questionnaires available to "objectively" estimate life quality. Usually these are used in research studies or to assess change and they should be applied to the individual with circumspection, because, clinically, the individual is the judge of their quality of life, not a scoring system or the HCP.

When learning about the patient and the problem to plan management:

Ask yourself, does the patient's quality of life inform management?

Frequently a problem impacts on patient's quality of life. For example:

- A seizure or an AMI, preventing the patient from driving causing them to not only lose their independence but also their job.
- Arthritis, angina or claudication preventing the patient from doing exercise, such as walking with their wife, or their job.
- Cervical spondylosis or carpal tunnel syndrome affecting a hobby, such as playing a piano or computer games.
- Not leaving the house because of the risk of incontinence.
- Pain may affect a patient's quality of life in many ways. For example, stopping the patient from undertaking activities they enjoy or from sleeping at night.
- Disability and dependence leading to low self-esteem and guilt.
- The condition may prevent the patient from achieving life goals and aspirations.
- The nature of the symptoms, such as a new onset of rectal bleeding or thoughts about a possible diagnosis, such as cancer, may cause profound anxiety.

Learning about a patient's quality of life indicates the impact a problem is having on the patient. This may be a proxy measure of severity and be used to inform risk benefit and the priority of management.

There are many factors that may influence the impact a problem has on a patient's quality of life including:

- The nature of the problem. Some symptoms, such as chest pain or breathlessness, have a greater impact on a patient than others, such as mild weakness or a change in bowel habit, because they are recognised alarm signals.
- Its severity. More severe symptoms tend to have a greater impact on a patient's quality of life than mild symptoms.
- The speed of onset or the duration. More acute symptoms tend to have a greater impact on a patient's quality of life than symptoms that have been present a long time and the patient has had time to adjust their lifestyle.
- Treatment.

- Responsibility. A problem caused by someone else may affect a patient's quality of life more than if it was self-inflicted.

A patient's quality of life may affect their assessment of benefit and risk. For example:

- When the patient's current quality of life is so poor that they are prepared to accept significant risks rather than stay the way they are.
- When a complication is likely to significantly adversely affect their quality of life, a patient may prefer to live with their symptoms and debility rather than risk an investigations or treatment.
- Many patients, particularly the elderly, worry more about how an illness, investigation or a treatment will affect the quality of life of a carer or family member, than of the outcome for them.

When quality of life is affected by the presenting problem, treatment is likely to result in an improvement. When it is dependent on other factors, such as obesity and mobility, changing a life choice may lead to an improvement. Treatment may be aimed at improving a patient's quality of life rather than treating the underlying problem. Occasionally, such as for patients with chronic or terminal conditions, specialist interventions may be indicated.

Use Information about the Patient's Functional Performance and Capability to Inform the Consultation

Functional performance describes the ability to undertake expected activities of everyday life. This can range from activities of everyday living, such as getting washed and dressed, to complex physical or mental work, such as those required of a surgeon. Talking with a patient about what they do with their time, their occupation, hobbies or exercise during the introductory conversation not only demonstrates an interest in the patient as a person but also is a proxy measure of their functional performance.

For most patients, their functional performance does not influence care and this early check is sufficient. However, when a clinical problem, such as breathlessness, arthritis, angina or claudication or faecal or urinary incontinence, is likely to impact on a patient's functional performance learning more is indicated with the aims of assessing the impact of the problem on the patient, to inform the benefit-risk balance, compliance with management, management choice and may influence the examination. It is unlikely to inform formulating a diagnosis. The questions to ask could include:

How do you spend your time?
What do you do during the day?
What is your job?
Do you have any hobbies or interests?
Can you climb up a flight of stairs?
Are you able to walk up a hill?
Can you work in the garden?

Patients with a sedentary lifestyle can be difficult to assess. For example, a patient who stays in their house through choice could have significant ischaemic heart disease yet have no symptoms because they do not exercise enough to induce angina. It may be appropriate to ask:

What stops you from doing more?
Why don't you do more?
Could you do more if you wanted to?
What would happen if you [...]?

When listening to the answers it is important to distinguish between current performance and past performance. It is not uncommon to be told by the patient what they could do previously rather than what can be done now.

Objective assessments may be indicated to measure performance against a standard or to provide a baseline assessment prior to an intervention. This could include watching a patient walk or climb stairs or by using a scoring system.

> Objective measures of function
>
> - The UK Functional Independence Measure (FIM). This scores essential daily activities including Selfcare, Sphincter control, Mobility, Communication, Psychosocial and Cognition on a score from 1 when total assistance is needed to 7 when fully independent.
> - Frailty scoring
> - Mental test scoring
> - Cardiac and pulmonary exercise testing
> - Pulmonary function tests
> - Cardiac "stress" tests, such as an exercise ECG

Ask yourself, how does their performance affect management?

A patient's functional performance may influence management. When functional performance is limited, it may increase the risk of a treatment, such as an operation. In which case, it is important to discuss the risks and benefits with the patient and consider whether their performance can be improved. When the functional performance is dependent on changing a life choice, the impact on risk likelihood or treatment options may be a motivation for the patient to change. If not, a limitation on treatment options may reduce the indications for investigations. For example, it would be inappropriate to subject a patient to an investigation to plan treatment when such a treatment is contra-indicated. Functional performance may also affect adherence and compliance. For example, a patient with limited mobility may not be able to attend an early appointment or a patient with an intention tremor may not be able to administer eye drops.

Ask yourself, does the patient's performance status affect the examination?

For some patients, the examination is an opportunity to assess functional performance. Usually, this is limited to observing the patient undertake simple tasks such as walking along a corridor or climbing a flight of stairs. Occasionally, signs, such as blood pressure, heart or respiratory rate may give additional information.

Use Information about the Patient's Wishes, Views and Beliefs to Inform the Consultation

For most patients their wishes, views and beliefs conform to expectations and can be assumed or confirmed by asking a few questions.

Is it OK if I organise [investigation]?
We recommend [treatment], is that alright with you?

It may become apparent while talking to the patient that they appear to know a lot about their problem or their wishes, views and beliefs about their problem or the care they want are likely to be different from what would be recommended. In which case, it may be appropriate to ask questions to learn more.

Have you thought about what [management] you want?
Can you please tell me what you think we should organise/do?

Ask yourself, how does the patient's wishes, views, and beliefs influence information exchange or management?

The aims of learning the patient's wishes, views and beliefs are to understand what is important to the patient to establish a working relationship and inform information exchange and management and to avoid potential future disappointment or upset. It is unlikely to influence the diagnosis or the examination. If the patient's wishes, views and beliefs are respected, management is more likely to be accepted and adherence and compliance with future care more likely.

A management option is usually only recommended when it is indicated to meet the aims. Many are derived from guidelines or are the recommendation of an MDT. Occasionally, the recommendations do not conform to a patient's wishes, views or beliefs. For example:

- Some patients do not want a particular investigation, such as a colonoscopy, or a treatment, such as chemotherapy, because they or a friend previously had an unpleasant experience or they are frightened of what is involved or the adverse effects.
- Some patients want a certain test or treatment, such as one they have read about previously or has been recommended by a friend. This may be inappropriate or contra-indicated.
- Some patients believe in "alternative" treatments or "natural" treatments, such as herbal or holistic remedies.
- Some patients have pre-determined views on their care; what treatment they want or do not want or limitations to their treatment. For example:
  o Patients dying from cancer or end stage organ failure may want palliative care rather than be subjected to investigations or treatment.
  o Some patients make advanced directives, stating they do not want to be resuscitated should they have a cardio-pulmonary arrest or have agreed a "treatment escalation plan".
  o A Jehovah witness will refuse any blood products.
- Occasionally, a patient's wishes, views and beliefs may affect their assessment of benefit and risk. For example:
  o When their current quality of life is so poor that they are prepared to accept significant risks rather than stay the way they are.
  o Some patients want symptom relief to improve their quality of life rather than treatment to increase longevity.
  o Some patients do not want a particular investigation or treatment because of the risks.
  o Some patients have an overly optimistic opinion of the likely benefit.

When a patient wants a management option that is not indicated, it may be appropriate to ask:

Why do you want [investigation/treatment]?
What makes you think [investigation/treatment] is right for you?

When a patient wants management that is not indicated or refuses management that is indicated and recommended and likely to be beneficial, this will need to be discussed carefully with the patient and the discussion and outcome documented to ensure there is no misunderstanding and that their views are respected. It may be appropriate to ask:

A [investigation] is the recommended investigation; can you please tell me why you do not want one?
This would normally be treated by [treatment]. Why do you not want [treatment]?

Use Information about the Patient's Hopes, Fears and Expectations to Inform the Consultation

For most patients their hopes, fears and expectations will conform to expectations. For example:

- Most patient's hope/expect to be helped, for a treatment, a good outcome or a good prognosis.
- Most patient's hope/expect to continue to work, play a sport or live independently.
- It is not uncommon for patients to have talked to other people or read about their problem and be scared about medical care or the outcome.
- Many patients have expectations about the treatment they will get, what the investigation or treatment will involve, the care they will receive or the outcome, such as their life expectancy, future functional performance or future quality of life.

Occasionally, a patient will have individual, more personal, hopes, fears or expectations. For example:

- A patient, may hope/expect to go to a wedding or live until the birth of a grandchild.
- The patient may be frightened they have cancer, about having to be injected with a needle or to come into hospital.

- A patient may have inappropriate or unrealistic expectations about the accuracy of an investigation or the efficacy of a treatment.

Similarly, the HCP will have their own personal, hopes, fears or expectations. For example:

- An HCP may focus on an outcome such as mortality or morbidity.
- An HCP may focus on life expectancy whereas a patient is frightened of losing their independence.

Hopes, fears and expectations are influenced by many factors including, demographic information, such as age and marital status, past experience and family medical history, psychological factors, the influence of media, lifestyle, quality of life, social support and friendships, religious beliefs, emotional, social and cultural opinions and personal values. Asking questions to learn about a patient's hopes, fears and expectations, and what is behind them, is indicated when it may influence care. The aims are to understand what is important to the patient, to establish a working relationship and inform management and prognosis and to avoid potential future disappointment or upset. It is unlikely to influence the diagnosis or the examination. The questions to ask could include:

What do you want?
How do you want to be helped?
What do you hope for?
What do you expect to happen?
What concerns you most?
What would be a good outcome/result?
What would be a bad outcome?
What worries you most?
What are your expectations?
Did you expect something else?
Is that what you expected?

More specific questions to ask are likely to be determined by the context. For example, when it is appropriate to learn more about a patient's life expectation the questions to ask could include:

How long do you hope to live?
What age would you like to live to?
Are your parents still alive? If not, *how old were your parents when they died? Do you think you will live as long?*
Do members of your family tend to live to an old age?
What would be a good age to live to?
Have you ever thought about when you might die?

Ask yourself, how does the patient's hope, fears and expectations influence management?

It is not uncommon for management to be influenced by a patient's hopes, fears and expectations. For example:

- An investigation may be undertaken to reassure a patient, such as when they are frightened that they may have cancer.
- A preliminary visit to the hospital may help reassure a patient who is frightened about going into hospital.
- Ask them how they can be helped if they have a phobia, such as agoraphobia or claustrophobia, or of needles. A lot of reassurance may be indicated or mitigating measures put in place.
- Patients may need re-assurance from friends or family when they are frightened that they will be an imposition on others.
- More information may be required by patients who are frightened about an investigation or treatment, who have inappropriate or unrealistic expectation, such as when an investigation will occur, a treatment started, the duration of treatment or the time to recover, or are unrealistically optimistic about the prognosis or their life expectancy.

It is important to ensure the patient's expectations align with what is likely because the patient's expectations are the benchmark against which the patient measures the HCP, the consultation and the outcome. For example:

- A patient may expect a cure, yet the only treatment available is to relieve symptoms.
- A patient may inappropriately expect to live many years.
- A patient may incorrectly believe a procedure is without risk and challenge.

A mismatch between a patient's hopes, fears and expectations and the reality should be managed to ensure the patient is informed and to avoid future misunderstanding. Managing expectations is the responsibility of the HCP but the consequences affect the patient and future care. If their hopes, fears and expectations are not aligned with reality they may be very disappointed.

Chapter 7
Learn and Understand Information about the Person as a Patient

Abstract

Most patients are fit with few medical conditions so asking about their medical background and safety concerns is undertaken as a quick check to ensure nothing relevant is missed and to complete the medical record. However, in some patients, such as those with a complex medical background, learning detailed information is indicated. Background medical information and safety concerns should always be documented, if only to record their absence.

Learning about the person as a patient includes asking questions about their previous and ongoing conditions and treatment, safety concerns and risk factors and preventative treatment. The medications the patient is taking should be listed separately in addition to being linked to the medical condition. Safety concerns include previous allergic reactions, non-allergic adverse reactions, infection risk to the patient or to others and bleeding or thrombosis risks.

The main aim of learning about the person as a patient is to inform management. Occasionally, it may help formulate a diagnosis, such as when the presenting problem could be a deterioration or a complication of an ongoing condition, an adverse reaction to treatment or a relapse or recurrence of a previously treated condition. Risk factors may influence the likelihood of a problem occurring, the differential diagnosis or likely cause. In addition, a patient is reassured when they know that the HCP is aware of their medical background and any safety concerns.

In conclusion, learning about the person as a patient is essential to understand the impact of background medical problems on the patient, to contextualize the problem and to ensure management can be undertaken safely.

Introduction

Learning about the person as a patient is an important part of the consultation. It helps establish a working relationship, reassuring the patient that the HCP knows about medical problems, informs management and may inform the diagnosis.

"Learn from yesterday, live for today, hope for tomorrow. The important thing is not to stop questioning"
Albert Einstein

Traditionally, in the section "past medical history" there was no distinction between previous and ongoing medical conditions or pre-disease states. Treatments were listed under the heading "drug history" and safety concerns were confined to listing allergies. This is no longer adequate. Many patients live with ongoing medical conditions that are managed but not cured. These should be distinguished from past conditions that are cured and are genuinely "past medical history" and are unlikely to be relevant to the presenting problem or patient care, and "pre-disease" states, that patients are at risk of, or likely to get in the future. Many different treatments are available, not just medications, and many treatments are used to treat a range of different conditions. Furthermore, an increasing number of patients are receiving preventative treatments or awaiting treatment. To avoid uncertainty, the condition and the treatment should be linked, in addition to listing current medications separately.

The meaning of taking drugs has changed. It is now widely used to describe risky substance use, including taking illegal substances. Therefore, the term medication should be used. Safety information includes not only a previous allergic reaction but also non-allergic adverse events and infection, bleeding or thrombotic risks. Ideally, the allergen should be specified together with a description of the allergic reaction, to validate the safety concern and as a measure of risk. Traditionally, drug taking and other potentially risky activities, such as drinking alcohol, smoking, taking supplements or eating an unusual diet were considered "personal and social" activities and included under the heading "personal and social history". Similarly, learning about hereditary diseases was considered under the heading, "family medical history". However, these are all risk factors for disease and should be discussed when learning about the patient and documented with other risk factors.

The aim of this chapter is to discuss the information to include when learning about the person as a patient and how this information can be used to help meet the aims of the consultation.

Determine the Aims of Learning about the Person as a Patient

Learning and documenting information about the patient is an important part of information exchange. The principal aim is to inform management planning, to ensure it is safe. In some patients, an aim is to inform formulating a diagnosis or prioritising a list of diagnoses. Occasionally, the aim is to reassure the patient that their medical background and safety concerns are known and being considered when caring for them. This is likely to help the working relationship and compliance and adherence with care. In summary, the aims of learning about the patient include:

- To exchange information:
  - To put the problem in context.
  - To learn and understand background medical information.
  - To understand the impact on the patient.
  - To document relevant information.
- To inform management planning:
  - To ensure management is safe and appropriate.
  - To ensure management is in context.
  - To prioritise management.
  - To assess:
    - The impact on the patient.
    - Future risk.
- To inform formulating a diagnosis:
  - To formulate or exclude a diagnosis.
  - To identify or exclude possible causes.
  - To prioritise a list of diagnoses.
- To help build a working relationship:
  - To reassure the patient.
  - To learn what the patient understands about their background medical information.
  - To increase the likelihood of adherence and compliance with future care.

Decide Whether Learning about the Patient Is Indicated

Learning important details about the patient, such as about ongoing medical problems, medications and safety concerns, is always indicated. However, there is no indication to learn about everything that has happened in the past. For example:

- Learning about an adult's vaccination history is rarely indicated. It is usually assumed that they received the normal vaccinations.
- Learning about the occasional previous infection, such as a viral illness or a skin infection is rarely indicated.
- Learning about a minor and well recognised medication adverse effect that is unlikely to change management is not indicated.
- Learning about a minor complication, such as thrombo-phlebitis at the site of an intravenous infusion is unlikely to be relevant to future care.

When to Document Information about the Patient

In general, information should be documented at the end of the consultation to avoid disrupting the flow of the conversation. However, it may be appropriate to document information about the patient contemporaneously because some information, such as lists of medications, the dose, frequency and mode of administration may be forgotten or prone to a transcription error.

Decide When to Learn about the Patient

The consultation should be managed flexibly. There is no pre-determined time when the focus should be on learning about the patient. The medical records and the introductory conversation will often indicate whether it is appropriate to learn about the patient early in the consultation or later, at an opportune time. If, as is often the case, there are no significant medical conditions, learning about the patient early on is simply a check for reassurance and the rest of the consultation can then focus on the problem. For example, it may be appropriate to ask early in the consultation:

Can I just check you have not had any significant medical problems?
Do you have any medical problems at the moment or are you awaiting an investigation for a medical problem?
Are you taking any medications or awaiting any treatment at the moment?

On the other, hand, when a patient has a complex medical background or when learning specific information about the patient is the aim of the consultation, such as to assess the response to treatment, learning detailed information about the patient at the start of the consultation may be indicated. When a patient presents with a new problem, learning about the patient is frequently undertaken after learning about the problem or, when the new problem is a visible or palpable abnormality, after examining the patient.

Learn and Understand Safety Information

Questions should be asked to learn and document any and all relevant safety information. The principal aim is to inform management planning, to ensure management is safe and appropriate. Occasionally, the aim is to inform formulating a diagnosis, to identify possible causes or to reassure the patient. The safety concerns to specifically consider in every patient include:

- A previous allergic reaction.
- A previous non-allergic reaction.
- An infection risk to the patient or to others.
- A bleeding risk.
- A thrombosis risk.
- In some patients there are additional safety concerns. For example:
  - Pregnancy.
  - Special needs, such as very fragile skin or bones.
  - An unstable cervical spine.

Usually, infection, bleeding or thrombosis risk and additional safety concerns only become apparent when learning about previous or ongoing medical conditions and treatments or when learning about the person or the problem. Occasionally, a check is indicated prior to recommending a management option.

Previous allergic reactions

Allergies are caused by the immune system reacting to an allergen, such as pollen, animal dander, mould, household chemicals, shellfish, nuts, gluten, insect bites, latex, or medications, such as penicillin or angiotensin converting enzyme inhibitors. They affect 1 in 4 people and are becoming more common. The consequences of an allergic reaction can be severe so it is essential that patients are specifically asked whether they have had a previous allergic reaction and the answer is clearly documented.

> **Information about previous allergic reactions is the most important safety information to document and consider when planning management**

The risk of an allergic reaction is determined from the medical records and by asking the patient. Patients more susceptible to allergens include:

- Children.
- People who have had an allergic reaction.
- When other family members have an allergy.
- Patients with a complex medical background.

The questions to ask could include:

Have you had an allergic reaction?
Are you allergic to anything?
Do you have any allergies?

It may be appropriate to ask about specific common allergens such as iodine, latex or medications.

Are you allergic to [iodine]?

When a patient states that they have had a previous allergic reaction:

Ask yourself, was it a genuine hypersensitivity reaction?

Questions should be asked about the reaction to confirm it was a hypersensitivity reaction and to determine the likely allergen, severity and type of reaction. For example:

What happened?
What were the symptoms and signs?
What was the reaction?
How severe was it?
What treatment was necessary?
How long did it last?
What caused it?
How quickly did it start?
Were there any lasting effects?
Who told you it was an allergic reaction?

When the allergic reaction occurs within seconds or minutes of exposure to an allergen it is a type I hypersensitivity reaction mediated by Immunoglobulin E (Ig E). The symptoms can be minor, such as a wheeze or a feeling of choking, widespread itching and a pale or red blotchy rash ("hives") or severe and life-threatening such as angio-neurotic oedema or anaphylactic shock.

Some hypersensitivity reactions are delayed, occurring several hours or even days after exposure. Delayed symptoms are usually relatively mild, such as colic, bloating, sickness or a change in bowel habit in response to a dietary allergen, but occasionally can be serious, such as toxic epidermal necrolysis (Stevens-Johnson syndrome) characterised by widespread blistering pustules in the skin and mucosae.

When listening to the patient's description it is important to remember some adverse reactions are frequently mistaken for an allergy. For example:

- Food intolerance. A non-immunological reaction to a food, usually caused by an enzyme deficiency. For example, cow's milk (lactose) intolerance, caused by low or absent lactase is characterised by bloating, colic and a change in bowel habit. These symptoms usually occur a few hours after ingesting the food.
- Sensitivity to chemicals. For example, to chemicals contained in perfumes, deodorants and air fresheners. Symptoms can include an itchy rash, patchy skin swellings, problems with breathing or migraines.
- Metal sensitivity. For example, to nickel. Symptoms can include an itchy rash or swelling at the site of contact.
- Medication "side effects". For example:
  - Urticaria with morphine
  - Diarrhoea with antibiotics
  - Headaches with nitrates
  - Myalgia with statins
  - A photosensitive reaction following amiodarone
  - Asthma with non-steroidal anti-inflammatory medications.

Ask yourself, how does a previous hypersensitivity reaction influence formulate a diagnosis?

When the presenting problem is likely to be a hypersensitivity reaction it is important to learn about the symptoms and signs to formulate a diagnosis and identify the allergen. Some patients present with a recurrence of a hypersensitivity reaction following re-exposure to the allergen. Patients who have had a previous a hypersensitivity reaction are at increased risk of being hypersensitive to another allergen.

When a delayed hypersensitivity reaction is suspected, the allergen is likely to be more difficult to identify because of the delay between exposure and onset of symptoms. Delayed type hypersensitivity reactions may be caused by a food product, such as peanuts, shellfish or gluten (a protein in wheat, barley and rye), or a medication. Questions that could be asked to identify a likely allergen include:

What do you think caused the reaction?
What were you doing before it started?
Do you think it could have been caused by [medication]?

Ask yourself, how does a previous hypersensitivity reaction influence management?

Information about a previous allergic reaction should always be considered when planning management.

Exposing a patient to a known allergen is contraindicated

When the presenting problem was likely to be an allergic reaction, the patient and close friends or family should be informed of the allergen and be given advice on avoiding the allergen and what to do if an allergic reaction occurs. For many lifestyle or environmental allergies treatment is aimed at relieving symptoms and damping the immune response. For example, the treatment of hay fever includes minimising exposure to pollen and treatments to alleviate the symptoms, such as an antihistamine to reduce itching, a decongestant, an inhaler for a wheeze or cough, eye drops for conjunctivitis or a nasal spray for rhinorrhoea. A minority of patients with severe allergies may need to carry adrenaline with them for emergency treatment. Some patients may benefit from referral to an allergy specialist to assess their allergy, to screen for common allergens or to provide additional information.

When an investigation or treatment is being considered as part of the management plan, it is important to ask whether they have had a previous reaction to a specific allergen associated with the investigation or a treatment. For example:

- If a patient is due to have an injection of intravenous contrast it would be appropriate to ask:

Have you ever had a reaction to iodine or a reaction when having an Xray?

- Before starting an antimicrobial medication, it would be appropriate to ask:

Have you ever had an allergic reaction to an antibiotic, such as penicillin?

Ask yourself, what signs should be looked for when examining the patient?

When a patient has had a previous allergic reaction, there are unlikely to be any signs to find on examination. When the presenting problem could be a hypersensitivity reaction the signs to look for include:

- A blanching rash, wheals or blisters
- Cutaneous scratch marks
- Tachycardia and hypotension
- Breathlessness and a wheeze

Previous non-allergic adverse reactions to a medication

A non-allergic adverse reaction, a "side effect", is an occasional unwanted and potentially harmful reaction to a medication. The medical records may include information about previous adverse reactions, but these are often incomplete and it is more important to ask the patient.

Have you had a reaction or side effect from any medication?
Have you had a bad experience with any medicine or procedure?
Has any medication previously caused unexpected symptoms?

When a non-allergic reaction is suspected, it is important to ask questions to learn more detail about the reaction to distinguish between an allergic reaction and a non-allergic adverse reaction.

Some non-allergic adverse reactions are an occasional minor problem, such as a loose bowel action when taking statins. Some are predictable side effect of the medication, such as constipation from taking opiates, urticaria when taking morphine, drowsiness while taking antihistamines or a cough while taking angiotensin converting enzyme inhibitors. Some adverse reactions are dose related, such as respiratory depression caused by morphine or hepatotoxicity from paracetamol, and others occur when the response to a medication is excessive, such as hypotension caused by hypotensive medication or hypoglycaemia after taking insulin. Some side effects occur after prolonged use. For example, taking steroids long-term can cause osteopaenia and osteonecrosis or bisphosphonates long-term may predispose to femoral fractures. A non-allergic adverse reaction may occasionally be severe, and even life threatening. For example:

- Bone marrow aplasia caused by immunosuppression medication, such as methotrexate.
- Acute pancreatitis caused by medication, such as thiazide diuretics, sodium valproate or sulphonamide antimicrobials.
- Rhabdomyolysis caused by simvastatin.
- A deterioration of asthma or renal function after taking NSAID's.
- An oculogyric crisis caused by metoclopramide.
- Malignant hyperpyrexia caused by succinyl choline or volatile anaesthetic mediations.

If there is a safety concern, it should be clearly documented and may inform the diagnosis, management and the examination.

Ask yourself, is a non-allergic adverse reaction likely to be relevant to the diagnosis?

In general, when the symptoms start shortly after taking a medication or after starting a new medication it may be a non-allergic reaction. If the patient is taking several medications or if there is a delay between taking the medication and the adverse reaction, the identification of the medication responsible can be difficult. Conversely, some patients claim a nocebo effect, when the patient believes the medication is making them feel worse or causing an adverse reaction when it isn't.

Ask yourself, is a previous non-allergic adverse reaction likely to influence management?

When the presenting problem is caused by an adverse reaction, changing the medication is usually sufficient. The change and reason for the change should be documented. The patient and close friends or family should be informed and be given advice on avoiding the medication in the future.

Before starting a new medication, it is appropriate to ask about previous non-allergic reactions to the medication or to the class of medicines being proposed.

Ask yourself, what signs should be looked for when examining the patient?

When a patient has had a previous adverse reaction, there are unlikely to be any signs to find on examination.

When an adverse reaction is suspected, the symptoms will indicate the signs to look for to confirm the diagnosis and assess the severity of the problem. Occasionally, the signs are diagnostic. For example:

- A fixed extreme upward stare, flexed neck, open mouth and tongue protrusion or painful jaw spasms are characteristic of an oculogyric crisis caused by metoclopramide.
- Pin-point pupils and bradypnea are characteristic of opiate toxicity.

Infection risk to others

When the presenting problem is caused by an infection, the patient harbours a chronic infection, or the patient is potentially an asymptomatic carrier, the risk to others is an important safety concern to be considered. The principal aim of assessing this risk is to inform management, such as when a specialist investigation, treatment or hospital admission is planned. Information about the risk a patient poses may be available from the medical records. For example:

- When a patient has recently been in hospital, they are at increased risk of being colonised by a pathogen such as MRSA, ESBL or C. difficile.
- Patients infected with a highly contagious pathogen such as Nora virus, COVID or influenza virus or a significant and difficult to treat pathogen, such as TB, Hepatitis, or HIV.
- A patient with chicken pox is a risk to pregnant women or fertile females who may be pregnant.

It may be appropriate to ask:

Have you been told you are an infection risk to others?
Have you recently been in hospital?
Have you ever been tested for MRSA?
Have you ever had TB, hepatitis or HIV?

If there is a safety concern, it should be clearly documented and may inform management and the examination.

Ask yourself, how does the infection risk to others influence management?

When a patient is an infection risk to others, the risk should be assessed and, when indicated, measures taken to reduce the risk. When the pathogen is uncertain, a microbiological test of a representative sample, such as skin, sputum, urine or faeces, may be indicated to identify a pathogen (Appendix 20).

When the patient is an infection risk, general measures to reduce the risk to others will depend on the context. In general:

- Inform likely contacts, including other HCPs.
- Minimize close contact with other people, and vulnerable people in particular.
- Avoid sharing enclosed spaces with others and avoid crowds.
- Consider whether lifestyle change is indicated, such as when there is a risk of transmitting a sexually transmissible disease or HIV.

Additional measures may be indicated in special circumstances, such as when attending hospital. These may include:

- Treat an infection or colonisation. For example, chlorhexidine body washes to reduce MRSA colonisation.
- Wearing personal protective equipment for people when close contact is unavoidable.
- Cleaning potentially contaminated surfaces.
- Isolating the patient.

A minority, such as those with a persistent or difficult to treat infection, may need to be followed up. The risks should be documented, together with mitigations and asking for specialist advice may be indicated.

Ask yourself, does the infection risk influence the examination?

The nature of the presenting problem will inform the signs to look for on examination. When the infection tends to spread through body fluids, such as HIV or Hepatitis B and C, the risk to the HCP during the examination is small unless an invasive procedure is undertaken. However, when the infection is highly contagious, such as COVID infection, protective measures are indicated before examining the patient.

Infection risk to the patient

The infection risk to a patient is an assessment based on information in the medical records, from previous or ongoing medical conditions and treatments and when learning about the person or the problem. Patients at an increased risk of catching infection include:

- During pregnancy.
- When malnourished, tired or stressed.

- While taking broad spectrum anti-microbial medication.
- When taking immuno-suppressing medication.
- When unwell due to cancer or a chronic illness.
- Patients with ongoing medical conditions, such as an auto-immune disease or DM.
- Following a splenectomy.
- When the barriers to infection are compromised. For example, open wounds, ulceration or burns.
- Following a recent admission to hospital. In-patients are at increased risk of colonization by a potential pathogen, such as MRSA or C difficile. The risk is increased the longer the patient spent in hospital and is influenced by factors such as the treatments they received.
- When a partner is infected by HIV or a close contact, such as a family member, is infected by TB.
- Following a recent visit to a country or area where an infectious disease is prevalent.

Occasionally, it is appropriate to ask a patient:

Are you prone to getting recurrent infections?
Are infections difficult to treat?
Has anyone in your family been told they have reduced resistance to infection?

If there is an infection risk, it should be clearly documented and may inform the diagnosis, management and the examination.

Ask yourself, is an infection risk relevant to the diagnosis?

An increased risk of infection may increase the likelihood of an infection causing the presenting problem. Patients may present feeling ill due to sepsis, with a superficial abnormality, such as cellulitis or abscesses, a functional abnormality, including breathlessness from a chest infection or dysuria from a UTI, pain, including neck or back stiffness from meningitis, joint pain from septic arthritis or abdominal pain from a liver abscess.

When the patient describes frequent and recurrent infections, persistent or severe infections, difficult to treat infections or atypical infections, they may have a weak immune system and an increased susceptibility to infection. In a child, unexplained delayed growth and development may indicate an underlying immune-deficiency disorder and an increased risk of infection.

Ask yourself, how can the increased infection risk be managed?

When there is evidence for an unexplained tendency to infections without an apparent explanation it may be appropriate to consider whether they may have a primary immunodeficiency disorder, such as B-cell, T-cell or complement deficiencies or defective phagocytosis, or a secondary or acquired immune-deficiency caused by DM or HIV. First-line investigations usually start with an FBC to measure the WBC count (Appendix 2). Most patients who are at increased risk of contracting an infection do not have an underlying abnormality and, if the results are normal, they can be reassured. If the WBC count is inexplicably abnormal, referral to a specialist may be indicated.

When a patient is at increased risk of contracting an infection, they should be informed and measures taken to reduce the risk. These could include:

- Change lifestyle. Healthy diet, exercise and good oral hygiene.
- Providing personal protective equipment, such as a face mask or condom, when close contact is unavoidable.
- Cleaning potentially contaminated surfaces.
- Minimize close contact with other people. Avoid crowds or enclosed spaces. Isolating and barrier nursing the patient in a clean air environment.
- Prophylactic treatment or vaccination. For example:
  o Penicillin prophylaxis prior to a splenectomy.
  o Antimicrobial prophylaxis when there is a risk of a bacteraemia during a procedure.
- Stopping immunosuppression medications.
- Boost immunity. For example, immunoglobulin treatment.
- Good wound care.

Ask yourself, does the infection risk influence the examination?

The nature of the risk will inform the signs to look for on examination. When a patient is susceptible to infection, the risk from the examination is usually small, but for some very vulnerable patients, such as those undergoing a bone marrow transplant, personal protective measures are indicated before close contact with another person.

Bleeding risk

Many presenting problems are caused by bleeding and an increasing number of patients are taking medications that increase the bleeding risk. In addition, some patients have a co-morbidity that compromises coagulation or a primary coagulopathy. People with an increased risk of bleeding include:

- Patients taking anticoagulant medications, such as aspirin, warfarin, heparin, edoxaban, daltiparin, ticagrelor or dabigatran.
- Elderly patients and patients who have taken steroids long term or previous exposure to radiotherapy have a tendency to bleed and bruise easily.
- Patients with co-morbidity. For example:
  o Liver failure.
  o Haematological malignancy, such as leukaemia or myelodysplasia.
  o Patients with an aneurysm, such as an AAA or a Berry aneurysm, or with an arteriovenous malformation (AVM).
  o Patients with a cancer adjacent to a named blood vessel.
  o A pancreatic pseudocyst.
- Patients with a clotting disorder, such as sickle cell disease, haemophilia, Von Willebrand disease or anti-phospholipid syndrome.
- Patients with family members who have a heritable clotting disorder.
- Malnourished patients, such as when Vitamin B12, Vitamin C or folate may be deficient.

For most patients, the risk of bleeding is an assessment based on the medications they are taking, information learnt from the medical records or from information about previous or ongoing medical conditions and family medical history. Occasionally, it is appropriate to ask a patient:

Are you prone to bleeding or bruising?
Have you ever had trouble stopping bleeding?
Has anyone in your family been known to bleed easily?

If there is a safety concern, it should be clearly documented and may inform the diagnosis, management and the examination.

Ask yourself, is a bleeding risk relevant to the diagnosis?

When a patient presents with overt bleeding, such as haematemesis, melaena, rectal bleeding, menorrhagia, haemoptysis, or haematuria it is likely there is an underlying abnormality nearby, such as a peptic ulcer, bowel cancer or a TCC. When a patient presents with an unexplained bleeding tendency, such as recurrent bleeding gums, recurrent nose bleeds or persistent bleeding following a cut or minor procedure, there is an increased likelihood that a primary clotting abnormality is the cause. Bleeding is usually an indication for investigations to identify the diagnosis.

A bleeding risk may be the cause of occult bleeding. Occult bleeding may present with feeling non-specifically ill, with a superficial abnormality, such as petechiae, bruising, a diffuse firm deep seated intra-muscular or intra-articular swelling, with a functional abnormality, such as breathlessness, a change in bowel habit or unilateral weakness, or with pain, such as a headache, neck or back pain, joint pain or muscle pain. For example:

- Vitamin B12 deficiency causing anaemia.
- Acute hypotension from a ruptured AAA.
- Widespread petechial haemorrhages caused by ITP.
- Intra articular haemorrhage in patients with sickle cell disease.

- Melaena caused by radiation colitis.
- Severe breathlessness may be "air hunger" in haemorrhagic shock.
- A sudden onset of a severe headache may be caused by a sub-arachnoid haemorrhage from a Berry aneurysm.

Formulating a diagnosis is usually dependent on investigations.

Ask yourself, how does the bleeding risk inform management?

Information about a bleeding risk should be considered when planning management for a patient who presents with overt or suspected occult blood loss, or when an invasive procedure is considered. For example:

- When a patient is on an anticoagulant, it may need to be stopped. However, anticoagulants are being taken for a reason, so stopping an anticoagulant should only be done when the indications, the benefits and risks have been carefully considered and discussed with the patient.
- Patients with a primary or unexplained coagulopathy should be referred to a specialist.
- Patients living on a limited diet, with liver disease or who have malabsorption, are at increased risk of vitamin deficiency, which may increase the risk of bleeding. Investigations to measure Vitamin C, Vitamin B12 and serum folate may be indicated in addition to measuring the FBC and clotting factors. Vitamin supplements may be indicated.

First line investigations to diagnose, exclude, screen for, or assess severity of a bleeding risk include measuring the platelet count and requesting tests of blood clotting (Appendix 2)
When the cause of the bleeding is unknown, such as for occult bleeding, investigations are indicated to diagnose the cause. The choice of investigation is determined by the presenting problem and likely cause. For example:

- Investigating haematemesis with an OGD to diagnose a cause, such as a Mallory Weiss tear, a gastric ulcer, angiodysplasia, oesophageal varices or cancer.
- Investigating haematuria with a urinary MC&S and cytology and a flexible cystoscopy to distinguish between a UTI, bladder TCC or a calculus.
- Investigating rectal bleeding with an endoscopy, CT scan or barium enema to distinguish between a solitary rectal ulcer, proctitis, diverticulitis or cancer.
- Investigating a headache with a CT scan.

When a patient presents with bleeding, management is usually aimed at stopping the bleeding, assessing the impact of the blood loss on the patient, replacing losses and determining the cause.
Measures to stop the bleeding are determined by the source of the blood loss. For example:

- Bleeding from a laceration or blunt soft tissue trauma will usually stop when continuous pressure is applied.
- A nose bleed can usually be stopped by firmly pinch the soft part of the nose for at least 10 mins or applying topical cocaine. Occasionally, referral to a specialist is indicated for packing, cautery or embolization.
- Bleeding from a fracture and the associated soft tissue injury will usually stop when the fracture is immobilized.
- Bleeding into a joint will usually stop when the joint space is filled with blood.
- Bleeding from a peptic ulcer may require an OGD and clipping a visible vessel, or cauterizing or injecting the ulcer base with adrenaline or a sclerosant.
- When the patient is taking an anti-coagulant, this may need to be stopped and, if possible, the coagulopathy reversed. For example:
  o Giving Vitamin K to a patient taking warfarin.
  o Giving protamine to reverse heparin.
  o Giving a platelet transfusion when a patient has thrombocytopaenia.
  o Giving Andexanet to reverse apixaban or rivaroxaban.

Learning about the symptoms, examining the patient, and the results of investigations are used to assess the severity of blood loss. Overt blood loss is very distressing and usually appears to the patient or witness, to be a lot. However, subjective estimations of the volume of blood lost and the rate of loss are unreliable. The physiological response of the body and the results of tests provide a more accurate measure of the severity of haemorrhage. First line tests to assess severity may include (Appendix 2):

- FBC.
- ABG.
- Serum electrolytes, urea and creatinine.
- ECG and serum troponin.

When the location of the cause of the bleeding is uncertain, further investigations, such as an angiogram, are indicated.

Blood transfusion indications are widely available and the HCP should follow local guidelines. In general, a transfusion is indicated in patients with active or acute bleeding or symptomatic anaemia when the haemoglobin is below 8g/dL.

A patient's bleeding risk should always be considered when planning an invasive procedure. When a patient has an increased risk of bleeding and an invasive investigation or procedure is indicated, management options include:

- Not doing the investigation or procedure.
- Accepting the risk of a bleeding complication and managing bleeding when it occurs.
- When the increased risk of bleeding is due to a medication, consider stopping the medication early enough for the bleeding time to return to normal. For example:
  o Stopping daltiparin for 1 day.
  o Stopping ticagrelor for 2 days.
  o Stopping warfarin for 5 days prior to the procedure or giving Vitamin K if the pre-procedure interval is reduced.
  o Stopping aspirin or clopidogrel for 7 days.
    When considering stopping an anticoagulant, published guidelines help make an informed assessment of the benefit and risk and mitigating measures indicated. For some patients, such as in a patient with a metal heart valve, bridging therapy may be indicated.
- Providing treatment to return the bleeding time to normal. For example:
  o Factor X treatment for haemophilia.
  o An infusion of cryoprecipitate, fresh frozen plasma or platelets.
- Specialist advice.

Management decisions to reduce the bleeding risk should be made after a careful consideration of the benefits and risks and with the informed consent of the patient.

Ask yourself, how does a bleeding risk inform the signs to look for when examining the patient?

It is unusual for the examination to inform an assessment of bleeding risk. Usually, signs are apparent only when the patient is anaemic or bleeding is overt.

When a clotting abnormality is suspected, signs to look for include petechiae, purpura or unexplained bruising.

Thrombosis risk

Patients at an increased risk of thrombosis include:

- Patients on thrombogenic medication. For example, the oral contraceptive pill.
- Recent trauma or surgery.
- Patients with a hereditary condition. For example, protein C deficiency.
- Patients with an acquired condition. For example:
  o Cancer.
  o A previous DVT or PE.
  o Immobility.
  o Dehydration.
  o Calf compression.

      o   inflammation.

When a patient presents with a thrombotic problem, such as a stroke, a DVT, a PE or an ischaemic leg, an increased thrombotic tendency should be considered in the differential diagnosis. If relevant, specific questions may be indicated. For example:

Have you had a stroke/DVT/PE?
Has anyone in your family been told they clot easily?

If there is a safety concern, it should be clearly documented and may inform the diagnosis, management and signs to look for.

Ask yourself, is a thrombosis risk relevant to the diagnosis?

Patients with a tendency to develop thromboses may present with:

- A visible or palpable abnormality, such as
  - o   A tender diffuse firm deep seated calf swelling from a DVT.
  - o   A swollen cyanosed limb.
  - o   A sub-cutaneous firm chord swelling from thrombophlebitis. If it is multifocal or migratory consider thrombophlebitis migrans.
  - o   Prominent abdominal veins from IVC or portal vein thrombosis.
- A functional abnormality, such as breathlessness from a PE or weakness from a stroke.
- Pain, such as:
  - o   Claudication or rest pain from an ischaemic limb.
  - o   Constant abdominal pain from mesenteric ischaemia.
  - o   Acute onset of calf pain from a DVT.
  - o   A bursting pain in the calf when taking exercise associated with a blue swollen leg from extensive DVT.

Ask yourself, how does a thrombosis risk inform management?

When a thrombosis is suspected, management is focused on investigations to confirm the diagnosis and treat the cause. For example:

- A Doppler USS to diagnose a limb DVT or arterial thrombosis.
- A triple phase CT angiogram to diagnose portal vein thrombosis.

When a thrombosis is suspected, formulating a diagnosis is insufficient, it is also important to consider a likely cause. When a patient is taking thrombogenic medication, such as the oral contraceptive pill, the indications, benefits and risks of the medication should be reviewed. When the cause is uncertain, investigations may be indicated to confirm the diagnosis and identify or exclude possible causes. Specialist investigations may be indicated when there is an unexplained tendency to thrombosis or a family history of thrombosis. First-line investigations are similar to when the patient has a bleeding risk and include, sending blood to measure the blood cell count and to assess clotting and clotting factors. Additional tests include measuring Protein C, Protein S, homocysteine, anti-phospholipid antibody and lupus anticoagulant.

Measures to reduce the thrombosis risk may include:

- Removing the underlying cause.
- Maintaining hydration.
- Providing an anticoagulant medication.
- Fitting graduated compression hosiery.

An increased risk of thrombosis may influence any investigations planned. For example:

- Not doing the investigation or procedure should be considered.

- Accepting the risk of a thrombotic complication.
- Stop a thrombogenic medication. For example, stop the oral contraceptive pill.
- Provide prophylactic treatment.

Management decisions can only be made after a careful consideration of the benefits and risks and with the informed consent of the patient. The patient and close friends or family should be informed.

Ask yourself, how does a thrombosis risk inform the signs to look for when examining the patient?

When a patient is suspected of having a thrombosis or thrombosis risk, signs should be sought to confirm the diagnosis, to look for a cause or exclude a cause and to assess severity. For example:

- The signs to look for when a DVT is suspected include a tender swollen calf, plantar flexion and a positive Homan's sign.
- The signs to look for when thrombophlebitis is suspected include a sub-cutaneous firm chord-like swelling.
- The signs to look for when IVC thrombosis is suspected include prominent abdominal veins in which the blood flows from the groin to the chest.
- The signs to look for when portal vein thrombosis is suspected include prominent abdominal veins in which the blood flows away from the umbilicus.
- Look for signs of a nearby infection.
- When cancer is a possible cause, look for a mass, lymphadenopathy or hepatomegaly.

Other safety information

In some patient's, other information may be a safety concern. For example:

- A Jehovah Witness is likely to refuse blood products.
- Legal advance directives may specify a patient's views on treatment, such as resuscitation, dialysis or parenteral nutrition.
- Pregnancy.
- A mental health condition that puts the patient or staff at risk.
- Dementia causing the patient to wander.
- A pattern of self-harm.

Learn about Medications being taken

The patient should be asked to list the medications they are taking and what medicines they have recently started, stopped or changed. For each medication the indication, the dose, mode of administration, frequency and a start/stop date should be reviewed and documented. The questions to ask could include:

Do you take any medications regularly?
What medications do you take?
What medication do you take occasionally?
Can you show me your medications?
Do you have a list of the medications you take?
Can I check when you take your medications?
What was the last medication you took?
When did you start taking the medication?
Has there been a recent change to your medications?

It is also important to learn about ongoing or pending treatment. The questions to ask could include:

Are you waiting for treatment?
Are you expecting to start a new treatment?

When learning and documenting the list of medications it is important to also check what they are treating. The questions to ask could include:

What do you take this [medication] for?
Why do you take...?
Do you take this for...?

The aims of linking medications with the indications are:

- To validate ongoing medical conditions. Linking the condition and the treatment provides a measure of internal validation. Some medications are used to treat a number of different conditions so the link should not be assumed. For example:
  o A beta-blocker may be used to treat hypertension, AF or anxiety.
  o Diazepam may be used as to treat anxiety, to help patients sleep or to relieve muscle spasm.
  o Amitriptyline may be used as an antidepressant or for pain relief.
  o Codeine may be used to treat pain, diarrhoea or coughing.
- To check all the medications are indicated.
- To ensure all important co-morbidity is learnt and documented.
  o Some patients omit to mention a medical condition but do remember the medication they take or the operation they had. For example:
    ▪ A patient taking aspirin may have forgotten to mention a previous TIA.
    ▪ A patient may forget they had an AMI but remember they are taking an anticoagulant medication following coronary artery stenting.
- To ensure all medications are learnt and documented. Some patients forget to mention a medication they are taking. Suspicion of an error of omission may come from the information about their past or ongoing medical conditions or from learning about the person or the problem. For example:
  o A patient who has occasional angina may forget to mention that they occasionally use a GTN spray.
  o A patient with GORD may forget to mention they take an antacid.
  o A patient with diarrhoea may not mention they have been taking loperamide.
- To identify what conditions are ongoing and untreated, what conditions are ongoing and being treated or awaiting treatment and what conditions are being prevented with treatment. For example:
  o Some patients are known to have gallstones but these are asymptomatic, having been found incidentally and have been left untreated.
  o Some patients are awaiting an operation or a therapeutic intervention.
  o Back pain and sciatica are frequently long term or recurrent conditions that may or may not be treated at any given time.
  o Many patients taking anti-hypertensive medication are no longer hypertensive.
  o Aspirin treatment to reduce the risk of a stroke in a patient with AF.
- To assess severity of a co-morbidity. For example:
  o Some medications are recognised second or third-line treatments or patients are on multiple medications for the same condition indicating therapeutic control is difficult. For example:
    ▪ Most patients with hypertension are successfully treated by taking medications such as beta-blockers, diuretics or calcium channel blockers. If the patient is on numerous medications or second or third-line anti-hypertensives it is likely their blood pressure is difficult to control.
  o Some conditions are not severe enough to need treatment. For example:
    ▪ An obese patient may have borderline DM but does not currently require treatment.

Ask yourself, are any of the patient's medications relevant to formulating a diagnosis?

There are many different ways a medication may cause a presenting problem.

- Some medications can make a patient feel unwell when they are being effective. For example, a low blood pressure in patients taking anti-hypertensive medication or antidepressants.
- The medication may cause an adverse reaction. The presenting problem is more likely to be caused by an adverse reaction when a new medicine has been started or the dose of a medicine has been changed or the

patient is taking many different medications. An adverse reaction is more likely when the medication has a narrow therapeutic range, such as insulin, warfarin, digoxin or lithium.

The clinical features of hypoglycaemia.

- Feeling unwell
- Confusion, disorientation and convulsions
- Feeling tired and weak
- Nausea
- Impaired consciousness and confusion
- Pallor
- Sweating
- Tachycardia

- Deranged salt and water homeostasis is a frequent abnormality caused by medications and may be the cause of the presenting problem. Maintaining a stable internal environment, homeostasis, is vital for normal cellular function. Most of the time, homeostasis maintains a stable environment because there are effective buffering and compensatory mechanisms and the organs and tissues have sufficient functional capacity or reserve so that they can continue to function or recover despite injury or insult. However, when these buffering and compensatory mechanisms are overcome, medically significant changes can occur. For example:
  o Diuretics, such as frusemide or amiloride, proton pump inhibitors (PPIs) and heparin may affect sodium, potassium and chloride concentrations.
  o Thiazide and loop diuretics, anti-epileptic drugs, bisphosphonates, long-term lithium use can cause hypocalcaemia.
  o Diuretics, mannitol, aminoglycosides and chemotherapy drugs may cause hypomagnesaemia.
  o Glucocorticoids, cisplatin, pamidronate may cause hypo-phosphataemia and phospho-soda laxative abuse may cause hyper-phosphataemia.
- Some medications, such as steroids, immunosuppression medications or stimulant laxatives, cause problems after prolonged use.

The clinical features of prolonged steroid use.

Symptoms
- Feeling unwell
- Tired, with disturbed sleep
- Weak and lethargic
- Depressed, irritable, poor concentration and forgetful
- Loss of libido, impotence and amenorrhoea
- Osteoporosis and osteopaenia
- Hirsutism, with baldness and brittle hair
- Thin skin and striae
- Weight gain
Signs
- Moon face and a buffalo hump (Cushingoid features)
- Overweight
- Cutaneous striae
- Hypertension

- Some medications, such as steroids, benzodiazepines, opiates, lithium and barbiturates, cause a problem when they are stopped too quickly.

Ask yourself, do the medications influence management?

For most patients, but not all, the medications they are taking do not influence management. When the problem may be an adverse effect of a medication or a medication is known to have relevant adverse effects, such as abnormal homeostasis, investigations may be indicated. For example:

- Measuring serum electrolytes and creatinine concentrations when a medication may affect salt and water homoeostasis or renal function.
- Measuring the blood sugar when the patient is taking insulin.
- Measuring the LFTs when the patient is taking immunosuppressant medication.
- Measuring the TFTs when a patient is taking amiodarone.

Management of the presenting problem may impact on the medications a patient is currently taking. For example:

- Some medications, such as an anticoagulant, need to be stopped before an invasive procedure can be undertaken.
- A change in the management of DM may be indicated to improve blood glucose control during treatment of an infection.
- When a new medication is indicated, it may interact with a current medication. For example:
  - Warfarin interacts with NSAIDs, calcium channel blockers, such as amlodipine and diltiazem and some antimicrobial medications, such as metronidazole and trimethoprim.
  - Statins interact with anti-fungal medications.
  - Phosphodiesterase inhibitors, such as sildenafil, interact with nitrates.
  - Steroids, benzodiazepines, tri-cyclic antidepressants, antihistamines, amiodarone, diltiazem, rifampicin, isoniazid and paracetamol interact with each other because they change the activity of CYP enzymes which affects their metabolism.
- Occasionally medications interact with food or supplements, such as antiarrhythmic medications interact with grapefruit and warfarin interacts with pineapple and St John's Wort.

In general, polypharmacy is associated with an increased risk of medication interaction. It is appropriate to discuss this with the patient before recommending a new medication.

The consultation is also an opportunity to review the medications being taken by the patient and, when possible, stop a medication (deprescribing) or reduce the dose. This can be challenging, because there is a tendency to maintain the status quo rather than risk a potentially difficult conversation with the patient.

Ask yourself, how do the medications a patient takes inform the signs to look for when examining the patient?

Occasionally, the medications a patient is taking inform the signs to look for when examining the patient. For example:

- The pulse and blood pressure when a patient is taking an anti-arrhythmic or antihypertensive medication, or a B-blocker.
- The air entry and wheeze when a patient is taking a bronchodilator.

Learn about Ongoing Medical Conditions (Co-Morbidity) and their Treatment

Learning about ongoing medical conditions (co-morbidity) and treatment is not only to document the information but also to determine whether the co-morbidity and its treatment are relevant to the diagnosis, management of the presenting problem or the examination. Questions that could be asked to find out about ongoing medical conditions include:

Tell me about any illnesses you have at the moment.
Do you have any other medical conditions?
I note you are being treated for [conditions], are there any others?

It may be relevant to ask about specific medical conditions that patients of their age and lifestyle frequently have but that they may not have mentioned, such as osteoarthritis, hypertension, DM, IHD, asthma or COPD. Ongoing medical conditions should be linked with their treatment both to ensure all conditions have been identified and the condition is fully understood.

When learning about ongoing medical conditions:

Ask yourself, is the information relevant to formulating a diagnosis?

An ongoing medical condition or its treatment may cause the presenting problem when it deteriorates or progresses or when a complication arises. For example:

- The new problem may be a deterioration or progression of a pre-existing condition. For example:
  o A heart attack may occur due to progression of IHD.
  o Rest pain caused by progressive peripheral vascular disease.
  o Inflammatory conditions, such as rheumatoid arthritis or inflammatory bowel disease tend to wax and wane.
  o Ulcerative colitis may deteriorate causing a toxic megacolon.
  o Structural abnormalities, such as Budd Chiari malformation or adhesional sub-acute bowel obstruction can progress.
  o Many neurological abnormalities, such as dementia, Parkinson's disease or motor neurone disease are progressive.
- The new problem may be a complication of the co-morbidity. For example:
  o A chest infection complicating COPD.
  o Diverticular disease may be complicated by a perforation, bleeding or a stricture.
  o A fistula or an abscess may develop as a complication of Crohn's disease.
  o A stroke may be a complication of AF.
  o A PE may be a complication of a DVT.
  o An arrhythmia may complicate a previous myocardial infarction.
  o Pain, swelling and deformity affecting one joint such as the hip or knee can cause problems in another joint due to compensatory changes in weight distribution, gait or posture.
  o Small bowel obstruction caused by adhesions from a previous appendicectomy.
  o Deteriorating vision due to diabetic retinopathy.
  o A patient with chronic inflammation is at risk of developing a range of different late complications including:
    ▪ Cancer. For example:
      • A bronchogenic carcinoma in a lifelong smoker with COPD.
      • An SCC arising within a Marjolin's ulcer.
      • Oesophageal adenocarcinoma arising within Barrett's oesophagus.
      • Gallbladder cancer arising within a porcelain gallbladder.
    ▪ Ulceration. For example, secondary to:
      • Chronic venous hypertension.
      • Vasculitis.
      • Peripheral arterial disease.
    ▪ Stricture formation. For example, secondary to:
      • Bowel ischaemia.
      • Radiation enteritis.
      • Crohn's disease.
      • Recurrent episodes of salpingo-oophoritis causing infertility.
      • Recurrent UTI's causing a urethral stricture.
    ▪ Scarring. For example, secondary to:
      • Recurrent pyelonephritis causing a scarred kidney.
      • NASH causing liver failure.
      • Nerve entrapment in scar tissue.
    ▪ A deformity. For example:
      • Osteomyelitis causing bone deformity.

- Osteo-, rheumatoid or septic arthritis causing joint deformity.
- The presenting problem may be caused by a treatment. For example:
  - When a treatment causes a side effect or an adverse reaction it may present as a new problem. For example:
    - Feeling ill with jaundice may be a complication of azathioprine treatment for Crohn's disease.
    - Haematemesis while taking a NSAID.
  - Some medications are known to cause late complications. For example:
    - Chronic steroid use can cause osteopaenia, presenting with a fracture.
    - Chronic opiate or benzodiazepine use can lead to dependency, or withdrawal symptoms when stopped too quickly.
    - Chronic laxative use can lead to severe constipation (a cathartic colon).

When the presenting problem is likely to be a consequence of a previous or ongoing medical condition it is important to link information about the problem with information about the patient. For example:

- A patient presents with central abdominal colic followed by bloating and vomiting likely to be caused by small bowel obstruction. A previous laparotomy and the absence of a hernia on examination means it is likely the obstruction is a late complication of pre-existing adhesions.
- A patient with Crohn's disease presents with biliary colic or cholecystitis caused by gallstones. The gallstones may be caused by terminal ileitis disrupting the entero-hepatic circulation of bile salts.

Occasionally, the patient incorrectly attributes their symptoms to a pre-existing medical condition and delays seeking help. For example, a patient may consider a new onset of headaches to be caused by their treated hypertension, an abdominal pain to be due to their Crohn's disease, a change in bowel habit is due to their IBS or a persistent new cough to their COPD.

The co-morbidity may be a risk factor for the presenting problem. For example:

- Hypertension or DM are risk factors for developing renal failure or a stroke.
- Resection of the terminal ileum is a risk factor for the development of gallstones.
- Pan-colitis, chronic ulceration, Barrett's oesophagus or lymphoedema are risk factors for cancer.

Ask yourself, does an ongoing condition or its treatment influence management?

There are many ways co-morbidity and treatments may affect management. For example:

- Multi-morbidity and polypharmacy, make management planning more complicated.
  - Multi-morbidity may be associated with functional limitations and a decreased quality of life or life expectancy which may influence the management benefit-risk balance.
  - Polypharmacy is associated with an increased risk of an adverse reaction, interaction or a complication, particularly when a new treatment is started.
- When a patient has ongoing co-morbidity, it is likely they are being managed by other HCPs within a pathway of care. If so, it is important to ensure everyone is informed when a new problem arises not only for their information but also because it may be necessary to coordinate care.
- Most published guidelines are for patients with a single condition. When a patient has co-morbidity recommendations from guidelines should be considered in context.
- When a management option needs pre-procedure preparation to be safely performed. For example:
  - Anticoagulants may need to be stopped prior to an invasive procedure such as an angiogram.
  - Pro-thrombotic medications, such as the oral contraceptive pill, may need to be reviewed because they may increase the risk of a DVT following surgery.
  - Fasting may affect the effectiveness of a medication.
  - Immunosuppressants need to be reviewed because they may increase the risk of infection and may delay healing.
- When a patient is near the end of their life, palliative care, focused on providing psychological and physical support and treatment to alleviate symptoms, may be indicated.
- Patients with co-morbidities may have had investigations performed recently or be awaiting an investigation. The results of a recent test may be relevant to the management of the presenting problem. For example:

o A normal recent chest CT scan makes lung cancer less likely.
o A normal recent abdominal USS makes an AAA or gallstones unlikely.

The consultation is an opportunity to re-assess an ongoing condition and its treatment. For example:

- When a patient with a pacemaker presents, it is an opportunity for a pacemaker check.
- When a diabetic patient presents, it is an opportunity to re-assess their diabetic control.
- When a patient has ongoing kidney disease it is an opportunity to re-assess their renal function.
- When a patient with cirrhosis presents it is an opportunity to re-assess liver function.

The consultation is also an opportunity to screen for disease progression or a recognised complication. For example:

- In a patient with Barrett's oesophagus or UC it may be appropriate to perform an endoscopy to re-assess severity or screen for dysplasia or cancer.
- In a patient with liver cirrhosis, it may be appropriate to measure LFTs and AFP to re-assess liver function and screen for liver cancer. When the patient is taking immune-suppression medications it may be appropriate to screen for asymptomatic hepatocellular damage.
- In a patient with cancer, it may be appropriate to measure cancer markers or undertake an imaging investigation, such as a CT scan, to screen for metastatic disease or recurrence in patients treated for cancer.

Occasionally, the consultation is the opportunity to start treatment for a pre-existing condition to reduce the risk of a complication or deterioration. For example:

- Prescribing statins to reduce the risk of heart disease.
- Anti-coagulation medication to reduce the risk of a stroke.
- Treat hypertension in a patient with type 2 DM.
- Recommend treating an inguinal hernia to prevent bowel obstruction.
- Recommend a sub-total colectomy to prevent cancer in a patient with multiple polyps or dysplasia.

Ask yourself, how does information about ongoing medical problems inform the signs to look for when examining the patient?

The aims of examining the patient include to assess change or the severity of the condition, the response to treatment or to screen for a complication. For example:

- When the patient is being treated for cancer, examine the site of the cancer to assess the response to treatment locally and elsewhere to screen for metastatic spread by looking for signs of lymphadenopathy, a pleural effusion, ascites or hepatomegaly.
- When the patient is being treated for heart failure, examine the pulse, blood pressure, JVP, heart and lungs and for peripheral oedema to assess the severity or the response to treatment.
- When the patient is being treated for a skin condition, such as eczema or psoriasis, the sites affected should be examined to assess severity, the response to treatment and for a complication such as infection.

Learn about Past Medical Conditions (Past-Morbidity) and their Treatment

Learning about past medical conditions and their treatment is not only to document the information but also to determine whether the past-morbidity and treatment are relevant to the diagnosis, management of the presenting problem or the examination. Questions that could be asked include:

Have you had any other illnesses in the past?
What illnesses or operations have you had before?
Have you ever been in hospital? If so, why?
Have you ever been seriously ill?

It may be appropriate to ask about specific medical conditions that a patient of their age and lifestyle may have had.

Have you ever suffered from [condition]?

It is also important to learn how the condition was treated to confirm they had a particular condition and to assess severity. Questions that could be asked include:

How was it treated?
What treatment did you have?

Occasionally a patient forgets information or does not realise its significance. This does not matter when it is unlikely to be relevant to the new problem or future care, such as mumps as a child, a fracture, a chest infection, a period of back pain or an episode of depression during a significant life event. However, the HCP should judge what is relevant or irrelevant and what to document.

There is a risk that information about a past medical condition may be inaccurate. For example, when a patient uses a pseudo-medical term or when the diagnosis was provisional, such as a diagnosis of a peptic ulcer being made clinically without evidence from a gastroscopy. When there is uncertainty, it may be appropriate to ask relevant additional questions to assess the validity of the diagnosis.

How was the diagnosis of [condition] made?
Did you have a [test] that proved the diagnosis?
How did {condition] affect you?

When reflecting on the information learnt, it is important to:

Ask yourself, is a past medical condition relevant to the diagnosis?

Treatment of a past condition may make a diagnosis unlikely. For example, a previous appendicectomy makes appendicitis an unlikely cause for abdominal pain or a recent successful cardiac stenting makes IHD unlikely. Conversely, a past medical condition may present as a new problem when it relapses, recurs or causes a late complication. For example:

- The new problem may be caused by progression, a relapse or recurrence. For example:
  o Arterial stenosis can deteriorate or an aneurysm enlarge.
  o Infection can relapse, such as EBV, malaria or HIV.
  o Biliary or renal colic may recur.
  o A DVT or cancer can recur.
- When a late complication occurs. For example:
  o An embolic complication may arise from longstanding AF or an aneurysm.
  o A pericolic abscess may complicate diverticulosis.
  o Small bowel strictures can arise from previous pelvic radiotherapy.
  o Osteo-arthritis in a joint can arise following an intra-articular fracture.
  o A ventricular aneurysm may be a complication of a previous myocardial infarction.
  o Gallstones may develop in a patient with terminal ileitis.
  o Acute pancreatitis may occur in a patient with known gallstones.
- When a late complication of the treatment occurs. For example:
  o Adhesions following an appendicectomy can cause a bowel obstruction.
  o Gallstones may develop in a patient who has had a distal small bowel resection.
  o Cancer may be a late complication following radiotherapy in childhood.
  o Chromium or cobalt-linked complications may occur in patients with metal-on-metal prosthesis.
- Some past medical conditions are a risk factor. For example:
  o Atherosclerosis, causing a previous AMI, is a risk factor for other problems, such as claudication.
  o Multi-focal cancer may be indicative of genetic instability or mutations in DNA mismatch repair genes, increasing the risk of another cancer.

Ask yourself, how can a past condition influence management?

A past condition may influence the choice of investigation or treatment of the presenting problem. For example:

- When the problem is a recurrence, patients usually expect management to be similar or if a treatment worked previously, it is likely to work again, and vice versa.
- A recurrent DVT or PE is likely to need lifelong anti-coagulation.
- Previous abdominal surgery may make further surgery more difficult because there are likely to be adhesions.
- If intubation for a general anaesthetic was difficult previously it is likely to be difficult again.

For some patients, the consultation is an opportunity to screen for an asymptomatic problem associated with past morbidity. For example:

- Measuring serum levels of cancer markers to screen for recurrence (Appendix 2).
- Perform an ECG to screen for a recurrence of AF, IHD or left ventricular failure.
- Request a liver USS in a patient with known gallstones to reassess the gallbladder or to screen for choledocholithiasis (Appendix 2)

Ask yourself, how can a past condition influence the examination?

In most patients, past morbidity does not influence the examination. It may be appropriate to look for signs associated with the past medical condition. For example:

- When the patient has had an operation, the scars should be consistent with the operation.
- When the patient has had a condition, such as an AMI or stroke, the examination may include looking for signs of atherosclerosis or an arrythmia.
- When the patient has been treated for cancer, the examination may include looking for signs of recurrent cancer.
- When the patient has had a previous hernia repair, it may be appropriate to look for signs of a recurrent hernia.

Learn about Risk Factors (Potential Morbidity) and Their Treatment

Learning about the patient includes not only learning about past and ongoing morbidity and its treatment and safety concerns but also about assessing the likelihood or risk of potential or future morbidity. A risk factor is a variable that is associated with an increased likelihood of a future problem. However, when the condition arises, the risk factor becomes the cause. The aims of considering or asking about risk factors are to inform the diagnosis, and in particular the likely cause of the problem, to help plan management and to inform the examination.

Variables that are generally recognised to be risk factors include demographic and genetic information, ongoing or past-morbidity, regularly inhaling tobacco smoke, being over or under-weight and consuming alcohol. Other risk factors to be considered include the patient's diet, environment and occupation and drug taking. For some risk factors, the association with a condition is so strong that they are considered disease precursors or a pre-disease state. In other words, it is not a question of whether the condition will arise, but when will it start.

Examples of pre-disease states

- Some genetic mutations. For example, Huntingdon's disease.
- Drinking excessive quantities of alcohol for long enough will lead to liver and/or pancreatic disease.
- Severe morbid obesity will lead to NASH.
- Acetabular dysplasia will lead to osteoarthritis.
- Untreated hypertension will lead to heart failure.

The clinical significance or consequence of the condition should it arise will influence the patient's perception of risk. Usually, the patient and the HCP have a similar understanding of the consequence should a condition develop but, because assessment of consequence is subjective, it may be different. For example, a smoker will continue to smoke despite the risks and the likely impact on life expectancy yet may refuse to have a vaccination because of a perceived risk of a complication. Therefore, it is usually appropriate to ask the patient rather than assume their perception of risk.

What are you most worried about?
Are there any risks that particularly concern you?
What would be the worst outcome for you?
Do you know what is likely to happen if you continue [risk]?
Do you know how [complication] is likely to affect you?

Demographic risks

Demographic information is a risk factor for many conditions and should be considered when formulating a diagnosis, planning management and before examining the patient. For example:

- Old age is a risk factor for many health problems, such as arthritis, diverticulitis, dementia or cardio-vascular disease, particularly when combined with sex. For example, in a female, the risk of breast or ovarian cancer increases with age.
- An unhappy marriage or partnership is a risk factor for many conditions including stress and emotional, psychological, physical or sexual abuse.
- Some conditions are more prevalent in certain ethnic groups.
- Many occupations expose a patient to additional risk factors.

Environmental risks

We are all exposed to environmental risks. For most patients, these are minor risks that are not relevant to patient care. However, when an environmental risk is relevant to the diagnosis or the cause of the problem it is appropriate to learn more about the risk. In which case, it would be appropriate to ask questions to determine the nature and extent of the patient's exposure. For example:

Tell me about your home.
Do you have an open fire?
Where do you work?
Do you live near a very busy road?

Examples of environmental risks

- Air pollution. The common pollutants patients are exposed to include:
  - Particulate matter, including diesel exhaust and an open fireplace or wood-burning stove. There is increasing evidence linking PM2.5 particles to many medical conditions, including respiratory, cardiovascular and inflammatory diseases and to mortality.
  - Airborne infection, mould in a damp and poorly ventilated building.
  - Volatile organic compounds and nitrogen oxides from vehicles.
  - Carbon monoxide from gas heaters: "weekend headache".
  - Chemicals, such as from cleaning products and air-fresheners.
  - Exposure to asbestos. This may occur in old buildings.
- Water pollution. The common pollutants patients are exposed to include:
  - Infection, such as Cholera, Campylobacter, Amoebiasis, Giardiasis, Legionella, Nora virus.
  - Chemicals, such as fluoride or pesticides.
  - Heavy metals, such as lead or arsenic poisoning.
- Sunlight.
- Surface contamination by viruses or other organisms.
- Exposure to ionizing radiation, such as radon exposure or from imaging investigations.

Ask yourself, could an environmental risk factor be relevant to the diagnosis?

The symptoms indicating the presenting problem is caused by an environmental risk are usually vague and non-specific. They include feeling ill and anorexia, pains, such as a headache, abdominal pain or muscle aches, symptoms of deranged function, including nausea, vomiting and diarrhoea or a wheeze and breathlessness, or a visible or palpable abnormality, such as a rash. Conditions caused by an environmental risk include, asthma caused by airborne pollution or gastroenteritis caused by a water borne infection.

Ask yourself, is an environmental risk factor relevant to planning management?

An environmental risk may influence the investigation of the presenting problem. For example, testing for the blood carboxyhaemoglobin concentration when carbon monoxide poisoning is suspected or testing for the blood lead levels when lead poisoning is suspected. A screening investigation may be indicated. For example, measuring the peak flow or performing lung function tests to assess the impact of air pollution or measuring FBC, Urea, creatinine and electrolytes and liver function tests to screen for secondary abnormalities. For most patients, managing an environmental risk is about managing their lifestyle to reduce the risk. For example:

- Carefully washing all food before cooking. Taking care what is eaten or drunk when abroad.
- Avoid drinking contaminated water.
- Not lighting a fire.
- Not cycling or walking along a polluted road.
- Improving the indoor ventilation to reduce smoke or radon exposure.
- Not frying food.
- Changing an occupation or a hobby.
- Changing another person's life choice. For example, a partner stopping smoking.

Ask yourself, how does an environmental risk inform the signs to look for when examining the patient?

Usually, an environmental risk does not influence the examination. However, the nature of the risk may indicate the signs to look for.

Occupational risks

For most patients their occupation does not pose a risk so is not a risk factor. For some, the risks associated with their occupations are risk factors and may influence the diagnosis, management or the examination. For example:

- Asbestosis is an occupational risk among construction workers, farmers, firefighters, insulation workers, plumbers, shipyard workers, mechanics, engineers and power plant workers.
- Exposure to radiation is an occupational risk among dentists, pilots, health care and nuclear workers.
- Heavy metal or chemical poisoning is an occupational hazard among e-cigarette smokers, engineers, decorators, mechanics, welders and chemical workers. For example:
  o Arsenic is used in the manufacture of pesticides.
  o Lead and cadmium are present in many batteries and solder.
  o Chromium is used in the manufacture of cars, glass and pottery.
  o Mercury was used by dentists and in the manufacture of many chemicals.
- Musculo-skeletal injury, such as a back injury or joint injury, is an occupational risk among manual labourers, factory workers, dockers, carers, sportsmen and women and extreme athletes.
- Repetitive strain injury is an occupational risk among sportsmen and women, secretaries and factory workers.

Ask yourself, is an occupational risk relevant to the diagnosis?

When learning about the problem, the differential diagnosis may include a condition known to be associated with or caused by an occupation. The nature of the occupation will indicate whether it is likely to be a cause.

Ask yourself, is an occupational risk relevant to planning management?

For most patients the occupational risk is low and unlikely to affect management. Occasionally, an occupational risk may influence investigation of the presenting problem. For example:

- An X-ray or bone scan to assess damage to a bone or joint, such as a stress fracture, or an MRI scan to assess soft tissue injury in an athlete.
- A CXR and pulmonary function tests in a patient with breathlessness who may have been exposed to asbestos or air pollution.
- A screening investigation may be indicated. For example:
  o A low dose CT scan to screen for cancer in a patient previously exposed to asbestos.
  o Blood tests for metal ions, such as chromium and cobalt.

An occupational risk may influence treatment. For example:

- Changing posture at work to help treat back pain.
- Changing the keyboard for a typist with repetitive strain injury.

When there is a risk, the problem should be discussed with the patient and it may be appropriate to obtain advice from an HCP with an interest in occupational health.

Ask yourself, how does an occupational risk inform the signs to look for when examining the patient?

For some patients, the nature of the risk may indicate the signs to look for. For example:

- To assess the power and range of movement of a joint when a repetitive strain injury is being assessed.
- A chest examination when a patient has previously been exposed to asbestos or coal dust.

Dietary risks

Dietary risks include eating contaminated or uncooked food, eating an unbalanced diet for a long period of time, taking dietary supplements to excess or inappropriately, inducing vomiting or laxative abuse. Eating contaminated or uncooked food is always a risk. For example:

- Eating uncooked meat may cause E. coli or Salmonella infection.
- Drinking unpasteurized milk may cause E. coli, Salmonella, Campylobacter, Listeria or Cryptosporidium infection.
- Eating uncooked shellfish may cause E. coli or norovirus infection.
- Eating lectins in uncooked beans can cause toxicity.
- Eating uncooked or re-heated rice can lead to Bacillus cereus infection.

Eating an unbalanced diet or taking supplements for a short time is unlikely to cause harm. However, some patients persistently eat a diet that risks harm. For example:

- A vegan diet is associated with a reduced bone mineral density, a risk factor for a fracture, and strict adherence to a vegan diet of fruit and vegetables, legumes, nuts, seeds, grains, and non-dairy products is likely to be deficient in iron and zinc, vitamins B12 and D, calcium and long-chain n-3 (omega-3) fatty acids.
- Diets, such as the keto diet, a low-carbohydrate diet, or the Paleo diet or a diet which includes highly processed food, are associated with different risks ranging from obesity, triggering an eating disorder to a deficiency.
- A very low-calorie diet may lead to rapid weight loss, sarcopaenia and metabolic abnormalities.

There are many different dietary supplements and homeopathic treatments available and people take them for many different reasons. For example, in response to advertisements, on the recommendation of friends or family, such as to treat a perceived dietary or vitamin deficiency, to allay fear or anxiety, such as St John's Wort, to improve a feeling of well-being, such as Ginseng, or for the management of chronic disease, such as turmeric for inflammation, calcium for osteoporosis or glucosamine for arthritis.

Dietary supplements often claim to include herbal or other "natural" products and are generally harmless except when the source is unregulated, the dose is uncertain, when it contains active ingredients that have biological effects in the body in susceptible individuals, when taken excessively or if combined.

Examples of dietary supplements

- Vitamins: Vitamin D and C in particular.
- Amino acids, such as glucosamine.
- Minerals, such as iron and calcium.
- Herbs, such as echinacea and garlic.
- Animal-based products, such as chondroitin sulphate or fish oil.
- Plants and plant-based products, such as:
  - Ginko.
  - Wild mushrooms.
  - Tea.
  - Ginseng.
  - St. John's Wort (Hypericum perforatum).
  - Bilberry.
  - Turmeric.
  - Evening primrose oil.
- Cranberry juice.
- Bacteria, such as probiotics.
- Enzymes, such as amylase and pepsin.

Inducing vomiting and laxative abuse or extreme exercise are abnormal behaviours that may be associated with a dietary risk. They are often associated with a mental health condition and may cause liver and renal disease, nutritional deficiencies, dehydration and metabolic abnormalities.

Ask yourself, is the patient's diet relevant to formulating a diagnosis?

Dietary risks may become apparent when learning about the person, but are usually only discussed when considering the cause of the presenting problem. When there is concern a patient's diet may be causing them harm, it would be appropriate to ask questions to determine whether it constitutes a risk. Questions that could be asked include:

Tell me about your diet
What do you normally eat?
Do you take any herbal medicines or supplements?

The symptoms and signs indicating diet may be relevant to the presenting problem include:

- Feeling ill, with fatigue and weight loss.
  - Patients who present feeling ill, tired and weak could have iron deficiency. It is the most frequent nutritional deficiency worldwide, being caused by a diet that does not contain dark leafy vegetables, red meat or eggs.
  - Feeling ill with fatigue, unexpected weight loss, confusion and short-term memory loss could be caused by thiamine (Vitamin B-1) deficiency. This is most frequently found in people drinking too much alcohol but can also occur in patients with anorexia, starvation, cancer, malabsorption or on dialysis.
  - Feeling ill with anorexia and weight loss, breathlessness, fatigue and weakness, dizziness and unsteadiness can be caused by pernicious anaemia (Vitamin B12 deficiency). Deficiency can occur in the elderly, vegans or in patients who have previously had gastric surgery.
- A superficial abnormality, such as pallor, mouth ulcers, bleeding gums, hair loss, brittle nails or erythema could be caused by folate or Vitamin C deficiency.
- A functional abnormality, including breathlessness, fatigue, lethargy and weakness, confusion, irritability, drowsiness, depression and poor concentration, or anorexia, nausea and vomiting could be caused by iron deficiency.

- Pain, including headaches, non-specific abdominal, muscle, bone or joint pains, or widespread atypical pains could be caused by calcium deficiency.

Some dietary supplements are known to cause specific abnormalities. For example:

- Atropa belladonna ("Deadly nightshade") has anticholinergic activity and may cause a headache, hallucinations, blurred vision and slurred speech and, in higher doses, seizures and death.
- St John's wort contains a monoamine oxidase inhibitor and inhibits the re-uptake of neurotransmitters such as serotonin, noradrenaline, glutamate and dopamine. It not only interacts with many medications, but also may cause a headache, anxiety, dizziness, fatigue, a dry mouth, a change in bowel habit and a rash, and, in higher doses, skin necrosis.
- Digitalis (such as from foxgloves) can cause confusion, visual disturbance, anorexia, nausea, vomiting and diarrhoea, and arrythmia's that may be fatal.
- Mushrooms. There are more than a million species of mushroom of which only about 10% are safe to eat. Eating unsafe wild mushrooms, such as those containing psychoactive compounds, such as psilocybin, can cause various symptoms including tiredness, skin rashes, nausea and vomiting, abdominal colic, diarrhoea, forgetfulness, dizziness, headache, anxiety, paraesthesia, delirium, seizures and hallucinations. Some may cause arrythmia's, liver and renal failure and be fatal.

Ask yourself, is the patient's diet relevant to planning management?

When a patient's diet is different, it may be a risk factor. Tests may be indicated to screen for a secondary problem. For example:

- A FBC and ferritin to screen for anaemia and changes to iron stores
- Measuring serum electrolytes, urea and creatinine to screen for abnormalities of water and electrolyte homeostasis.
- Measuring liver function tests, including measuring blood protein, and lipids.
- Measuring vitamin, folate and trace element blood concentrations to screen for a deficiency.

A dietary risk factor may influence treatment of the presenting problem. For example:

- When there is a risk of a drug interaction. For example, warfarin interacts with St John's Wort.
- If the risk is identified early enough a change in lifestyle, stopping homeopathic supplements or taking food or vitamin supplements may be sufficient.
- In some patients it is appropriate to discuss referral to a dietician, a psychiatrist or a specialist team.

When a patient's diet is causing harm, it is the responsibility of the HCP to ensure the patient is informed and, not only to recommend measures to mitigate or treat the problem, but also to try to help them change their diet. However, it is important to remember that it is the responsibility of the patient to change.

Information about the person and the patient and having a good rapport with the patient may help ensure the context, the timing, the tone and the method of the conversation about change are appropriate. In general, the right time to bring about change is when the patient is receptive and if it is discussed in context of something the patient says or a health problem. Telling the patient may bring about a meaningful change but a non-directive approach is more likely to be successful. Ask permission to raise the concern, use questions to identify the barriers to change and then to help the patient identify solutions for themselves. For example,

Can we talk about your diet?
Is it OK if we talk about your diet and what it is doing to you?
Do you know the risks?
Did you know your [problem] was caused by your diet?
Do you know what might happen to you if you don't change?
What is likely to happen if you carry on with this diet?
What will you do now?
What can you change?

Frequently, dietary problems are caused by a lack of awareness or self-belief. A lack of awareness or knowledge that their diet is harmful or could have caused a particular problem is possible despite the information available in the media.

Ask yourself, how does a dietary risk inform the signs to look for when examining the patient?

The nature of the risk influences the signs to look for on examination.

Genetic risks

Inherited chromosomal abnormalities or mutations in a gene or, rarely, in mitochondrial DNA may be a risk factor. Information about genetic risk may be available from immuno-histochemistry of tissue samples or genetic tests, but for most patients, age, ethnicity and information about other family members are used clinically as proxy measures of genetic risk. Questions that could be asked include:

Are there any illnesses that affect members of your family?
Have any other family members had [condition]?

Ask yourself, is a genetic risk factor relevant to formulating a diagnosis?

When a young person presents with a problem that is atypical for their age it may be caused by a genetic mutation. For example:

- The differential diagnosis of a persistent cough and recurrent chest infections in an adolescent includes cystic fibrosis.
- The differential diagnosis of recurrent excessive bleeding from minor wounds or extensive bruising following minor injury in a young person includes haemophilia.
- Cancer in a young person may be associated with a genetic mutation.

The genetic diversity between ethnic groups affects the prevalence of some problems. For example:

- The risk of DM is higher in patients from South Asia.
- The risk of heart disease is increased in patients from Asia, Africa or the Caribbean.
- Korean Americans have a low incidence of breast cancer.
- Hispanic females have a lower risk of developing lung cancer.

Patients are at increased risk if a close relative has a gene mutation (called an index mutation) or a hereditable condition. For many heritable conditions the site of the genetic mutation, the proximity and number of family members affected and the co-existence of other risk factors, such as environmental or lifestyle risk factors, influences the probability of the condition developing.

Examples of common hereditable conditions

- Type 1 neurofibromatosis, tuberous sclerosis, Huntingdon's disease, Marfan syndrome, polycystic kidney disease, or APC or BRCA 1 and 2 gene mutation are autosomal dominant genetic conditions.
- Cystic fibrosis, sickle cell anaemia, thalassaemia or Tay-Sachs's disease are autosomal recessive genetic conditions.
- Duchenne muscular dystrophy, haemophilia or fragile X syndrome are X chromosome linked genetic conditions.
- Statin-induced myopathy, encephalopathy, epilepsy, lactic acidosis or optic atrophy are disorders caused by mutations in mitochondrial DNA.

However, it should be remembered that many conditions that affect other family members occur by chance and are not caused by a heritable genetic mutation or are weakly associated with multiple genetic mutations (polygenic). For example, most cancers and metabolic abnormalities, auto-immune disease, cardiovascular disease or mental health conditions.

Ask yourself, how does a genetic risk affect management?

For most patients the genetic risk is low, and it is unlikely to affect management.

When a genetic risk may influence management, a screening test may be indicated. In the future, it is likely a better understanding of genetic or molecular causes of disease and increased availability and reduced cost of genetic testing will change the way risk is assessed. Genetic testing can be performed on any DNA containing sample, such as blood, urine, saliva or a pathology specimen. Most genetic tests have a sensitivity and specificity approaching 100% for a known index mutation, such as a mutation identified in another family member. If a known index mutation is not found, the probability of not developing the disease is almost 100%. When an index mutation is unavailable, the probability is variable, and even when present, not all patients will develop a condition or it is uncertain when it will arise.

Examples of screening tests.

- Regular colonoscopies to screen the colon for polyps, dysplasia or cancer in first degree relatives of a patient with bowel cancer or who have an APC (adenomatous polyposis coli) gene mutation.
- Performing regular OGDs, colonoscopies and abdominal MRI scans to screen for polyps or dermoid cysts in a patient with FAP.
- Requesting a mammogram to screen first degree female relatives of a patient with breast cancer.
- Performing regular breast MRI and transvaginal USS scans to screen the breast and ovaries of patients with a BRCA 1 or 2 gene mutation.
- Requesting a genetic test.

As with other screening tests, there are many potential pitfalls of performing a genetic test for screening. The variable penetrance of a genetic mutation means the lifetime risk of developing the condition is often variable. In addition, genetic tests may have unintended or unexpected personal, social and financial consequences for the patient.

Increasingly treatments are available to reduce the risk of a condition developing when there is a genetic risk. When the patient's lifestyle or diet is likely to compound a genetic risk, it may be appropriate to recommend a change.

Examples of treatments that may reduce risk.

- A colonoscopic polypectomy to reduce the risk of bowel cancer developing.
- A colectomy in an FAP patient to prevent colon cancer developing.
- A mastectomy in a patient with the breast cancer gene (BRCA1 and 2) to prevent breast cancer developing.
- An oophorectomy in a patient with the BRCA1 and 2 gene to prevent ovarian cancer developing.

Ask yourself, how does a genetic risk inform the signs to look for when examining the patient?

Occasionally, a genetic risk will inform the signs to look for on examination. For example:

- When a female has a genetic risk of breast cancer, examination of the breasts may be indicated.
- When a patient has a genetic risk of bowel cancer an abdominal and rectal examination may be indicated.
- When an infant has a risk of a hereditable condition appropriate signs should be looked for.

Risks from ongoing or past-morbidity

Essentially, all ongoing or past medical conditions are also risk factors for other conditions, because, with every medical condition there is a risk of a complication or a secondary problem developing. For most problems the risk is low and it is unnecessary to document the medical condition as a separate risk factor. On the other hand, when the risk is high or consequential the risk should be considered to be a risk factor and it may be relevant to formulating a diagnosis, planning management or the examination.

Ask yourself, is the medical risk factor relevant to formulating a diagnosis?

The nature of the ongoing or past-morbidity or its treatment will indicate whether the problem has the potential to recur or relapse and what late complications may arise. These should be considered when learning about the problem to formulate a diagnosis.

> Examples of when ongoing or past morbidity is a risk factor for the presenting problem.
>
> - Hypertension is a risk factors for the development of heart failure.
> - AF is a risk factor for a stroke.
> - DM is a risk factor for renal failure or retinopathy.
> - Hyper-cholesterolaemia is a risk factor for atherosclerosis.
> - Resecting the terminal ileum is a risk factor for gallstones.
> - Chronic inflammation, such as pancolitis or a chronic ulcer is a risk factor for cancer.
> - GORD is a risk factor for Barrett's oesophagus.
> - Steroid medication is a risk factor for fragility fractures.

When a condition is effectively treated it may still be a risk factor. For example:

- When a patient treated with an anti-hypertensive medication is no longer hypertensive, the risks associated with hypertension are reduced but the underlying risk factor, namely atherosclerosis remains.
- When GORD is treated with a PPI the symptoms may resolve but the risk of metaplasia may persist.

Ask yourself, is the medical risk factor relevant to planning management?

Management may be influenced by a medical risk factor in many different ways. A medical risk factor may influence investigation of the presenting problem. For example:

- A patient with chronic pancreatitis is at risk of developing exocrine insufficiency. When the patient presents with pale, offensive diarrhoea investigations, such as measurement of faecal fat, are indicated to diagnose steatorrhea.
- Crohn's disease or a previous right hemicolectomy is a risk factor for gallstones. When the patient presents with upper abdominal pain an USS may be indicated.

An additional out-of-program screening test, or a screening test for an asymptomatic problem associated with a co-morbidity or a treatment may be indicated.

When an ongoing medical problem is a risk factor for a recurrent problem or a future complication, management may be aimed at reducing or preventing the risk. For example:

- Anticoagulating a patient with AF to reduce the risk of a stroke.
- Removing the gallbladder during the same admission after an attack of gallstone pancreatitis to reduce the risk of a recurrence associated with a 5% mortality.
- Repairing an asymptomatic inguinal hernia because of the future risk of a complication.
- Performing a bowel resection for a dysplastic polyp that is likely to become malignant.

A medical risk factor may influence treatment of the presenting problem. For example:

- A risk of multiple intra-abdominal adhesions may be a relative contra-indication to a further operation.
- A risk of osteoporosis or metastatic cancer may change the treatment of a long bone fracture.

Examples of tests frequently performed on asymptomatic patients to screen for a potential problem (Appendix 2).

- Measurement of blood glucose in patients with ongoing medical conditions, such as renal or liver failure, or taking medications that could affect glucose metabolism, such as insulin or metformin. The aim is to screen for hypo- or hyper-glycemia.
- Measurement of serum sodium and potassium chloride, urea and creatinine concentrations in patients with ongoing medical conditions, such as liver or renal disease, congestive cardiac failure or DM or insipidus, or taking medications that are nephrotoxic, such as phenytoin, sulphonamides or aminoglycosides or that could affect salt and water balance, such as a diuretic, heparin or a proton pump inhibitor. The aim is to screen for deranged salt or water balance, kidney injury and to assess protein metabolism and liver function.
- Measurement of plasma transaminases and alkaline phosphatase to screen for asymptomatic hepatocellular damage in patients with cirrhosis, congestive cardiac failure, diabetes insipidus or the nephrotic syndrome, or who take medications, such as carbamazepine, macrolide antibiotics, statins, sulphonamides or immunosuppressants. In general, although they are non-specific tests, a change in the blood level from a previous baseline or a significantly abnormal result in an at-risk patient is likely to indicate hepatocellular damage.
- Measurement of blood lipids to screen for hyperlipidaemia in patients with DM, metabolic syndrome, cardio-vascular, renal or liver disease or when taking some medications, such as anti-viral medications, steroids or tamoxifen or to assess response to treatments, such as statins.
- An ECG to screen for a cardiac electrical abnormality, such as an arrythmia or IHD, in patients with ongoing or past medical conditions, such as previous AMI or stroke.

Ask yourself, how does a medical risk inform the signs to look for when examining the patient?

Occasionally, the risk associated with an ongoing or past-morbidity influences the examination, such as when there is a risk of a complication from atherosclerosis or a risk of a metabolic problem. Usually, the nature of the risk will indicate the signs to look for, but when the problem is asymptomatic the examination may include looking for signs of a possible problem.

Risks from inhaling tobacco smoke

Regularly inhaling tobacco smoke, whether as a primary smoker or as a second-hand smoker, is a risk factor for numerous medical conditions including cancer, and pulmonary and cardiovascular disease. At the start of the consultation, it is usually obvious when a patient is a smoker. If there is uncertainty, questions that could be asked include:

Do you smoke?
Have you ever smoked?
Does anyone in your family smoke?
If they smoke ask:
How many do you smoke each day?
How long have you smoked?

The risk from smoking increases with the duration and severity of the exposure. For example, the lifetime risk of cancer developing in a patient who has smoked since they were 20 years of age is about 15%. Stopping smoking freezes the risk at the level set when they stopped so that:

- A patient who smoked for 10 years when they were young has a 2% risk of developing lung cancer
- A patient who smoked for 30 years before stopping has a 6% risk of developing lung cancer

Ask yourself, how does a smoking habit affect the diagnosis?

When learning about the problem, the differential diagnosis may include a condition known to be associated with or caused by the patient smoking. For example:

- Breathlessness and a wheeze likely to be caused by asthma.
- Breathlessness likely to be caused by heart or lung disease.
- Leg pain likely to be caused by peripheral vascular disease.
- Chest pain likely to be caused by coronary artery disease.

Ask yourself, how does a smoking habit affect management?

A heavy smoker is at high risk of a complication, such as lung cancer. If the patient is 55-74 years of age and otherwise in good health a low dose CT scan may be indicated. A nodule is suspicious if it is >5mm or a new nodule when compared with a previous scan, a CXR is not sufficiently accurate to screen for cancer because the sensitivity is <50% for early signs, such as detecting a <1cm peripheral lung lesion, segmental pulmonary collapse or consolidation or mediastinal widening. On the other hand, a CXR may be indicated if there are symptoms, such as feeling ill, breathlessness or a persistent cough with the aim of excluding a diagnosis such as a pneumonia or a pleural effusion. The sensitivity and specificity of a CXR for the diagnosis of clinically suspected pneumonia ranges from 70-90% and for detecting a moderate to large pleural effusion is >95%.

For all patients who smoke, it may be appropriate to help them stop smoking. It is the responsibility of the HCP to ensure the patient is informed and to try to help them stop but it is the responsibility of the patient to stop.

Learning about the person and the patient and establishing a good rapport with the patient may help ensure the context, the timing, the tone and the method of the conversation are appropriate. In general, the right time to bring about change is when the patient is receptive and if it is discussed in context of something the patient says or a health problem. For example:

- Reflecting on something the patient says can be an opportunity to introduce change:

Earlier, when you were talking about…
I heard you say…

- Agree with something a patient says and introduce the topic of change:

Yes, it is likely your breathlessness is caused by smoking. Would you like to talk about it?

- When asking about a smoking habit, asking permission to focus on their habit.

Would it be OK if we talked about…?
Can we talk about…?
What do you think about…?
Would now be a good time to talk about…?
Do you want to know…
Would you like to hear/know…?

- Discussing the results of a test or the diagnosis may be an opportunity to discuss stopping smoking:

I have the results of the [test/biopsy/operation] would you like me to explain them to you? What do you think brought this about?
Have you thought what could be have caused the problem to arise?
What do you think might have caused your [problem]?

- Discussing the risks from a treatment may be an opportunity to discuss stopping smoking:

Smoking greatly increases the risk of a complication following your operation. Have you thought about stopping?

The method used to help the patient stop smoking should be appropriate to the patient and the context. Traditionally, directive methods are tried. For example:

- Telling the patient.

You must stop smoking.

- Scaring patients with warnings or threats about what might happen.

If you don't stop smoking you will get cancer.

- Reasoning: using statistics.

If you carry on smoking you have a 15% chance of dying from lung cancer.

- Begging patients

Please try to stop smoking.

- Emotional blackmail

You must stop smoking if you want to see your children grow up.

- Bribery

If you stop smoking, we will do your operation.

- Hoping

I am sure you will be able to stop.

Being direct, rarely brings about meaningful change. A non-directive approach using questions to first identify the barriers to change and then to help the patient identify solutions for themselves is more likely to be successful. Frequent barriers to stopping smoking include a lack of awareness, motivation or self-belief.

A lack of awareness or knowledge that smoking is harmful or could have caused a particular problem is possible despite the information available in the media. Questions to ask to raise awareness could include:

What is smoking doing to you?
Do you know the risks if you continue to smoke?
Do you know what might happen to you if you continue to smoke?
Do you know what damage smoking does to you?
What is likely to happen if you carry on smoking?
Did you know your [problem] was caused by smoking?

Patients will stop smoking if they want to. It may be appropriate to ask questions to determine whether or not motivation is a barrier:

Why do you choose to smoke?
What is preventing you from stopping smoking?
Do you want to stop?
How badly do you want to stop?
Do you know about the benefits of stopping?

A lack of self-belief may be a barrier. Questions to ask could include:

Do you think you can stop?
What is stopping you trying?
Have you tried to stop before? If not, why not? If so, what happened?
What happened when you tried to stop previously?
Do you know of other people who have stopped?

The aim is then to move from focusing on the problem and the barriers, which often seem too big to resolve, to focusing on solutions which are achievable.

When a lack of knowledge is the barrier, sharing information to increase their knowledge and understanding will raise awareness. Questions to ask could include:

Would it help if I explained what harm smoking can cause?
Would you like more information about the problems caused by smoking?
When a lack of motivation is a barrier:

What would increase your motivation to stop?
What would help you stop smoking?
Can we talk about the benefits of stopping?

When the patient lacks self-belief, the aim is to move from negative thoughts, such as blame, guilt, inadequacy or failure, to positive, problem-solving thoughts. Questions to ask could include:

How did other people manage to stop?
What would give you more confidence to stop?
What could you do differently?
What would help you to stop?

Small changes are more likely to be successful than a sudden major change. Questions can be asked to help the patient identify small changes that are achievable and therefore more likely to be successful. Questions to ask could include:

When do you smoke most? What could you change?
What could you do to make it more difficult to reach for a cigarette?
Do you carry your cigarettes around with you?
List what makes you smoke.

Some stop-smoking strategies are well known.

Examples of "stop-smoking" strategies

- Throw away all your cigarettes.
- Make the cigarettes difficult to access.
- Display positive distracting messages in key places.
- Write down your reasons for stopping and display them in prominent places.
- Tell everyone you are stopping. Enrol help from friends and family.
- Focus on strategies that worked before/for others, such as a keeping busy, a hobby or exercise.
- Develop coping strategies or distractions when the craving returns.
- Join a friend or a self-help group.

Some patients need help from the health service, i.e., helping the patient help themselves. Services that may be available include:

- Nicotine replacement treatment.
- Counselling.
- Supervision by an HCP.

The risk and conversation should be documented.

Ask yourself, how does a smoking habit inform the signs to look for when examining the patient?

Usually, a smoking habit does not influence the examination. However, when a patient is at risk of a complication, such as COPD, cardio-vascular disease or cancer, relevant signs should be looked for, such as clubbing, cyanosis, crepitations, a wheeze, hypertension, a murmur, a bruit, hepatomegaly or lymphadenopathy.

Risks associated with the patient's weight

At the start of the consultation and when learning about the person it is usually obvious when the patient is significantly over- or under-weight. The risk of harm from being under- or over-weight is proportional to the deviation from the reference range. A BMI 15-18.5 kg/m^2 is underweight and <15 kg/m^2 severely underweight, and a BMI 30-39.9 kg/m^2 obese and >40 kg/m^2 severely obese. The BMI has a high specificity of >90% for obesity but a low sensitivity at 50% because BMI does not distinguish between lean and fat mass. Visceral obesity assessed using waist circumference or waist: hip or height ratios, may be a better measure of obesity for some patients. The aim of making an assessment of a patient's weight is to inform management, as a baseline, and occasionally it is relevant to formulating a diagnosis or the examination.

Ask yourself, is the patient's weight relevant to formulating a diagnosis?

Obesity is a risk factor for many conditions including osteoarthritis, GORD, fatigue, sleep apnoea, cancer, cardio-vascular disease and metabolic syndrome. The risks associated with obesity frequently compound one another. For example, obesity, hypercholesterolaemia and hypertension individually and collectively increase the risk of heart disease. At the other extreme, anorexia may cause vitamin and trace element deficiency, hypoglycaemia, electrolyte abnormalities and kidney failure, anaemia, heart disease, osteoporosis, amenorrhoea and infertility.

Most patients are overweight as a result of their lifestyle: they eat more than they need, the nutrients in the food they eat are in the wrong form, or the food they eat stimulates more eating, such as eating a lot of highly processed food. Some obese patients have an underlying condition, such as depression, hypothyroidism, insulin resistance, Cushing's syndrome, polycystic ovary syndrome or take medications such as steroids, antidepressants, antipsychotic and anti-epileptic medications that contributes to their obesity. Patients who are underweight may have an underlying psychological or behavioural condition such as anorexia, stress or anxiety. A few are malnourished because of malabsorption, short gut syndrome or small bowel disease, such as Crohn's disease, or increased catabolism, such as cancer, chronic sepsis or thyrotoxicosis.

Ask yourself, is the patient's weight relevant to management planning?

Morbid obesity or anorexia may influence management planning because they cause some problems, increase the risk of many problems and are associated with increased mortality. Obesity may present procedural difficulties, such as gaining venous access or being too heavy to lie on a table or too wide to go through a scanner. When patients are morbidly obese or anorexic screening tests may be indicated. For example:

- BGL measurement to screen for DM in an obese patient and for hypoglycaemia in an anorexic patient.
- Measurement of blood lipids to screen for hyperlipidaemia in obese patients. The reference level is dependent on many factors including age, gender, lifestyle, genetics and ethnic group.
- Measurement of serum transaminases and perform a liver USS to screen for NASH in a morbidly obese patient. An early diagnosis of NASH is important because it is an independent risk factor for liver fibrosis. NASH is suspected if there is evidence of persistent hepatocellular damage and hepatic steatosis and an absence of other causes of liver disease, such as alcohol excess, hepatitis or auto-immune liver disease. Typically, in NASH, ALT levels are persistently raised <3 fold and exceed AST levels. An USS may indicate steatosis and exclude other causes of liver disease. However, the sensitivity for steatosis is about 50% and the specificity about 75%. A normal AST and the absence of steatosis is reassuring with a negative predictive value of >95%.
- Measurement of the blood haemoglobin concentration (reference range in males 140-175 g/L and 125-155 g/L for females) and haematinics may be indicated to screen for anaemia in an anorexic patient. Anaemia associated with a low MCV (reference range 80-96 fL/red cell), MCHC (reference range 33.4-35.5 g/dL) and MCH (reference range 27-31 pg/cell) indicate low iron stores (microcytic hypochromic anaemia). Anaemia associated with a high MCV (megaloblastic anaemia), MCH and MCHC is indicative of Vitamin B12 and/or folate deficiency. Anaemia associated with a normal MCV and MCHC (normochromic, normocytic anaemia) is

indicative of chronic disease. A high haematocrit (reference range 40-54% in males and 36-46% in females) may indicate deranged water balance.

- Measurement of serum sodium (reference range 135-145 mmol/L) and potassium (reference range 3.5-5.5 mmol/L) chloride (reference range 96-106 mmol/L), urea (reference range 2.5-7.8 mmol/L) and creatinine concentrations (reference range 62-115mol/L in men and 53-97 in women) may be indicated in patients with anorexia or DM. An abnormality may indicate deranged salt or water balance or kidney injury.

Initial management may focus on changing a life choice, such as a dietary or activity change. As with helping a patient to stop smoking a step-wise approach may help:

- Choose the right time when there is a good rapport and the patient is receptive.
- Ensure the discussion is appropriate and in context.
- Ask permission.
- Choose the right method.
- Identify solutions and strategies.
- Provide help and support.

Ask yourself, how does a patient's weight inform the signs to look for when examining the patient?

Measuring the patient's weight and height to determine their BMI may be indicated as a baseline or to assess change. In some patients, upper arm skin fold thickness or waist: hip or waist: height ratio may be measured.

Usually, a patient's weight does not influence the examination except when there may be an underlying condition or to look for signs of a complication. It should be recognised that the examination is often more challenging in obese patients, some signs are difficult to assess, such as pulse and blood pressure and deep-seated abnormalities, such as an intra-abdominal mass, are likely to be missed. Conversely, in a very thin patient, a normal organ may be easily felt and considered to be abnormal.

Risks from excessive alcohol consumption

When alcohol consumption is low or moderate it is not generally considered to be a risk factor. Indeed, there is a J shaped association between mortality and alcohol consumption because a low consumption reduces the risk of some conditions, such as heart disease, a stroke or DM, but the likelihood of medical, physical, psychological and social problems increases as the consumption increases.

Alcohol consumption is usually measured in units per day. The number of units in any drink can be calculated by multiplying the percent alcohol by volume (ABV) by the volume and dividing the result by 1000.

1 unit = (ABVxvolume)/1000

For example, 500mL of 5% beer contains 2.5 units of alcohol.

Alcohol consumption is considered hazardous when consumption regularly exceeds 3 units per day in women and 4 units per day in men. Questions that could be asked include:

Do you drink alcohol?
How much do you drink each day?

If so:

How long have you been drinking?
What alcohol do you drink normally?
What time of the day do you start drinking?
Can you go without alcohol for several days at a time?

When the reliability of a patients account of their alcohol consumption is uncertain relevant information may be obtained from the patient's medical records or from family or friends.

Ask yourself, is the patient's alcohol consumption relevant to the diagnosis?

When learning about the problem, the differential diagnosis may include a condition known to be associated with or caused by the patient drinking excessive quantities of alcohol. Binge drinking may cause acute toxicity with confusion, vomiting, and seizures, aspiration or injuries. People who regularly drink excess alcohol over many years may present with a variety of problems. Excess alcohol consumption is a risk factor for many medical conditions including a mental health condition, dementia, liver cirrhosis, chronic pancreatitis, cancer of the breast, mouth, throat, oesophagus, liver and bowel, infertility and impotence or cardiovascular disease.

Symptoms that could indicate excess alcohol consumption.

- Feeling ill, with anorexia, nausea, fatigue and weakness. For example:
  - From anaemia
  - From thiamine deficiency or malnutrition
  - With early onset dementia
- Acute and severe abdominal pain, such as from acute pancreatitis or persistent abdominal pain, such as from chronic pancreatitis
- Symptoms of deranged function, For example:
  - Social and behavioural changes, such as neglecting responsibilities, poor work performance, anxiety and aggression
  - A tremor
  - Jaundice from liver cirrhosis
  - Fatigue, weakness, giddiness, anxiety and memory loss from thiamine deficiency
  - Confusion, ataxia and visual disturbance (caused by oculomotor problems) from Wernicke's encephalopathy
  - Infertility and impotence
  - A headache from hypertension
  - Breathlessness from heart failure
  - Weakness from a stroke
- A visible or palpable abnormality. For example:
  - Abdominal distension from ascites
  - Spider naevi

Symptoms that could indicate withdrawal from excess alcohol consumption.

- A headache
- Blurred vision
- Dizziness, sweating
- Irritability, anxiety or insomnia
- Dry mouth
- Muscle or abdominal pains
- Anorexia, nausea and vomiting
- Diarrhoea

Ask yourself, is the patient's alcohol consumption relevant to management planning?

For most patient's, their alcohol consumption is low or moderate and does not affect management. Should a patient appear to be intoxicated it may be appropriate to take blood to measure the blood alcohol concentration. When a patient drinks alcohol to excess, investigations to screen for a complication may include:

- Measure the blood haemoglobin concentration and haematinics to screen for anaemia or polycythaemia.
- Measure serum urea, creatinine and electrolytes to screen for deranged salt or water balance, kidney injury and abnormal protein metabolism.
- Measure LFTs to screen for hepatocellular damage.

The patient should be told when their consumption is excessive and an attempt should be made to help them stop. As with helping a patient to stop smoking a step-wise approach may help:

- Choose the right time when there is a good rapport and the patient is receptive.
- Ensure the discussion is appropriate and in context.
- Ask permission.
- Choose the right method.
- Identify solutions and strategies.
- Provide help and support.

Ask yourself, how does an alcohol risk factor inform the signs to look for when examining the patient?

Usually, a patient's alcohol consumption does not influence the examination. When there is a suspicion that they drink alcohol to excess the signs to look for would include, agitation, twitching, shaking, sweating, palmar erythema, a liver flap, spider naevi, hepatomegaly or dull abdominal distension.

Risks from drug taking

Drug taking describes the act of taking a chemical, a drug, that has not been prescribed by an HCP or is taken for a purpose different from that which was intended or is taken in excessive quantities or in an abnormal way. The chemical may or may not be legal and may or may not be addictive.

Drugs commonly taken.

- Amphetamines ("speed or phat").
- Cannabis ("dope, hash, weed, pot or skunk").
- Cocaine and crack cocaine ("coke, white, snow or sniff").
- Ecstasy ("beans, pills or doves").
- Heroin ("smack, junk, brown, gear or skag").
- Ketamine ("special K or super K").
- Khat.
- LSD ("acid or trips").
- Piperazines ("smileys, pep twisted or happy pills").
- Alpha-methyltryptamine (AMT).
- Benzodiazepines ("roofies or downers").
- Steroids ("roids or smart drugs").
- Magic mushrooms ("shrooms or mushies").
- Aerosols, glues and solvents.

Drug taking is most prevalent in the 18-25-year-old age group. Some patients declare when they are taking drugs but usually a habit or an addiction are only disclosed when the HCP has gained the confidence of the patient. For this reason, any questions regarding drug use are best asked opportunistically, after gaining a patients' trust and then in a discreet and sensitive way. The questions to ask include:

Do you take drugs?
Have you ever taken drugs?

If so:

When did you last take drugs?
What drugs do you take?
How often do you take drugs?

There may be relevant information from the patient's medical records or from family or friends.

Whatever the circumstances, drug taking is risky behaviour and may cause medical, family, social and financial problems. The short- and long-term medical effects and the severity are influenced by the type of drug, the frequency, the amount taken and its purity, the duration and the susceptibility and tolerance of the patient. Early on, drug taking is a lifestyle choice, but, later, as a consequence of repeated exposure, persistent brain changes drive an overwhelming need to continue to take drugs; it is then an addiction.

Ask yourself, is the patient's drug consumption relevant to the diagnosis?

Drugs can affect different people in different ways and different drugs cause different symptoms and signs. When learning about the problem, the differential diagnosis may include a condition known to be associated with taking a drug. Patients may present:

- Feeling ill, with fatigue, exhaustion and anorexia or mental health conditions, such as depression, paranoia or hallucinations.
- With pains, including, headaches and abdominal pains.
- With symptoms of deranged function. For example:
  - A change in behaviour or extremes of behaviour, such as anxiety, sadness, dishonesty, aggression, irritability or agitation or increased energy and confidence and a loss of inhibitions.
  - Insomnia.
  - Impaired learning and intellectual performance, causing a deterioration in memory, judgment and decision-making.
  - Withdrawal from friends and family.
  - Problems with work, social, and family life, leading to a loss of employment, friends and divorce.
  - Blurred vision.
  - Dizziness.
  - Sweating, dry mouth, and muscle aches.
  - Nausea, vomiting, and diarrhoea.
- With a visible or palpable abnormality, such as a tremor, shaking or twitching.

The symptoms and signs may indicate the drug taken. For example:

- Anxious aggressive behaviour, irritability, twitchiness, tremor, with nausea and vomiting, headaches and dizziness, palpitations, tachycardia and dilated pupils are characteristic of cocaine, amphetamine or ecstasy.
- Euphoria, detachment, drowsiness, nausea and vomiting with pin-point pupils are characteristic of heroin.

Ask yourself, is the patient's drug consumption relevant to management?

A drug habit always affects management.

- Toxicology tests are indicated in all patients suspected of taking drugs.
- Investigations to screen for an asymptomatic complication, such as a metabolic abnormality or a chronic infection, may be indicated.
- Adherence and compliance with care is often unpredictable and unreliable.
- Gaining venous access in an intravenous drug user is likely to be difficult.

It is the responsibility of the patient to stop but it is the responsibility of the HCP to ensure they are informed and to try to help them stop. As a minimum, the patient should be told of the risks and the conversation documented. As with helping a patient to stop smoking a non-directive approach is more likely to be successful:

- Choose the right time when there is a good rapport and the patient is receptive.
- Ensure the discussion is appropriate and in context.
- Ask permission.
- Choose the right method.
- Identify solutions and strategies.
- Provide help and support. Addiction is often managed by specialists within a rehabilitation program.

Ask yourself, is the patient's drug consumption relevant to the examination?

Usually, a drug habit does not influence the examination, but, in some patients, an examination to look for signs of drug taking may be indicated, such as needle puncture marks, absent or thrombosed superficial veins.

Participation in a screening program

Screening is offered to people at increased risk of developing a particular condition. The aim is to detect a treatable condition early, before it becomes a significant problem. Screening may be undertaken for an individual on the basis of personal risks or as part of a national screening program. The medical records may indicate when a patient is in a screening programme. If there is uncertainty, it may be appropriate to ask.

Have you been asked to have a screening investigation, such as [investigation]?
Have you recently had a screening investigation?
When did you last have [investigation]?

If the patient has had a screening investigation, it would be appropriate to ask:

What was the test?
When was it done?
What was the result?

Examples of national screening programs.

- Pre-conception screening for genetic abnormalities. For example, cystic fibrosis, fragile-X syndrome, sickle cell disease.
- Pre-natal screening, including an USS, AFP chorionic villous sampling or amniocentesis.
- Hearing tests in new-born infants.
- Cervical cancer screening in young females.
- Breast cancer screening in middle aged or elderly females.
- Bowel cancer screening in the middle aged or elderly.
- AAA screening in the elderly.
- Prostate screening in elderly men.
- Screening for retinopathy in patients with DM.
- Screening for lung cancer in patients with previous exposure to asbestos.
- Screening for liver cancer in patients with cirrhosis.

If a patient has not had a screening test that they were eligible for, it may be appropriate to ask:

Did you get invited to have [investigation]?
Why didn't you have [Investigation]?

This may give an insight into their beliefs and likely compliance or adherence with future management.

Ask yourself, is their participation in a screening program relevant to the diagnosis?

Patients in a screening program are participating because of their increased risk. This should be considered when formulating a diagnosis. Alternatively, some patients will have had a recent investigation. The results of this may exclude some diagnoses.

Ask yourself, is their participation in a screening program relevant to planning management?

When a patient is already within a screening program, an "extra", "out of program", screening test may be indicated to provide additional information or to assess change relevant to the management of the new problem.

Examples of when an "out of program" screening test may be indicated.

- A CT scan may be indicated to exclude cancer recurrence in a patient who presents with a new problem but is already getting regular CT scans to detect cancer recurrence within a screening program.
- Measurement of serum cancer markers, such as PSA, CEA, CA125 or AFP to assess cancer progression or to screen for metastases or recurrent cancer in patients who have been or who are being treated.
- An abdominal USS may be indicated to re-assess the diameter of a AAA, a measure of the likelihood of rupture.
- An OGD may be indicated to re-assess dysplasia in Barrett's esophagus.
- Blood tests and eye tests may be indicated to re-assess renal function and retinopathy in a diabetic patient.
- In patients with chronic UC a colonoscopy may be indicated to re-assess disease severity or to detect dysplasia or cancer.

Ask yourself, is their participation in a screening program relevant to the examination?

The indications for their involvement in a screening programme may inform the signs to look for in the same way as the examination is influenced by ongoing morbidity.

Chapter 8
Learn and Understand Information about the Problem

Abstract

Learning about the problem is usually a pre-requisite to formulating a diagnosis and planning management. When the patient presents feeling ill, with pain or with symptoms of deranged function learning about the problem is usually the main focus of the consultation and is undertaken early in the consultation. When the patient presents with a visible or palpable abnormality, learning about the problem is undertaken while examining the site of the problem or after. The principal aims of learning about the problem are to formulate a diagnosis or a list of possible diagnoses, to plan management, in conjunction with information about the person and the patient, and to inform the signs to look for when examining the patient.

When a patient presents with a new problem, the headline information and the patient's description may include trigger words or phrases, "red flag" symptoms or indicate a disease pattern or a short list of possible diagnoses which inform the questions to ask to confirm or exclude a suspected diagnosis, to inform management and the examination. When the differential diagnosis is long or uncertain, questions should be asked to learn and understand the problem; to learn when and how the problem started, the onset, to determine if there has been any change, to determine the main symptom(s) and associated symptoms, to assess the severity of the problem and to learn about the location of the problem, the character and aggravating and relieving factors to formulate a diagnosis, or to determine the likely location of the abnormality causing the problem, the type of problem and a likely cause as a bridge to formulating a descriptive diagnosis or a limited list of possible diagnoses. Together this information should be used to inform management and the examination.

In conclusion, the quality and quantity of information learnt about the problem determines the likelihood a true diagnosis will be made and relevant management planned and sign sought.

Introduction

Listen to your patient, he is telling you the diagnosis.

(Sir William Osler FRS FRCP 1849-1918)

The traditional approach to learning about the problem is for the HCP to ask a predetermined sequence of questions to find out the presenting "complaint", and the "history of the presenting complaint". Patients usually describe their symptoms chaotically, and the traditional aim of the HCP is to make sense of the answers and to structure the information into a standard format. It is traditional for the "subjective" history to then be followed by an "objective" examination, in which each system is examined in turn in a standard way and documented accordingly. The information is used to complete a proforma, summarized and a differential diagnosis and management plan proposed. The traditional approach is rarely used by clinicians who have learnt that asking questions to learn and understand information about the problem should be undertaken to meet the aims of the consultation, usually to formulate a diagnosis, plan management and inform the examination, and be influenced by the available information and the patient.

Gathering information, understanding and interpreting the information to meet the aims should go hand in hand from the moment of first contact to the end of the consultation. The HCP should know why they are asking a question and how they will use the information learnt. Not all questions asked are of equal importance, but each answer should be used to understand the problem better. A knowledge of medicine and the basic sciences and method should be used throughout the consultation to know what questions to ask and to understand and interpret the available information.

Learning the necessary information is not a passive process, relying on the patient to be forthcoming with relevant information, but an active one, in which the HCP is actively seeking answers to pertinent questions, listening carefully and thinking. The HCP should know why they are asking a question and how they will use the information learnt. Gathering information and considering the differential diagnosis, management and the signs to look for should be concurrent from the moment of first contact to the end of the consultation.

Occasionally, the patient's description of their problem includes pathognomonic symptoms or fits a pattern indicating a likely diagnosis. This then informs the questions to ask, and the signs to look for and management. However, for most problems, the diagnosis is unclear. In which case, questions should be asked to learn and understand the problem to determine the location of the abnormality, the type of problem and the likely cause. The symptoms and possible diagnoses inform management options and the signs to look for on examination, and the differential diagnosis, management options and the examination findings should inform additional questions to ask.

The aim of this chapter is to describe how learning about the problem should be used to meet the aims of the consultation. Examination methodology is discussed in the next chapter.

Determine the Aims of Learning about the Problem

The aims for most people presenting with a new problem or a change in a pre-existing problem are to formulate a diagnosis, plan management and to inform the examination. When a patient presents for a follow up consultation, such as following an investigation, a lot of information is already known but asking additional questions about the problem may be indicated to assess change, usually to inform management. When a patient presents following a screening test that has revealed the likely diagnosis, learning about the problem is undertaken to identify any relevant symptoms, and, if present, confirm they are consistent with the likely diagnosis. Giving the patient an opportunity to talk about their problem also reassures them that they are being listened to, gives them hope that they will be cared for and helps build a working relationship. Relevant information about the problem should be documented in the health care record. In summary, the aims of learning about the problem include:

- Information exchange:
  - To learn and understand available information.
  - As a baseline assessment.
  - To inform learning about the person and the person as a patient.
  - To inform the examination.
  - To document relevant information.
- To formulate a diagnosis:
  - To confirm a diagnosis.
  - To make a diagnosis.
  - To exclude a diagnosis.
  - To determine the location of the abnormality causing the problem.
  - To determine the type of problem.
  - To determine the cause.
  - To screen for:
    - Another abnormality.
    - A secondary abnormality.
    - A complication.
- To help plan management:
  - Of the problem.
  - Of the symptoms.
  - Of the diagnosis.
  - To assess:
    - The local problem.
    - The impact on the patient.
    - Future risk.
- To help build a working relationship:
  - To reassure the patient.
  - To learn what the patient understands about their medical conditions.
  - To increase the likelihood of adherence and compliance with future care.

Decide Whether Learning about the Problem Is Indicated

Learning about the problem is indicated:

- When the patient presents with a new problem,
- When the patient presents with a change in an ongoing problem,
- When the patient is referred from another HCP,
- When the patient is seen following a screening investigation,

- When the patient is seen as a follow up consultation,

Learning about the problem may **not** be indicated when:

- It is unnecessary. For example, when all relevant information is already known or the problem has resolved,
- Confidentiality cannot be guaranteed,
- The patient is unable to give a reliable account of their problem,

Not learning about the patient should be a deliberate decision and the reasons documented unless they are obvious. Learning about the problem is contraindicated when the patient refuses permission.

Decide When to Learn about the Problem

The context of the consultation, the patient and the nature of the presenting problem determine when to learn about the problem.

When the HCP has not previously met the patient, when a patient is challenging or difficult or has a complex medical background, learning about the problem usually follows learning about the person and the person as a patient. This helps establish a working relationship and puts the problem in context, ensuring the patient is treated as a person with a problem (Figure 49).

When a patient presents with a new problem, feeling ill, a new pain or symptoms of a deranged function, or as a follow up consultation to assess change, learning about the problem is usually the initial focus of the consultation. When the presenting problem is a visible or palpable abnormality, examining the problem is usually the initial focus of the consultation (Figure 50).

Figure 49: A figure illustrating when to learn about the problem when meeting a new patient for the first time.

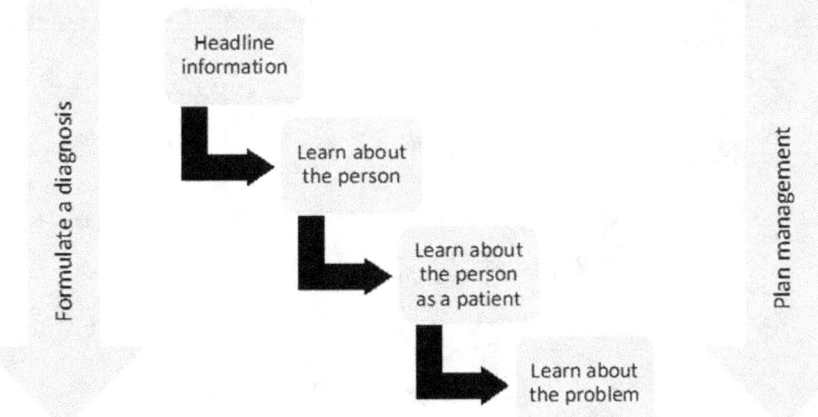

Figure 50: A figure illustrating when to learn about the problem when the patient presents with a new problem.

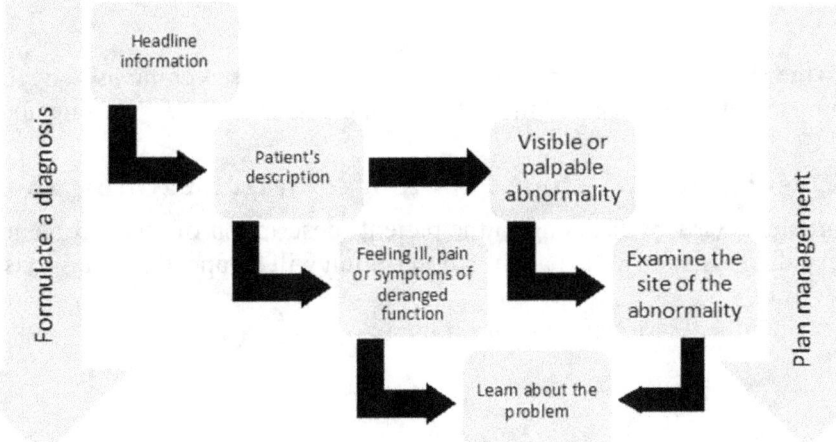

When the presenting problem is a visible or palpable abnormality, questions are asked to learn and understand more about the problem while examining the patient or after. For example:

- When a patient presents with an itchy blistering rash affecting the scalp or elbows the rash should be examined as the location and signs may be characteristic. If the signs are characteristic of dermatitis herpetiformis, questions can then be asked not only about the rash but also to find out about associated symptoms that may support the diagnosis. For example:

Have you been feeling unwell and tired?
Have you lost weight?
Have you had diarrhoea?

- A patient who presents with a localized uncomfortable pilonidal swelling should be examined as the location and signs may be characteristic. If the signs are characteristic of a pilonidal sinus, questions can be asked to learn about the problem. The questions to ask could include:

Have you had any previous episodes of swelling?
Has it ever been very painful or tender?
Has it discharged?

When the consultation follows an investigation, learning about the problem usually follows sharing information with the patient, such as the results of the investigation or the reason for the referral (Figure 51).

Figure 51: A figure illustrating when to learn about the problem when the patient is seen following an investigation or a previous consultation.

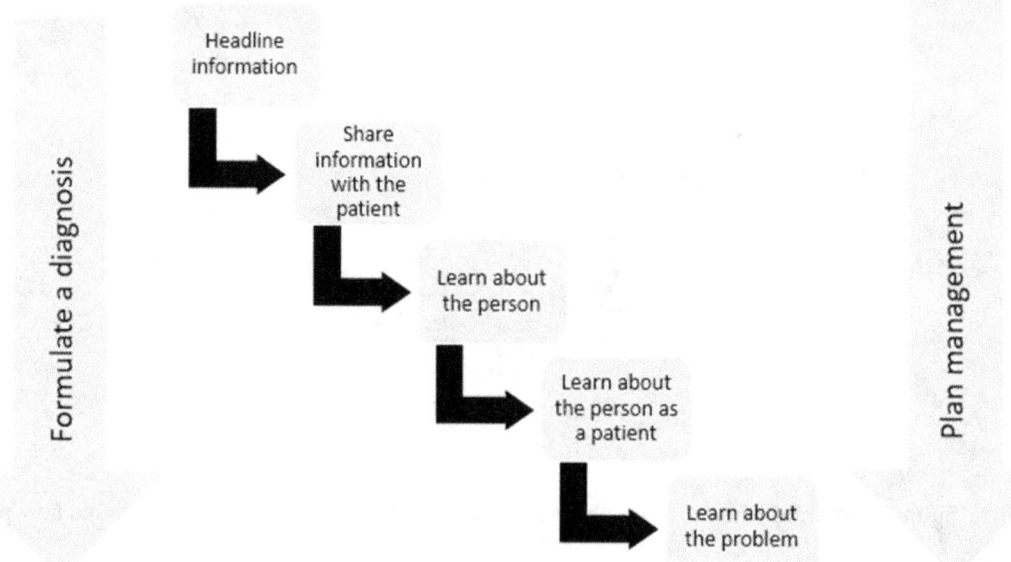

If the patient is new to the HCP, such as when they are seen following a screening investigation or following referral from another HCP, learning about the person and the patient usually also precedes learning about the problem.

Use the Patient's Description of Their Problem to Start Learning about the Problem

Learning about the problem starts by listening to the patient' description of their problem. When the diagnosis is uncertain or the differential diagnosis long, the patient's description will signpost the questions to ask first to learn and understand the problem.

While listening to the patient's description of their problem:

Ask yourself, what is the likely diagnosis or list of possible diagnoses?

The patient's description may include trigger symptoms or symptoms that indicate a diagnostic pattern. Trigger symptoms refer to any symptoms that indicates a likely diagnosis. They can include a pathognomonic symptom or a "red flag" symptom. This will inform the questions to ask or signs to look for to confirm the diagnosis and inform management.

Examples of trigger symptoms:

- Painless cloudy vision is characteristic of a cataract, painful tunnel or halo vision is characteristic of glaucoma and visual floaters or flashes of light suggests a retinal detachment.
- Vertigo and tinnitus are characteristic of Meniere's disease.
- Unexplained hyperpigmentation is characteristic of Addison's disease.
- "Rice watery" stool is characteristic of cholera.
- A painful clicking feeling or a catch at the base of the finger when bending or straightening the finger is characteristic of "trigger finger".
- An adult whose fingers turn white and feel cold with severe pain when exposed to cold and then become red and throb when re-warmed is likely to have Raynaud's syndrome (Auguste Gabriel Maurice Raynaud, a French doctor).

Examples of "red flag" or "alarm" symptoms:

- Unexplained weight loss of >5% over <6 months is an alarm symptom for cancer.
- Haemoptysis in a patient >40 years of age is an alarm symptom for lung cancer.
- An unexplained change in bowel habit in a patient >60 years or rectal bleeding and a change in bowel habit in a patient >50 years are alarm symptoms for colorectal cancer.
- Painless visible haematuria in a >45-year-old is an alarm symptom for transitional cell cancer of the bladder.

When the patient's description of their problem matches a diagnostic pattern, the information should be interpreted with the other headline information to inform the questions to ask to complete a pattern. For example:

- When a middle-aged patient presents with breathlessness on exertion and on lying down (orthopnoea) it may be caused by heart failure. The questions to ask to complete the pattern could include:

Do you suddenly wake up at night feeling very breathless (paroxysmal nocturnal dyspnoea)?
Do you prefer to sleep in a chair at night?
Do you have to pass water frequently at night (nocturia)?
Are you putting on weight?

- When a middle-aged patient presents with recurrent attacks of severe upper abdominal pain lasting a few hours or several days at a time the diagnosis is likely to be biliary colic. The questions to ask to complete the pattern could include:

Does the pain come and go in waves?
Could you find a comfortable position?
Was it as severe as having a baby?
Was it associated with a feeling of nausea and upper abdominal bloating?
Did it spread anywhere?
Do you know what brought it on?

- A middle aged, obese patient who presents with recurrent episodes of a "burning" retrosternal chest pain is likely to have gastro-oesophageal reflux disease (GORD). It may be appropriate to ask:

Is the pain retrosternal or more on one side?
Is it worse at night or on lying down or after meals?

Do you regurgitate bitter tasting fluid?

An incomplete pattern of symptoms does not necessarily exclude a diagnosis.

Some patients think they know the diagnosis and include it in their description of the problem. This may be because they have experienced the problem before or they may have talked to friends or family or they have researched the problem prior to the consultation. When this occurs, it remains important to ask questions and examine the patient to confirm the symptoms and signs are consistent with the diagnosis. When the pattern of symptoms indicates a likely diagnosis, this should be used to inform the signs to look for and management.

When there are no trigger symptoms or a diagnostic pattern is not recognised, the patient's description together with demographic information and other information learnt about the person and the patient may indicate a short list of possible diagnoses. Questions can then be asked to confirm or exclude each diagnosis ("diagnosis-hypothesis testing"). For example:

- When a middle-aged patient presents with a severe headache lasting several hours the differential diagnosis includes stress, migraine and a sub-arachnoid haemorrhage. It is important to exclude a sub-arachnoid haemorrhage (SAH). The initial questions to ask could include:

Did it come on suddenly?
How bad was it?
Have you ever experienced a similar headache before?
What were you doing before the headache started?
Did you feel weak or collapse?

When migraine is the working diagnosis additional questions may be indicated to support the diagnosis

Have you had it before?
Do you also feel sick when you get the headaches?
Do you avoid bright light?
Have you noticed if anything brings the headaches on, such as cheese or wine?

- When a teenage Libyan patient presents with severe pains in different joints the differential diagnosis includes sickle cell disease, juvenile arthritis or leukaemia. Given their Libyan ethnicity, it is important to exclude sickle cell disease. The initial questions to ask could include:

Have you had a fever or a rash?
Are the pains worse in cold weather?
Have you had pains elsewhere, such as in the chest or abdomen?
Has anyone commented that you have appeared slightly yellow?
Have your glands ever become swollen?

- When an elderly patient who has drunk a lot of alcohol over many years presents with chronic diarrhoea the differential diagnosis includes cancer, colitis and pancreatic exocrine deficiency from chronic pancreatitis. Given the history of alcohol consumption chronic pancreatitis is likely and the initial questions to ask could include:

What colour are your stools?
Are the stools difficult to flush away?
Is the smell very offensive?
Do you have any abdominal bloating?
Have you been losing weight?
Have you had any abdominal or back pain?
Have you noticed any blood or slime in your stools?

- When a middle-aged obese man presents with recurrent central chest pain the differential diagnosis includes GORD and angina. The initial questions to ask include:

Does the pain feel like a burning pain or is it more of a constant ache or tightness?
Does it spread anywhere, such as to your shoulder or upper arm?
What makes it worse? Can you walk up hills?
What makes it better?

When the differential diagnosis is long or the diagnosis uncertain, the patient's description is used as a springboard to asking questions to learn and understand the problem (Figure 52).

Figure 52: Illustrating how the patient's description leads to asking questions to learn and understand the problem

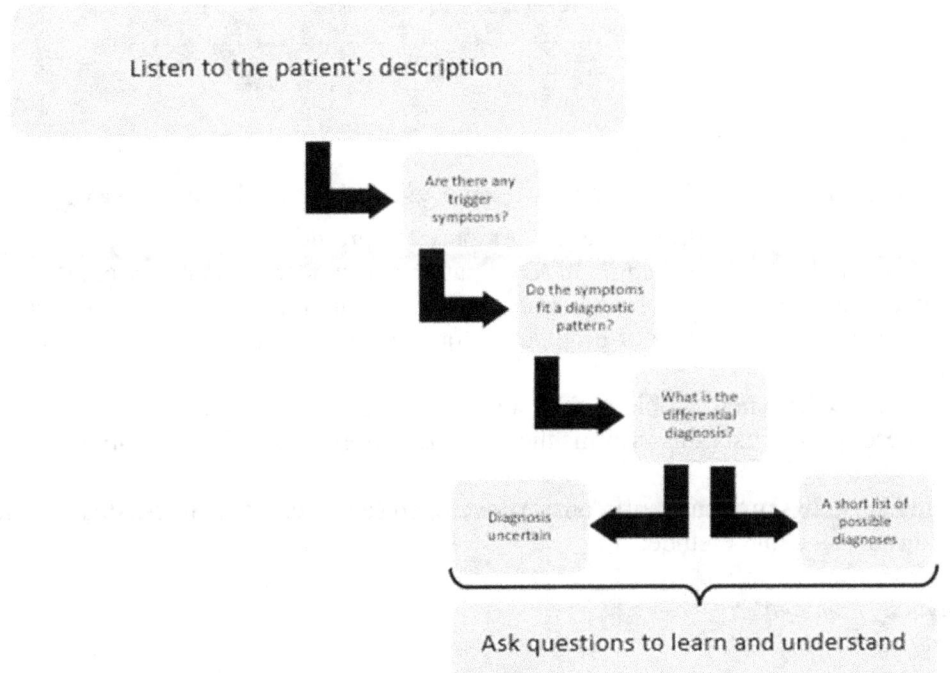

Ask Questions to Learn and Understand the Problem

The patient's description is a springboard to asking questions to learn and understand the problem. Before asking a question, it is important to ask yourself, "What is the aim of the question?", because questions should be asked to meet an aim, not as a ritual. When a diagnosis is likely, or the list of possible diagnoses short, questions are asked to confirm or exclude each diagnosis: this is "diagnosis-hypothesis" testing. When there is diagnostic uncertainty, the principal aims are to determine the likely location of the abnormality causing the problem, the type of problem and the likely cause to determine the likely diagnosis or a list of possible diagnoses, to inform management and the signs to look for on examination (Figure 53). Frequently, the answers to a question meet several aims.

There is no set question that should be asked first, or set order to asking questions. The questions to ask and order they are asked will be influenced by the headline information, the aims of the consultation, information from the patient, the emphasis the patient places on some symptoms, and other factors, such as intuition. In general, learning to understand starts with an open question based on the patient's description. Occasionally, such as when there is a need to clarify something a patient says, it starts with a closed question.

When the patient presents with a new problem it is usual to first learn about the onset and duration of the problem. This may then lead onto asking about any change in the symptoms. When the patient is seen as a follow up to a previous consultation, it is usual to first learn about any change. When a patient has a severe problem and is clearly distressed, it is usual to show empathy by asking them about its severity, and then to ask about when it started and how it was at the outset.

Figure 53: A figure outlining the information to use and questions to ask yourself when learning to understand.

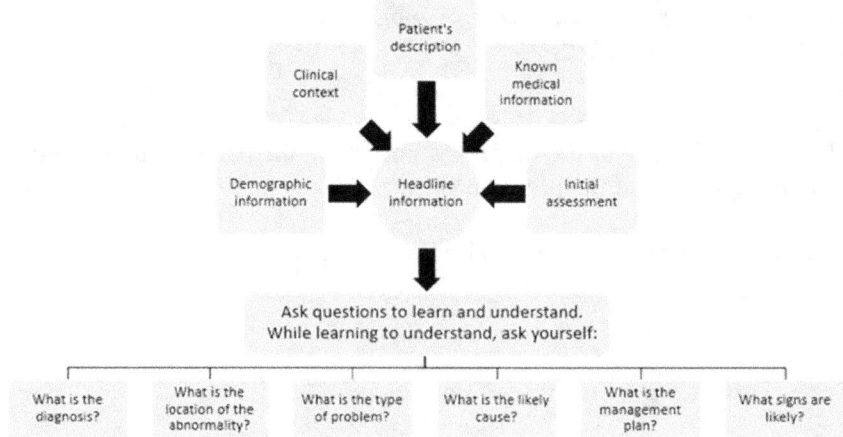

Ask questions to learn about the onset and duration of each symptom

The principal aims of learning about the onset and duration are to provide a timeframe for learning about the problem and for learning about and understanding change. In some patients, a sudden or acute onset or a short duration of their symptoms, together with the location of the problem and other headline information, may indicate a likely diagnosis, the location of the abnormality and the type of problem, inform management or the signs to look for on examination based on probabilities.

When a patient presents with a new problem, they may include information about the onset and/or the duration of their problem in their description. If so, this informs the initial questions to ask. For example:

- A 65-year-old man may say "I suddenly (onset) developed severe chest tightness this morning (duration)." The initial questions to ask could include:

What do you mean by "sudden"?
What were you doing at the time?

- A 25-year-old patient may say "I have had a really uncomfortable headache for several days (duration)." The initial questions to ask could include:

Did it start suddenly or has it been gradually getting worse over the last few days?

- A 50-year-old female may say "My abdominal cramps have got so bad over the last few months (duration) that I often have to lie down in bed." The initial questions to ask could include:

How did they start?
Did they start suddenly or gradually get worse over time?

If the duration was not mentioned, or is unclear, it may be appropriate to ask:

When did [symptom] start?
Can you tell me when it started?
How long have you been getting [symptom]?
Have you been ill for a few days, a few weeks or a few months?
Do you remember when you last felt well?
Were you well [chose a notable date, such as last Christmas]?

Usually, the patient will describe the onset, i.e., how quickly it started, if it started suddenly or acutely but only mention the duration if it came on gradually. If the onset was not mentioned, or it is unclear, it is important to ask questions to determine whether it started suddenly, in a matter of minutes, acutely, when it developed over several hours or days, or gradually, when it developed over several days or weeks. It may be appropriate to ask:

> *How quickly did [the symptom] start?*
> *Did it start suddenly or develop over minutes, hours or days?*
> *What were you doing when it started?*

If the patient cannot remember the onset or can't describe the onset, it is likely to have been gradual.

When learning about the duration it is usually sufficient to ask questions to distinguish between an acute problem that has been present for several hours or days, a sub-acute problem, that has been present for several weeks or months and a chronic problem that has been present for more than 3 months.

When symptoms have been present for a long time, it may be appropriate to ask:

> *Why have you presented now?*

There are many reasons why a patient presents late in the course of their condition. For example:

- The problem, such as a pain, is mild or the symptoms non-specific.
- The patient considered the problem, such as a pain to be a "normal" pain. For example, mistaking pleurisy for a musculo-skeletal pain.
- The patient hoped it would resolve.
- The patient did not consider the symptoms important.
- The symptoms may be embarrassing. For example, dyspareunia or anal pain.
- The patient may not want another family member to know they have a problem.
- The symptoms are only now affecting their life, such as when a self-employed worker only presents when it affects their work or a carer when they can no longer carry on.
- The symptoms are having an impact on a previously diagnosed problem, such as when a patient with pre-existing COPD presents when their coordination affects them using an inhaler.
- When there has been a change.

Some patients present because a problem has recurred after an interval without the problem. Patients usually mention when the problem is recurrent. If not, it may be appropriate to ask:

> *Is this the first time you have had these symptoms?*
> *Have you had this problem before?*
> *Is this similar to previous times?*

A minority of problems have a tendency to recur at regular intervals. In other words, they have a periodicity. If the differential diagnosis includes a condition likely to recur at regular intervals it would be appropriate to ask:

> *When does [the problem] recur?*
> *Have you noticed if it recurs [every day], [every week] or only in the [summer/winter]?*

An increasing number of problems are managed rather than cured. For many patients, there are periods when the patient is relatively well, in remission, and other times when the condition gets worse; a relapse. Usually, the patient will state when it is a relapse or it becomes clear when learning about change.

When the problem started suddenly or acutely, is recurrent or a relapse, the patient may mention a possible cause or precipitating factor. This may be diagnostically important. For example:

- Sudden severe chest pain precipitated by excessive exertion or stress may indicate an acute myocardial infarction.
- A sudden onset of unilateral superficial chest pain during vigorous coughing may be caused by a broken rib or a pneumothorax.
- A sudden onset of constant severe abdominal wall pain while straining to lift a heavy object may indicate a muscle injury, causing a rectus sheath haematoma.

- Retrosternal burning pain after swallowing food or liquid that is too hot or after swallowing a chicken bone indicates an oesophageal burn or laceration.
- Vomiting or retching followed by severe and persistent retrosternal chest pain may be caused by a ruptured oesophagus (Boerhaave's syndrome).
- Nausea, vomiting and/or diarrhoea may be caused by ingesting contaminated food or liquid.
- Dysuria and urinary frequency following intercourse may be caused by a UTI.

A suggested cause should be interpreted with caution because it may be incorrect or misleading. Nevertheless, the information may confirm how quickly the condition started or when the condition started and may give some insight into what the patient is concerned about. If the cause is not included in the patient's description it may be appropriate to ask:

What do you think caused your [problem]?
What were you doing when [the problem] started?
Is there anything that could have caused your [problem]?
Do you know what caused your [problem]?
Do you know why the [problem] started?
Do you know what brings on a recurrence?
Is there anything you avoid doing or taking because you think it brings on [symptom]?

When a particular diagnosis is suspected it may be appropriate to ask about recognized precipitating factors. For example:

- When a patient presents with recurrent attacks of severe pain in the right upper quadrant of the abdomen, likely to be biliary colic, the questions to ask could include:

Is an attack brought on by eating certain foods, such as cream, fried foods or pastries?
Do you avoid eating some foods because they bring on the pain?

- When a patient presents with recurrent severe headaches, likely to be migraine, the questions to ask could include:

Is an attack brought on by flashing lights or stress?
Do you avoid eating some foods, such as cheese, or wine, because they bring on the headache?

It is important to distinguish between a cause, or precipitating factor and an aggravating factor. A precipitating factor brings on or causes the problem whereas an aggravating factor makes a problem worse. For example:

- A patient who presents with severe chest pain during exertion may have angina or an AMI. If the pain started suddenly, for the first time, when they were undertaking exercise and persists despite resting, an AMI is more likely and the exercise is the precipitating factor. If the pain is worse whenever they exercise and better when resting, angina is more likely and exercise is an aggravating factor and resting a relieving factor.
- A patient who presents with a persistent severe anal pain and anal bleeding after passing a constipated stool is likely to have suffered anal trauma, whereas a patient who gets increased anal pain and passes more blood when opening their bowels may have an anal fissure.

When learning about the onset and duration:

Ask yourself, what is the likely diagnosis?

Information about the onset together with the headline information may indicate a likely diagnosis based on probabilities or pattern recognition. For example:

- When a patient presents with pain in the leg:
  - A sudden onset of leg pain in an elderly patient is characteristic of a femoral artery occlusion.

- o An acute onset of pain in the calf in a young female may be a DVT.
  - o Pain that has been coming and going for months in a middle-aged obese man may be claudication.
- When a patient presents with difficulty passing urine:
  - o A sudden onset of anuria is likely to be caused by bladder outflow obstruction, such as from a blood clot.
  - o An acute or sub-acute onset persistent for several weeks may be caused by renal failure.
  - o Chronic and increasing difficulty passing urine in an elderly man is likely to be caused by bladder outflow obstruction, such as from prostatic hypertrophy.
- When a patient presents with unilateral partial loss of vision:
  - o A sudden onset is likely to be caused by a retinal artery embolus.
  - o An acute or sub-acute onset persistent over several weeks in an elderly patient may be caused by glaucoma.
  - o A chronic deterioration over many months in an elderly patient may be caused by a cataract.
- When a patient presents with breathlessness and a wheeze:
  - o A sudden onset is likely to be caused by a hypersensitivity reaction.
  - o An acute onset over several days is likely to be caused by a chest infection.
  - o Symptoms that have been present for many months or years are likely to be caused by bronchitis.
- When a patient presents with dysphagia:
  - o A sudden onset is likely to be caused by a food bolus sticking in the oesophagus.
  - o A sub-acute onset persistent over several weeks in an elderly patient is likely to be caused by cancer.
  - o If it has been present for many years, it is likely to be caused by a benign stricture or a motility problem.
- When a patient presents with diarrhoea:
  - o An acute onset of watery diarrhoea is likely to be caused by infective colitis.
  - o A gradual onset persistent over several weeks may be cancer or colitis.
  - o Symptoms that have been present for many months or years may be caused by coeliac disease or colitis.
- When a patient presents with constipation:
  - o An acute onset of absolute constipation is likely to be caused by large bowel obstruction.
  - o A gradual onset persistent over several weeks may be cancer.
  - o Symptoms that have been present for many months or years may be caused by slow transit constipation.

Symptoms that are recurrent or relapse may also indicate a likely diagnosis. Conditions that typically are recurrent or relapse include sciatica, reflux oesophagitis, interstitial cystitis, biliary colic, irritable bowel syndrome, migraine or seizures. Some conditions tend to recur at regular intervals. For example:

- Conditions linked to a diurnal rhythm, such as Pel-Ebstein fever in Hodgkin's lymphoma, a fever associated with Stills disease, malaria or tick- or louse-borne relapsing fever.
- Conditions linked to the menstrual cycle, such as mid-cycle (ovulatory) or menstrual abdominal pain, endometriosis, polycystic ovary syndrome, depression, migraine or irritable bowel syndrome.
- Seasonal conditions, such as depression or hay fever.

Some conditions are known to relapse. Conditions that typically are prone to relapse include arthritis, asthma, Crohn's disease, polymyalgia, giant cell arteritis, EBV infection ("glandular" fever), or cancer.
A precipitating factor may indicate a likely diagnosis. For example:

- A recurrent headache starting when tired or stressed is likely to be a tension headache.
- Recurrent headaches after eating cheese or drinking alcohol are likely to be caused by migraine.
- A sudden onset of dysphagia while eating a chicken meal is likely to be caused by a chicken bone that gets stuck in the oesophagus.
- A sudden onset of constant retrosternal chest pain while profusely vomiting and retching is likely to be caused by a ruptured oesophagus.
- A sudden onset of breathlessness following sitting still on a long journey may be caused by a pulmonary embolus.
- A sudden onset of chest wall pain while vigorously coughing is likely to be caused by a broken rib.
- A sudden onset of chest pain precipitated by excessive exertion or stress is likely to be caused by an AMI.
- Profuse vomiting, diarrhoea and cramping abdominal pains after going out for a meal at a restaurant may be caused by gastroenteritis.

- Not passing urine following a hernia operation is likely to be caused by acute urinary retention.
- Abdominal wall pain and swelling occurring after lifting something heavy is likely to be caused by a muscle injury.
- Constipation following starting codeine or an opiate is likely to be caused by the medication.
- In an elderly patient, groin pain that started suddenly after a fall may be caused by a femoral neck fracture.

When the diagnosis is uncertain:

Ask yourself, what is the likely location of the abnormality, the type of problem and the likely cause?

In general, when a problem starts suddenly or acutely the location of the problem is likely to be the location of the abnormality and is likely to be caused by a circulatory, structural or neurological type of problem or by non-infective inflammation. Symptoms from infection, metabolic problems or cancer do not usually start suddenly. For example:

- A sudden onset of weakness or numbness on one side of the body indicates a primary neurological abnormality likely to be caused by a circulatory type of problem, such as a cerebral embolus or haemorrhage.
- A sudden unexplained loss of vision in one eye is likely to be caused by a circulatory type of problem affecting the eye, such as a retinal artery occlusion.
- A sudden onset of left sided chest pain is likely to be caused by a primary cardiac abnormality, such as IHD.
- A sudden onset of complete dysphagia is likely to be caused by a structural oesophageal abnormality, such as a foreign body.
- A sudden onset of pain in the flank is likely to be caused by a primary abdominal structural problem, such as ureteric colic.
- A sudden onset of abdominal pain is likely to be caused by a primary abdominal abnormality. It may be a circulatory problem, such as ischaemic bowel, a noninfective inflammatory problem, such as acute pancreatitis or a perforated peptic ulcer, or a structural problem, such as small bowel obstruction.
- A sudden onset of pain in the leg is likely to be due to a circulatory abnormality affecting the femoral artery or a deep vein, such as a femoral artery occlusion or a DVT.
- An acute onset of feeling ill is likely to be caused by, a primary neurological abnormality, such as, a seizure.
- An acute headache is likely to be caused by a primary neurological abnormality, such as a tension headache or migraine, or a circulatory type of problem, such as a sub-arachnoid haemorrhage.
- An acute onset of vomiting and diarrhoea is likely to be caused by an inflammatory problem affecting the gastro-intestinal tract, such as gastro-enteritis.

In general, problems that develop gradually over hours or days are usually caused by an infection, such as a chest or urinary tract infection.

Feeling ill or symptoms of deranged function, such as breathlessness or a change of bowel habit, often develops insidiously, over weeks or months. In such patients, the speed of onset or duration does not distinguish between a primary and secondary problem or indicate the likely type of problem. However, the initial symptoms may indicate the likely location of the abnormality or whether the abnormality is primary or secondary to a problem elsewhere.

Ask yourself, how can information about onset and duration inform management?

Information about the onset and duration may influence the priority and choice of management option. For some problems that start suddenly and present shortly after their onset, urgent investigations or treatment may be indicated. For example:

- A sudden onset of unilateral weakness in an elderly patient being treated for AF is likely to be caused by an embolic stroke. An urgent CT scan may be indicated to confirm the diagnosis and determine the likely cause.
- When an elderly patient, who previously had an AMI and a stroke, presents with a sudden onset of pain in the leg it is likely to be caused by a femoral artery occlusion. An urgent angiogram may be indicated to confirm the diagnosis, identify the cause of the occlusion and enable urgent reperfusion treatment.
- In an elderly patient, who has had a weak urinary stream for many months, lower abdominal pain and acute anuria is likely to be caused by bladder outflow obstruction. Urgent catheterization may be indicated to restore renal function.

Problems that start gradually and have been present a long time are less likely to need urgent investigations or treatment. However, occasionally, urgent investigations and treatment is indicated, such as when reserve function has been exhausted and organ failure is imminent.

Ask yourself, how can information about onset and duration inform the examination?

The onset and duration do not usually inform the examination although it is important when examining the patient to ensure the signs are consistent with the apparent duration of the problem. When the problem has been present a long time, it may be appropriate to look for signs to assess the impact on the part affected, the patient or to check for signs of an asymptomatic complication or secondary problem.

Ask questions to learn about a change in the symptoms

The aims of learning about change are to determine whether the problem has deteriorated or progressed, or is a complication, secondary problem or a new problem has arisen and to decide on the main symptom(s) (Figure 54). When the patient presents soon after the start of the problem or there is a single symptom it is unlikely the problem will have changed. However, this should not be assumed. Therefore, unless the patient describes a change in their symptoms, it is appropriate to check:

Have your symptoms changed?
Are your symptoms the same now as they were at the beginning?

When change is possible, the questions to ask could include:

What changed?
What was the first symptom?
Could you tell me what has happened from the beginning?
Tell me what you first noticed?
Which symptom occurred first? What happened next?
When did [symptom] start?

Figure 54: Illustrating the questions to ask yourself when there has been a change in the symptoms.

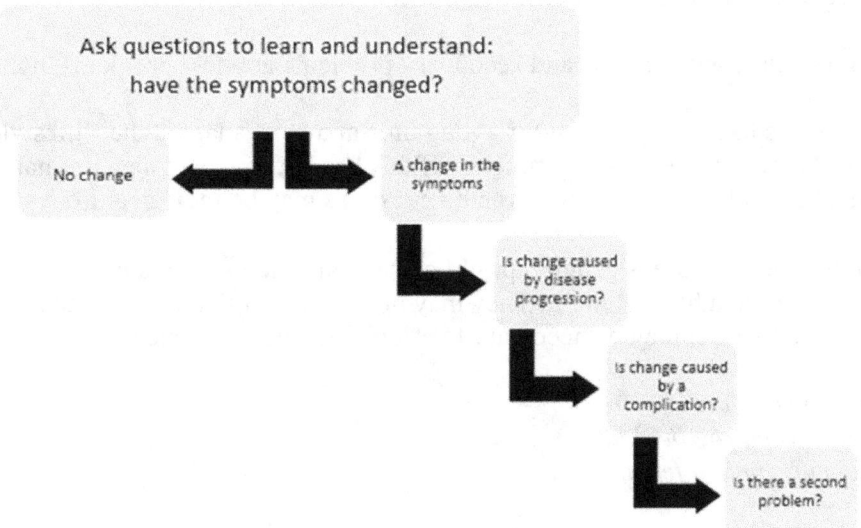

Disease progression is part of the natural history of the condition. It may be manifest as a change in severity, a change in the location or extent of the symptoms, or the development of new symptoms. Often the change in the symptoms caused by disease progression is diagnostic. For example:

- When chest tightness on exertion, likely to be caused by IHD, now stops the patient from walking to the shops, the angina is deteriorating.
- When central abdominal pain, likely to be caused by acute appendicitis, moves to the right lower quadrant, the inflammation is localizing, part of the natural history of appendicitis.
- When severe leg pain, likely to be caused by a femoral embolus, is followed by numbness and loss of power, the ischaemia is progressing.

A complication is a new problem caused by the initial problem. For example:

- Severe constant crushing central chest pain in a patient with longstanding angina indicating an acute myocardial infarction, a complication.
- Right upper quadrant abdominal pain, tenderness and a fever likely to be cholecystitis, severe generalized peritonitis likely to be acute pancreatitis or the development of jaundice, following previous episodes of upper abdominal colic, indicate a complication of gallstone disease.
- Sudden onset of severe deep seated abdominal and lumbar back pain from a ruptured AAA after a period of less severe constant back pain is a complication.
- Localized or generalized peritonitis after a period of upper abdominal pain caused by perforation of a peptic ulcer is a complication.
- Mid-gut abdominal colic and vomiting in a patient with a tender irreducible femoral hernia indicate the hernia is complicated by small bowel obstruction.
- Fever, hot and cold sweats and rigors in a patient with loin to groin colic indicating pyelonephritis complicating ureteric obstruction or in a jaundiced patient indicating ascending cholangitis complicating choledocholithiasis.
- A momentary loss of consciousness and recovering unilateral weakness in a patient with pre-existing AF indicating a TIA is an embolic complication of the AF.

A secondary problem is a reversible physiological response to the problem. For example:

- Profuse vomiting may cause dehydration and hypovolaemia, a secondary problem. Should renal failure caused by acute tubular necrosis develop, this is a complication.
- Acute confusion secondary to sepsis.
- Episodes of lower abdominal colic from diverticular disease, becoming a constant severe inflammatory pain in the right lower quadrant and a fever indicating acute diverticulitis, a secondary problem. If the bowel perforates forming an abscess or causing appendicitis, this is a complication.

Unlike disease progression, complications and secondary problems are new problems, not always associated with the problem.

Occasionally, a patient has had their problem for a long time and have adapted their lifestyle to reduce the severity of a problem or the risk of a recurrence of the symptoms. If this has become the "new normal", they may not mention the change. If change is likely but not mentioned, targeted questions may be indicated. For example:

- When a patient has heart failure, sleeping upright on several pillows or in a chair may seem "normal" to them and they are no longer breathless at night. They may not remember that the change in their behaviour occurred to avoid feeling breathless. It may be necessary to ask closed questions such as:

What happens when you lie flat?
Do you feel breathless when you lie flat?
Have you ever woken up at night feeling breathless?

It is not unusual for patients to present with multiple symptoms, but it is unusual for patients to have two or more unrelated new problems. When the initial and presenting symptoms seem unrelated or are inconsistent there may be more than one problem. For example:

- A patient may present with a reducible groin hernia and a change in bowel habit. They may think the hernia has caused the change in bowel habit. However, the hernia has been present a long time, and, on examination is small, soft, non-tender and disappears on lying flat. Therefore, it is likely the change in bowel habit is a new problem and the hernia is a longstanding co-incidental problem.

- An acute exacerbation of back pain after moving furniture without any other symptoms is more likely to be due to a musculo-skeletal injury or osteoarthritis than the 3cm AAA identified on a recent screening USS.

When more than one problem is likely it is necessary to ask questions to learn about each separately.
When learning about change:

Ask yourself, what is the likely diagnosis?

When there is evidence of disease progression the pattern may indicate a likely diagnosis. For example:

- A sudden onset of severe pain in the limb, followed by numbness, then weakness and eventually paralysis in the leg is likely to be caused by progression of ischaemia. The severe pain is caused by hypoxia from the initial arterial occlusion. When the hypoxia leads to cell death the function of the affected tissues deteriorates. Nerves are more sensitive to hypoxia than muscle and skin.
- In a young adult constant pain, tenderness and guarding in the right lower quadrant of the abdomen is likely to be caused by acute appendicitis. If the patient started with central abdominal colic 24 hours previously and then the pain moved to the right lower quadrant and changed, this diagnosis becomes more likely. The reason for this change is that acute appendicitis classically starts as midgut pain from a faecolith impacted within the lumen of the appendix. Then when the obstructed appendix becomes inflamed, the inflammation irritates the adjacent somatically innervated parietal peritoneum. In some patients, the inflammation causes a localized ileus, a type of functional small bowel obstruction, causing upstream, mid-gut intestinal colic, nausea and vomiting.
- An intermittent perianal spotting of pus following a burst perianal abscess is likely to be a perianal fistula. The abscess was initially caused by a sinus from an infected anal gland. Once the abscess burst, and if the sinus remains patent, there is an abnormal connection between the anal gland in the anoderm and the skin, a perianal fistula.

A complication or a secondary problem may also be evidence in support of a likely diagnosis. For example:

- When a patient presents feeling ill, breathless and has swollen ankles, it is likely they have heart failure. However, if they first had a flu-like condition, then they started to get increasingly breathless and noticed their feet and ankles swelling it is likely an initial viral condition is complicated by the development of heart failure due to either pericarditis or myocarditis.
- In an elderly patient with Parkinson's disease, a head injury or a fracture following a fall is likely to be a complication of their impaired balance, gait and bradykinesia.
- When a patient presents with acute confusion it is likely to be secondary to another problem. If, on asking questions about early symptoms and a change in the symptoms it becomes apparent that the patient first developed loin to groin colic and then developed a fever before becoming confused and unwell. The sequence of events would indicate the acute confusion was secondary to septicaemia, a complication of an infected obstructed urinary tract.
- When a patient presents with rectal bleeding and constipation it is likely the patient will highlight the rectal bleeding. However, if the constipation started first and was associated with straining the rectal bleeding is likely to be a secondary problem from, for example, a haemorrhoid or an anal fissure.
- When a patient presents with haematemesis, the blood in the vomitus is likely to be highlighted by the patient. However, if the blood appeared in their vomitus after a period of vomiting and retching, it is likely to be a secondary to the retching, i.e., a Mallory-Weiss tear.
- When a patient presents with lower abdominal colic and a constant pain in the left lower quadrant of the abdomen made worse on moving, they are likely to highlight the colic as it will be the dominant symptom. However, if the inflammatory pain in the left lower quadrant started first and the colic arose later it is likely the colic is secondary to a localized ileus caused by acute diverticulitis.

When the diagnosis is uncertain:

Ask yourself, how can change inform the likely location of the abnormality, the type of problem and the likely cause?

For some problems, the symptoms of change and their relative onset may not be diagnostic but can help localize the abnormality causing the problem, determine the type of problem and likely cause. For example:

- Lower abdominal colic and anuria following a period of time with a poor urinary stream, hesitancy and terminal dribbling is characteristic of bladder outflow obstruction. This is a structural type of problem likely to be caused by an enlarged prostate.
- Severe back pain followed by urinary or faecal incontinence is a neurological type of problem likely to be caused by a prolapsed intervertebral disc.
- Upper abdominal colic followed by increasing jaundice, pale stools and dark urine over several days is likely to a structural problem caused by choledocholithiasis.
- Sub-acute episodes of upper abdominal colic followed by effortless vomiting of undigested food, starting within a few minutes of eating food, usually indicates gastric outlet "obstruction", a structural problem likely to be caused by cancer.
- Lower abdominal colic followed by diarrhoea with blood and mucus indicates a colonic inflammatory problem likely to be UC.
- Absolute constipation followed by lower abdominal colic is likely to be caused by a colonic structural type of problem, such as cancer.

Ask yourself, how can information about change inform management?

When a problem is changing the nature of the change and the rate of change may inform the management priority. For example, a problem that is rapidly progressing is likely to be in need of urgent management. Conversely, when change indicates the problem is resolving, this may also affect management. For example:

- When the sudden onset of severe pain and weakness in the limb is reducing and the limb function is now returning, it is likely the initial limb ischaemia is resolving as the limb is re-perfused.
- When the headache and unilateral weakness are improving or have resolved the diagnosis is a TIA rather than a stroke.
- When the abdominal pain from suspected acute appendicitis is reducing it is likely the faecolith causing the appendicitis has cleared or the inflammation is being "walled-off" by the body's inflammatory response. A follow up assessment or CT scan is indicated.
- When a peri-anal pain and swelling feels better and heals up after the swelling has burst and discharged pus no further treatment is indicated.

Sometimes management of the complication or the secondary problem is a high priority that takes precedence over the original problem. For example:

- When septicaemia is a complication of a UTI, the septicaemia should be diagnosed and treated as a priority. Septicaemia may cause secondary hypovolaemia, so preventing hypovolaemia is also a priority.
- When an arrythmia causing heart failure is a complication of an AMI, the arrythmia should be diagnosed and treated as a priority.
- When there is a risk of compartment syndrome following a crush injury or a burn to a limb, emergency fasciotomies may be indicated.

Sometimes management is aimed at preventing a complication or secondary problem. For example:

- When a patient is vomiting and unable to drink, intravenous fluid replacement therapy may be indicated to prevent secondary renal failure.
- When a patient has an impacted ureteric stone in a solitary kidney, placement of a stent or a nephrostomy tube may be indicated to prevent renal failure.
- When a patient has closed loop large bowel obstruction from cancer, stenting or defunctioning the bowel may be indicated to reduce the risk of perforation.

Ask yourself, how can information about change inform the examination?

The nature of the change will determine the signs to look for.

Ask questions to determine the main symptom and associated symptoms

The principal aim of deciding on the main symptom is to determine which symptom will be the focus of asking questions to learn about the problem. Other symptoms are associated symptoms. Identifying the wrong main symptom may lead to misunderstanding and misinterpretation, the wrong diagnosis and the wrong management plan.

The main and associated symptoms together may describe a pattern indicating a likely diagnosis, the likely location of the abnormality or the type of problem. Targeted questions can then be asked to confirm or exclude the diagnosis (diagnosis-hypothesis testing).

When there is a single symptom, this is the main symptom. However, it is appropriate to check for associated symptoms by asking:

Is [symptom] your only symptom or have you any others?
Have you any other symptoms?
Is anything else wrong?
You've told me about [symptoms], is there anything else?

When there is more than one symptom, the dominant or most severe symptom highlighted by the patient, or the symptom that started first is likely to be main symptom. Other symptoms are associated symptoms. When there has been a significant change in the symptoms indicating either the development of a complication or of a new and separate problem, there will be more than one main symptom. Similarly, when the description includes a "red flag" symptom, this should be considered to be another main symptom so that a high-priority diagnosis, such as cancer can be considered. The method of determining the main symptom is best illustrated with an example:

- When a patient presents feeling unwell, with abdominal pain, anorexia, nausea, weight loss, constipation, bloating and pain, the main symptom may be unclear. It is likely the patient will highlight their pain, as this is distressing and a recognised alarm signal. Indeed, it may be the reason the patient has presented. However, it is important to ask yourself, is this the main symptom?
  o When a patient presents with an acute onset of severe abdominal pain and then develops constipation and bloating, feeling unwell, anorexia and nausea, the pain is the main symptom and the others are associated symptoms.
  o If the patient has felt unwell for several weeks and then became anorexic, developed constipation and felt nausea and abdominal bloating and then, more recently, started getting pain, feeling ill is the main symptom and the other symptoms are associated symptoms. The pain is likely to be caused by constipation, a secondary problem.
  o If the patient first became constipated and then, a few days later, developed abdominal pain and started to feel unwell, with anorexia, nausea and bloating, the constipation is the main symptom and the pain and other symptoms are associated symptoms. The pain and vomiting are likely to be caused by large bowel obstruction, a complication.
  o Weight loss may be a clinically significant "red-flag" symptom. Questions should be asked to ensure this is not an important symptom.

When a particular diagnosis is suspected or is part of a short list of possible diagnoses, it may be appropriate to ask about specific associated symptoms to look for a pattern or to check for a "missing symptom" that may not have been mentioned. For example:

- When a patient presents with seasonal breathlessness it is likely to be caused by "hay fever". It may be appropriate to ask:

Do you get a wheeze?
Do you get itchy eyes or a runny nose?
Do you have an unproductive cough?

- When a patient describes recurrent severe headaches behind one eye, they may have cluster headaches. It may be appropriate to ask:

Do your eyes water when you get the headaches?
Does your nose feel congested?

- When a young female presents with vaginal discharge it is likely to be caused by pelvic inflammatory disease. The questions to ask could include:

Have you had any pelvic or supra-pubic pain?
Do you get pain during intercourse (dyspareunia)?

- When a patient presents with recent onset of jaundice it is likely to be obstructive jaundice. It would be appropriate to ask:

Has your skin felt itchy?
Have you noticed your urine being darker or browner than normal?
Has the colour of your stools changed?

- When a patient presents with diarrhoea, it is likely to be caused by colonic inflammation. It would be appropriate to ask:

Have you passed any blood or mucus?
Have you felt sick or been sick?
Have you had any abdominal pains?

- When an elderly man presents with increasing difficulty passing urine, it is likely to be caused by an enlarged prostate. It may be appropriate to ask:

Has the stream been getting increasingly weak?
Is there a delay between wanting to go and the stream coming?
Do you continue to dribble urine at the end?
Do you feel you need to go again shortly after?

The absence of associated symptoms may exclude a diagnosis or make some diagnoses unlikely.
When learning about associated symptoms:

Ask yourself, what is the likely diagnosis?

The pattern of symptoms may indicate a likely diagnosis. The information should be interpreted with the other headline information to inform the questions to ask to complete, confirm or exclude a pattern. For example:

- A tremor, muscle fasciculation, paraesthesia in the extremities and around the mouth, itching, coarse hair, brittle nails and dry skin indicate a diagnosis of hypocalcaemia.
- Loud snoring at night and periods of apnoea, followed by loud deep breathing is characteristic of sleep apnoea. It is normally noticed by a sleeping partner. Patients feel tired all the team and readily fall asleep during the day.
- Jaundice associated with feeling tired, weak, lethargic and breathless is likely to indicate haemolytic anaemia.
- Breathlessness associated with palpitations, agitation and irritability, poor concentration, hyper-activity, weight loss, twitching and increased sweating, is likely to be secondary to thyrotoxicosis.

When the diagnosis is unclear:
Ask yourself, what is the likely location of the abnormality, the type of problem and the likely cause?

The associated symptoms may indicate a likely location of the abnormality causing the problem. For example:

266

- Jaundice associated with an itchy skin, dark urine and pale stools indicate a hepato-biliary abnormality, such as choledocholithiasis or cancer.
- Breathlessness associated with a wheeze and an unproductive cough is likely to be caused by an airway abnormality, such as asthma or a hypersensitivity reaction.
- Diarrhoea, associated with blood and mucus or lower abdominal pain is likely to be caused by a colonic abnormality, such as colitis or diverticulitis.
- Pain associated with a limited range of movement, stiffness and swelling affecting a joint suggests an intra-articular abnormality, such as osteo- or rheumatoid arthritis.

Alternatively, the associated symptoms may help distinguish between a primary abnormality at the site of the problem and a problem secondary to an abnormality elsewhere. For example:

- Feeling ill with associated neurological symptoms or behavioural symptoms, such as when the patients' mood appears low or depressed or when the patient describes odd, irrational thoughts (delusions) or hallucinations, indicate a primary brain abnormality. Feeling ill associated with a fever, breathlessness and sweating is likely to be secondary to a fever. Other associated symptoms may indicate a likely cause, such as urinary frequency and dysuria indicating a urinary tract infection.
- Breathlessness associated with a productive cough is likely to be caused by a primary lung abnormality. Breathlessness associated with palpitations or bilateral swollen ankles is likely to be secondary to a cardiac abnormality.
- A headache associated with visual disturbance is likely to be caused by a primary brain abnormality. A headache associated with vague or non-specific symptoms, such as feeling unwell, lethargic, irritable, weak, with anorexia, nausea and constipation is likely to be secondary to a systemic illness, such as renal failure.

The associated symptoms may indicate the likely type of problem or cause. For example:

- Abdominal pain associated with nausea, vomiting, abdominal distension and constipation is likely to be caused by intestinal obstruction, a structural problem.
- Feeling ill, associated with anorexia, lethargy and a fever is likely to be caused by inflammation.
- Progressive painless jaundice in an elderly patient associated with anorexia and weight loss is likely to be caused by cancer.

Ask yourself, how can the associated symptoms inform management?

It is not uncommon that investigations are indicated to confirm or exclude the cause of an associated symptom and treatment to alleviate an associated symptom. For example:

- When a patient presents with vomiting, associated blood in the vomitus may be an indication for an OGD to exclude an ulcer or other abnormality.
- When a patient presents with breathlessness associated with swollen ankles, liver function tests may be indicated to exclude hypo-proteinemia caused by liver disease.
- When a patient presents with breathlessness associated with a wheeze, treatment with a bronchodilator may be indicated to relieve symptoms.
- When a patient presents with abdominal pain associated with constipation, treatment with a laxative to relieve symptoms may be indicated while awaiting investigations.
- When a jaundiced patient has urticaria, treatment with an antihistamine may be indicated to relieve symptoms.

Ask yourself, how can the associated symptoms inform the examination?

When there are associated symptoms, the examination may include looking for additional signs to confirm or exclude a diagnosis or to inform management. For example:

- Carefully listening to the chest during expiration for a wheeze.

267

- Performing a neurological examination to exclude peripheral neurological signs in a patient with a behavioural change.

Ask questions to learn about the severity of the problem

The principal aims of learning about the severity of the problem are to assess the risk to the patient or the impact on the patient, and to inform management. Occasionally, severity may inform the diagnosis, indicate the likely location of the abnormality, the type of problem or indicate the signs to look for during the examination.

When a patient describes their problem, they usually include information about severity. This is often sufficient and there is no need to ask additional questions. For example:

- An 80-year-old female may say "The ache in my knee when I walk has now become so bad that I cannot leave the house (severity), and spend most of my time sitting in a chair."
- A 65-year-old man may say "I suddenly developed severe (severity) chest pain this morning."
- A 16-year-old female may say "I suddenly developed severe bloody diarrhoea 10 days ago and have to go to the toilet every hour (severity)."
- A 32-year-old man may say "I have been feeling so ill that I haven't been to work (severity) for the last few weeks."
- A patient may say "I have been feeling increasingly ill since Easter and no longer have the energy to go out (severity)."

When information about severity is not included, may be misunderstood or misinterpreted, or should be quantified, it is appropriate to ask questions to learn about the severity of the problem or the severity of a symptom. The questions to ask could include:

Can you tell me how severe it is?
How bad is it?
What do you mean by [severity]?

Sometimes, the patient's description indicates the initial questions to ask. For example:

- A 75-year-old man may say "I have had increasing difficulty swallowing since Easter so can now only drink liquids and have lost weight (severity). " The initial questions to ask could include:

What happens when you eat solid foods?
How much weight have you lost?

- A 25-year-old patient may say "I have had a really bad (severity) headache for several days." The initial questions to ask could include:

What do you mean when you say it is "really bad"]?
Do you mean it is worse than normal or different from a normal headache?
How bad, on a scale of 0 to 10?

- A 50-year-old female may say "My abdominal cramps have got so bad over the last few months that I often have to lie down in bed (severity)." The initial questions to ask could include:

Are there times when you are pain free?
Are the cramps as bad as having a baby?

- A 32-year-old man may say "I have become very (severity) breathless over the last few months." The initial questions to ask could include:

Is it all the time?
Has it been getting worse?

What does it stop you doing?

When a patient grades their severity, for example, describing it as "mild", "moderate", or "severe", this may need clarification. It may be more meaningful to suggest a comparison. For example:

Is your breathlessness as bad as running up a hill?
Is the pain as bad as [having a baby] or [a broken bone]?

An ongoing or previous condition may set a "severity benchmark". For example:

Is the pain as bad as the renal colic you had before?
Is the breathlessness as bad as when you had a chest infection?

When monitoring change, it may be appropriate to try to determine a reliable and reproducible severity assessment. For some symptoms severity can be measured. For example:

- On a range of 0 to 10, when 0 = no pain and 10 = the worst pain ever experienced?
- The severity of symptoms such as breathlessness can be measured by the distance walked before stopping to rest.
- Bowel function can be measured by defaecation frequency, such as hourly or every couple of weeks, and stool consistency, using, for example, the Bristol stool chart.
- When a patient says they can't eat anything, weight loss can be used as a measure of severity. Weight loss can be measured in kg, as a percent change in body weight, a change in the body mass index (BMI) or by the fit of clothing.
- Using a validated severity scoring tool.

Examples of validated severity scoring tools
<ul><li>The "generalized anxiety disorder" questionnaire.</li><li>The PHQ-9 questionnaire assesses the severity of depression.</li><li>Glasgow coma score to assess the level of consciousness.</li><li>Mental test score to assess the severity of mental impairment.</li><li>Dementia score as part of an assessment of the severity of dementia.</li></ul>

Severity not only refers to the severity or the symptom but also to the impact on the patient. For example, when the problem prevents the patient from working/shopping/reading/driving or is associated with a significant change in behaviour, such as when depression is affecting work and lifestyle, it may be severe. The questions to ask to assess the impact on the patient could include:

How has it affected you?
What does it stop you doing?
What would you like to do that you can't do now?

It may be appropriate to ask more specific questions such as

How much are you able to do before you feel you need to rest?
Does it affect your [ability to work or care for another]?
Does it affect your [lifestyle, sports or hobbies]?
Do you sleep more than normal?
Do you have difficulty concentrating?

A problem is also severe when a complication or secondary problem develops or is likely to develop. The patient's description and the differential diagnosis indicates the initial questions to ask. For example:
- When a patient with an arrhythmia, such as AF, presents with increased breathlessness it may be complicated by heart failure. The questions to ask could include:

Is your breathlessness less when you sit up?
Have you felt your ankles are swollen at the end of the day?

- When a patient presents with acute dysuria likely to be a UTI, it would be considered severe if septicaemia has developed. The questions to ask could include:

Have you had a fever?
Have you ever felt hot and cold all over, shaking uncontrollably?

When severity can be measured it is objective and likely to be reproducible. On the other hand, when the assessment is subjective, severity may be influenced by many variables, including the context, the person and previous or ongoing conditions, the nature and location of the problem, and the onset, and is prone to inter-observer variability.

The context and the person, such as their constitution, expectations and attitude to their problem, may influence their perception of severity. For example:

- Pain from a sports injury may be ignored at the time.
- When a highly trained athlete feels a little breathless the problem may be severe.
- A person who has many commitments is more likely to present only when their problem is serious.
- Some patients, such as the elderly, young children or those caring for others, may downplay their problem for various reasons, such as pride, reticence, concern for others, culture or social pressure.
- Some people have a high tolerance to pain and others a low tolerance or high sensitivity to pain.
- Symptoms may be exacerbated by fear or anxiety. Conversely, an agoraphobic patient may present only when their problem is severe.
- Some patients profess to be in severe pain yet can be observed behaving normally when distracted, such as sitting comfortably while reading a magazine or texting/talking on their mobile phone.
- A patient may emphasise the severity of their problem to seek attention or because they want help.
- Some people mimic being in severe pain in the hope that they will be given opiates.

Previous or ongoing conditions or their treatment may influence the assessment of severity. For example:

- When a patient is unable to describe the severity of their problem, such as those with dementia, autism or another mental health condition, severity may be indicated through a change in behaviour. For example, when in pain the patient may exhibit increased agitation, grimace, increase or decrease vocalizations, self-harm or be aggressive towards others. Other family members or their care workers, who know them well, usually recognize these changes.
- When a patient cannot "feel" pain because the normal pain pathways are disrupted, such as those with spinal cord or brain damage, symptoms such as sweating, tachycardia and nausea may indicate they should be in severe pain.
- Medications may influence severity. For example, pain severity can be difficult to assess when a patient takes analgesics regularly or a pulse rate, when a patient is taking a beta-blocker.
- A deterioration in a longstanding problem, such as an exacerbation of diarrhoea in a colitic, may not be considered abnormal. A "normal" bowel habit may be very abnormal for a normally constipated patient. It may indicate a new problem such as bowel cancer.
- A small change in an already breathless patient who has minimal respiratory reserve, such as a patient with pulmonary fibrosis, may be a severe deterioration.

Information about the symptom, such as onset, duration, associated symptoms, location and character may also influence the assessment of the severity of a symptom or the severity, i.e., seriousness, of a problem. For example:

- A problem that presents acutely tends to be considered more severe than a problem that has been present for a long time. However, some problems can progress or deteriorate slowly and imperceptibly so the patient presents late, when the symptoms are severe. For example, metabolic conditions, such as DM, liver or renal failure, or neurological conditions, such as dementia or Parkinson's disease.
- Chest pain is more worrying, and therefore likely to be thought to be more "severe", than limb pain.

- An ache in the knee joint, worse on moving is likely to be considered a more serious problem than a constant unremitting boring ache in the thigh because it affects the patient's mobility.
- A constant abdominal pain is generally thought by a patient to be a less severe problem than a colic.
- Pain may be considered to be a more severe problem than deranged function. For example, abdominal pain is likely to be considered a more serious problem than a persistent change in bowel habit.

Associated symptoms may influence severity assessment. For example, a fever associated with rigors or blood associated with diarrhoea may imply the problem is more severe.
While learning about severity:

Ask yourself, what is the diagnosis?

The severity assessment does not normally inform formulating a diagnosis unless the symptoms are severe and start suddenly or acutely and are considered together with the location. For example:

- Sudden severe unilateral facial pain is typical of trigeminal neuralgia.
- A sudden onset of severe chest pain is likely to be caused by an AMI.
- A sudden onset of severe breathlessness is likely to be caused by an acute hypersensitivity reaction, a PE or a pneumothorax.
- A sudden onset of severe loin to groin pain is likely to be caused by ureteric colic.
- A sudden onset of severe abdominal pain is likely to be caused by biliary or renal colic, acute pancreatitis or ischaemic bowel.
- A sudden inability to pass urine is likely to be caused by bladder outflow obstruction.
- A sudden onset of a severe headache is likely to be caused by a sub-arachnoid haemorrhage or a migraine.
- An acute onset of severe testicular pain in a young man is likely to be testicular torsion.
- Acute severe bloody diarrhoea is likely to be caused by colitis.
- An acute onset of global profound weakness is likely to be caused by Guillain-Barré syndrome

When the diagnosis is uncertain:

Ask yourself, what is the likely location of the abnormality, the type of problem or the likely cause?

When the problem is severe, the patient will usually present acutely and the location of the problem is usually the location of the abnormality causing the problem. For example:

- A severe headache is likely to be caused by a primary brain problem.
- Severe left sided chest pain is likely to arise from the heart.
- Severe pain on inspiration is likely to arise from the pleura or rib cage.
- Severe generalized abdominal pain is likely to be caused by an abdominal problem.
- Severe back pain is likely to arise from the back.

Acute severe symptoms may also indicate the likely type of problem or cause. For example:

- Feeling seriously ill is likely to be caused by an infection, a metabolic problem, such as renal or liver failure or a neurological type of problem, such as depression When acute breathlessness is severe it is likely to be a circulatory type of problem, such as a PE, heart failure or acute haemorrhage ("air hunger") or a structural problem, such as a pneumothorax.
- When a patient presents with acute severe chest pain the likely type of problem is either a circulatory problem, such as angina, acute myocardial infarction or aortic dissection, an inflammatory problem, such as pleurisy or a structural problem, such as a ruptured oesophagus
- When acute abdominal pain is severe it is likely to be a non-infective inflammatory problem, such as acute pancreatitis, a perforated peptic ulcer or gall bladder or a ruptured ectopic pregnancy, a structural problem, such as ureteric or biliary colic, or a circulatory problem, such as ischaemic bowel.

While learning about severity:

Ask yourself, what is the management plan?

Investigations are frequently used to assess severity (Appendix 2). For example:

- Blood tests to measure the impact on homeostasis or the severity of inflammation or organ damage. For example:
  - An Hb to assess the severity of anaemia.
  - Measuring the WBC, CRP or ESR to assess the severity of the inflammatory response.
  - Serum blood glucose to assess the severity of glycaemia.
  - Liver or renal function tests to assess the severity of organ damage.
  - Measuring the creatine kinase level to assess the severity of muscle damage, such as in rhabdomyolysis.
- Measuring the blood oxygen saturation to assess hypoxia.
- Arterial blood gas (ABG) measurement to assess the severity of deranged gas transfer and acid-base homeostasis, such as in patients with deranged pulmonary or renal function.
- Measuring 24-hour ambulatory blood pressure to assess the severity of hypertension in a patient with headaches.
- An echocardiogram to assess the severity of heart failure.
- A Doppler USS to assess the severity of occlusive peripheral vascular disease.
- A CT scan to assess the local severity and stage of bowel cancer.
- A barium swallow to assess the severity of an oesophageal stricture.
- Pulmonary function tests to assess the severity of breathlessness.
- An echocardiogram to assess the severity of valvular or arterial stenosis.

The severity assessment is usually used to inform management. For example, severity may inform:

- The management priority: the timing of an investigation, treatment or a follow up consultation. When the problem is severe, it is likely the patient should be managed urgently. For example:
  - Severe chest pain may be investigated by an urgent ECG and measurement of blood troponins if an AMI is suspected.
  - A severe headache may be investigated with an urgent CT scan if a subarachnoid haemorrhage is suspected.
  - When sepsis is suspected urgent antibiotic treatment should be started before awaiting the results of investigations.
  - When a patient is in severe pain, such as from ureteric colic, urgent analgesia may be indicated so that they can hold a meaningful conversation.
  - Oxygen supplementation or a bronchodilator may be needed for a very breathless or wheezing patient.
  - Priority may also influence the choice of management. For example, when a PE is suspected, anticoagulation should be started before the results of investigations are available, and some investigations, such as a VQ scan, may not be available in an appropriate time frame.
- Whether to investigate or not and the choice of investigation.
- Whether to treat or not and the choice of treatment.

However, severity does not always determine priority. For example, recurrent severe headaches likely to be caused by tension or a migraine, or severe pain in the knee following a twisting injury do not normally require emergency investigations and although, urgent symptomatic treatment may be indicated, urgent definitive treatment is not. Conversely, some patients in mild pain may be very ill and emergency treatment indicated. For example:

- A persistent mild headache, neck pain, fever and alternating episodes of feeling hot then cold and shivering or uncontrolled shaking (rigors) for several days, may be caused by meningitis. Antibiotics should be started urgently.
- A constant mild generalized abdominal pain in a patient who has become increasingly unwell over several days may be caused by peritonitis. An urgent CT scan is indicated.
- Longstanding mild abdominal pain with anorexia and unexplained progressive weight loss may be caused by cancer. An urgent CT scan is indicated.

- A patient who has mild breathlessness may be seriously ill when, for example, it is due to metabolic acidosis from renal failure. Urgent blood tests are indicated.
- A patient who presents with a slight change in bowel habit may be about to obstruct from a locally advanced cancer. An urgent CT scan or colonoscopy may be indicated.
- A patient who presents following a transient unilateral weakness may be about to have a stroke. An urgent CT scan is indicated.

When the problem is severe, there is often an increased risk of an asymptomatic complication or secondary problem. In which case, screening investigations may be indicated. For example:

- Blood tests to screen for an abnormality of water and electrolyte homeostasis in a patient with severe diarrhoea (Appendix 2).
- Arterial blood gas measurement to screen for acidosis in a hyperglycaemic patient (Appendix 2).
- Blood tests to screen for a deficiency of trace elements and vitamins in a patient with severe Crohn's disease (Appendix 2).

Occasionally, admission to hospital for observation to assess severity or for treatment may be indicated. For example:

- When it would otherwise be difficult to assess severity or the available information is unreliable or confusing.
- When a patient is apparently in severe pain despite being on numerous analgesics. Supervised management may be indicated.

While learning about severity:

Ask yourself, how can severity inform the examination?

The aim of the examination may be to assess severity. For example:

- Measure the temperature, heart rate, blood pressure and respiratory rate in a febrile patient.
- Look for cyanosis or clubbing, or use of the accessory respiratory muscles in a breathless patient.
- Look for signs of secondary spread of cancer.
- Assess muscle wasting and power in a patient with motor neuron disease.
- Assess muscle spasticity in a patient with multiple sclerosis.

Severity assessment may affect the conduct of the examination, such as when a part of the body is very tender it should be examined carefully, with sensitivity, to avoid causing undue pain and distress. Usually, the examination will start by focusing on the site of the problem. However, the examination may include looking for associated or systemic signs to assess the impact on the part of the body affected or on the patient. For example:

- Measuring the pulse, blood pressure and assessing skin turgor to assess the severity of dehydration secondary to vomiting.
- Assessing walking, coordination and muscle power in a patient following a stroke.

Ask questions to learn and understand what pain means to the patient, and aggravating and relieving factors

Pain is an unpleasant sensory and emotional experience that can affect wellbeing, quality of life, behaviour and function. It is a universally recognised alarm signal that serves many different functions. Pain tells us about normal body functions, such as lower abdominal or pelvic colic when feeling the need to defaecate, lower abdominal pain when the bladder is full, mid-cycle ("ovulatory") abdominal pains or "period" pains during menstruation. Pain also tells us when we have been overdoing it, such as headaches when stressed or tired, heartburn or abdominal discomfort after overeating or muscle aches and pains after strenuous exercise. Pain tells us when to stop before causing harm, such as to let go of a hot plate or to stop walking before a blister develops and to avoid doing things that may cause harm, such as to avoid picking up a hot plate or clutching a rose stem. Pain tells us when we have hurt or injured ourselves, such as when we get a cut, a bruise or a muscle strain. Pain that is different, more severe, atypical, unexplained, recurrent, more frequent or persistent tells us there is something wrong with our body.

A "sharp" pain, such as from a laceration, pleurisy or a broken bone, abdominal cramp or colic, a bursting pain, such as compartment syndrome or phlegmasia caerulea dolens or a boring pain, such as a headache or from an infiltrating cancer is generally recognised to be a pain, whereas some "pains" are not thought of as a "pain" by the patient. For example:

- A dull ache from a bruise, a muscle strain, an arthritic joint, a headache, an ear "ache", or from claudication.
- Chest tightness, a crushing sensation, a heaviness or an ache.
- Abdominal or pelvic heaviness, discomfort or bloating.
- A burning sensation, such as heartburn, proctitis or dysuria.
- A pulsating or throbbing sensation, such as migraine or giant cell arteritis.
- An abnormal sensation, such as pins and needles, paraesthesia, neuralgia, dysesthesia, hyperaesthesia or allodynia.
- Photophobia or tinnitus.

Questions should only be asked to learn about the character of the pain, aggravating and relieving factors when the information is likely to help formulate a diagnosis, determine the likely location of the abnormality, the type of problem or the cause of the pain or to inform management. The patient's description of their problem may indicate the initial questions to ask. For example:

- A 25-year-old patient may say "I have had a really uncomfortable headache (character) for several days and prefer to lie down in a dark room (relieving factor) because I don't like bright light (aggravating factor)." The initial question to ask could include:

Tell me about your headache
Describe your headache
What does the headache feel like?
How would you describe the headache?
Can you tell me more about the headache?

When the patient has difficulty describing their pain, it may be helpful to compare the pain with an "every day" pain felt at that location. It may be important to use the right words when to describe a pain. For example:

Does the pain feel like...

➤ *A cut or a bruise?*
➤ *A headache?*
➤ *Discomfort after swallowing a hot drink or too large a food bolus?*
➤ *Heartburn?*
➤ *Chest tightness when undertaking strenuous exercise?*
➤ *Pain from inspiring very cold air?*
➤ *Pain from retching?*
➤ *Colic of gastroenteritis, constipation or diarrhoea?*
➤ *Bloating after a full meal?*
➤ *An exertional "stitch" in the abdomen?*
➤ *Sigmoid or rectal "colic" when needing to pass stool?*
➤ *Intestinal colic caused by gastroenteritis?*
➤ *Mid-cycle ovulatory pain?*
➤ *Menstrual pain?*
➤ *A full bladder?*
➤ *Wanting to go to toilet?*

When the pain is an everyday pain, such as a headache or a joint pain, it is important to find out what is different about their pain this time. It may be appropriate to ask:

What is different about this pain?
Does the pain feel atypical?
Does the pain feel like you have a problem with your [site]?
Why do you think it is different from a previous [pain]?

The patient may state in their initial description what makes the pain better or worse. If they don't, or it is unclear is appropriate to ask. For example:

When do you get the pain?
What makes the pain worse?
What do you do when you get pain?
What do you do to relieve the pain?
What makes the pain better?
It may be appropriate to ask questions about specific aggravating or relieving factors. For example:

- When the patient presents with leg pain:

Can you walk to the shops?
Can you walk upstairs?
Is the pain worse when you walk quickly or up a hill?
Is it worse when you stand up?
Is the pain relieved by rest?
Is the pain better when your leg is raised up?
Does sleeping in a chair help the pain?

- When the patient presents with abdominal pain:

Do you get the pain after eating?
Do you get the pain before going to the toilet?
Do you find moving around, laughing or coughing more uncomfortable?
Do you prefer to rest or move around when you get the pain?

When learning about the character of the pain:

Ask yourself, what is the likely diagnosis?

The character, aggravating and relieving factors together with headline information and the location of the problem may indicate a diagnostic pattern. For example:

- A burning retrosternal pain aggravated by swallowing hot food and helped by swallowing saliva or some drinks, such as milk or antacids is likely to be GORD.
- Central or left sided chest tightness, an ache or feeling a weight inside, aggravated by exercise and relieved by rest is likely to be angina.
- Unilateral sharp chest pain, aggravated when the patient takes a deep breath, is likely to be caused by pleurisy.
- A sudden onset of cramping pain felt in the lumbar region, flank and groin on one side, is likely to be ureteric colic. The pain is helped by moving around or being curled up although the patient has difficulty finding a comfortable position.
- A sharp pain in the knee aggravated by straightening the knee when walking up and down stairs is likely to be a meniscal injury.
- A severe aching pain in the lower limb stopping the patient from walking or weight bearing yet worse on lying down is likely to be caused by ischaemia.
- A sharp pain in the elbow increased on extending the hand at the wrist, making a fist or gripping an object such as a door handle, is likely to be caused by lateral epicondylitis or "tennis elbow".
- Severe atypical unilateral facial pain is likely to be trigeminal neuralgia.

- Recurrent headaches, brought on by drinking alcohol or eating cheese is likely to be migraine.
- Chronic constant, unremitting dull aching pain in a bone, in the absence of significant trauma, may indicate a bone metastasis.

When the diagnosis is uncertain or the list of possible diagnoses long:

Ask yourself, what is the likely location of the abnormality, the type of problem and the cause of the pain?

When the diagnosis is uncertain, the character, aggravating and relieving factors should be used to determine whether the pain is a somatic pain, neuralgia, referred pain or an autonomic pain (Figure 55). This is a bridge to determining the location of the abnormality causing the problem and the type of problem to reduce the list of possible diagnoses, to inform management and the signs to look for.

Figure 55: An overview of the questions to ask yourself when learning about the character of the pain.

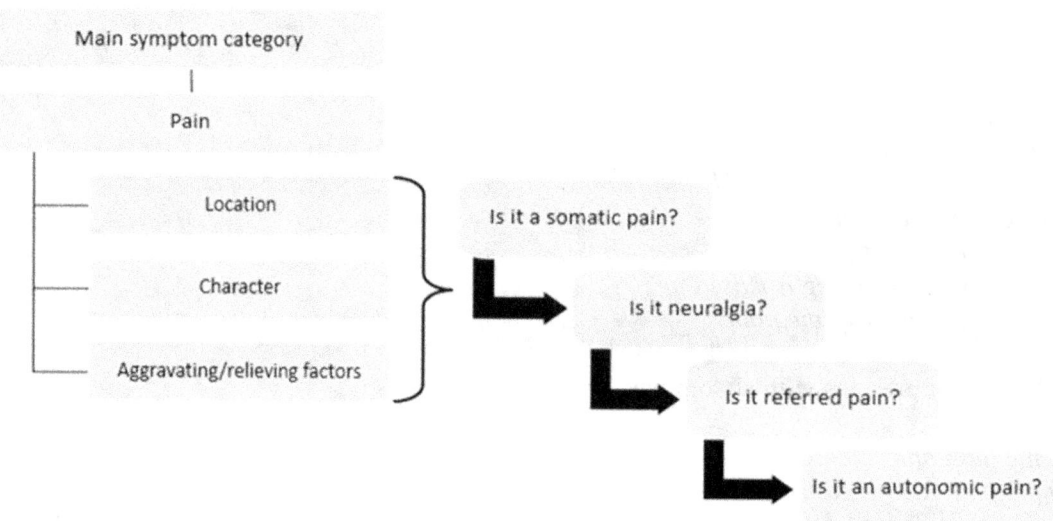

When the character of the pain is typical for the site and can be localized by the patient it is likely to be a somatic pain. The pain may be aggravated by direct pressure or using the site affected. Most "everyday" pains affecting the limbs or the trunk superficially, such as from cuts, burns, pressure or injuries are "somatic" pains arising from a receptor or bare nerve ending in the skin or the sub-cutaneous soft tissues, the bones or joints, the parietal pleura or peritoneum at the site indicated and carried by general somatic afferent nerves. The character of the pain indicates the receptor stimulated.

> **A pain that can be localized and feels superficial and typical for the site is likely to be a somatic pain from an abnormality nearby**

If somatic pain is suspected it may be appropriate to ask:

Does the pain feel sharp, like a cut, or a burning pain?
Does the pain feel like a bruise or an ache?

When the pain is precisely localized, the site should be examined as there may be a visible or palpable abnormality. For example, signs of inflammation, such as folliculitis or cellulitis or a structural abnormality, such as a sebaceous cyst. When there is no abnormality to see or feel, then the structure affected will indicate the likely diagnosis. For example, pain along the line of a tendon is likely to be tendinitis, a sharp unilateral chest pain aggravated by inspiration is likely to be pleurisy.

When the pain feels superficial but is atypical for the site, such as a burning or tingling pain or "pins and needles" and affects a specific point, an area, such as a dermatome or an area innervated by a named sensory nerve, it is likely to be "neuralgia". Neuralgia occurs when the afferent nerve is irritated, inflamed or damaged at some point.

276

> **A superficial pain that feels atypical for a precise site or an area is likely to be "neuralgia" from an abnormality affecting a sensory nerve.**

If neuralgia is suspected it may be appropriate to ask:

Does the pain feel unusual, like "pins and needles" or a burning pain?
Does the pain feel as though it is superficial, near the skin, or deep-seated?
Is it affected by certain movements, such as twisting or bending your back or posture?
Do you have any weakness anywhere?

When describing their pain, the patient may point to a specific point on their body or rub an area affected by the pain. On examination, there may be a visible or palpable abnormality, such as a sub-cutaneous mass or a nearby scar. When the neuralgia is precisely localized, it is likely to be caused by a structural problem, such as scarring, inflammation, such as shingles, a neurological problem, such as a neuroma, or cancer or rarely glomus tumour. Localized somatic pain or neuralgia is unlikely to be caused by a circulatory, neurological or metabolic type of problem.

When somatic pain or neuralgia is multi-focal, determining what each site has in common is likely to indicate the type of problem or a possible diagnosis. For example, poly-arthralgia may be caused by osteo-arthritis or an auto-immune problem, such as rheumatoid arthritis, widespread or multifocal muscle pains by an auto-immune problem, such as poly-myalgia, fibromyalgia, dermatomyositis, polymyositis, SLE or poly-myalgia rheumatica, widespread or multifocal neuralgia affecting different parts of the body may be caused by a peripheral neurological abnormality, such as poly-neuritis or poly-radiculopathy.

When neuralgia affects an area, it is likely to be caused by an abnormality affecting the afferent nerve or dorsal nerve root. In which case, it is a "referred somatic pain" and the location and area affected should be examined to determine the likely site of the abnormality. Referred somatic pain may be aggravated by pressure, percussion or movements that stretch or pinch the afferent nerve along its course. For example, leg extension in sciatica, hand extension or flexion in carpal tunnel syndrome or pressure on the ileo-inguinal nerve from tight clothes or certain postures.

> **A constant atypical superficial pain affecting an area is likely to be referred "somatic pain" from an abnormality affecting the afferent nerve.**

When the patient finds it difficult to describe their chest, abdominal, pelvic or back pain or describes a deep-seated constant dull ache, a feeling of discomfort or heaviness, a tightness, a weight, an uncomfortable bloating, a feeling of fullness or a colic or gripping pain it is likely to be an autonomic pain arising from visceral nociceptors, which include free nerve endings, mechanoreceptors and spindle cells that respond to stretch or tension or specialized sensory receptors that respond to chemicals, homeostatic changes, cell damage or imminent damage. It is often difficult for the patient to localize the pain and they may indicate the site with a vague hand gesture, by making a fist over the site or by rubbing the area.

> **A deep-seated trunk pain that is difficult to describe or localize is likely to be an autonomic pain from an internal viscus**

Distinguishing between a colic, an "inflammatory" pain and an atypical autonomic pain will indicate the likely location and type of problem causing the pain (Figure 56).

A deep-seated, often severe, gripping or aching abdominal, flank, groin or retrosternal pain which feels very uncomfortable and makes the patient move around or double up trying to find a comfortable position is typical of colic. Classically, the pain starts suddenly and is intermittent, occurring in attacks or waves which peak and subside within a few minutes (crescendo-decrescendo) with a more constant background discomfort between attacks. Sometimes, the pain is a more constant ache with occasional episodes when the pain is more severe. During an attack of colic, patients may feel sick and appear pale, grey, breathless and sweaty.

> **Colic is characterized by waves of deep-seated abdominal or retrosternal pain causing the patient to try to find a comfortable position.**

The questions to ask to confirm the pain is colic include:

Does the pain come and go in waves?
Are there times when the pain is a lot worse for a short period of time?
What do you do to get comfortable?
Do you prefer to move around because of the pain?

Figure 56: An overview of the questions to ask yourself when an autonomic pain is the main symptom

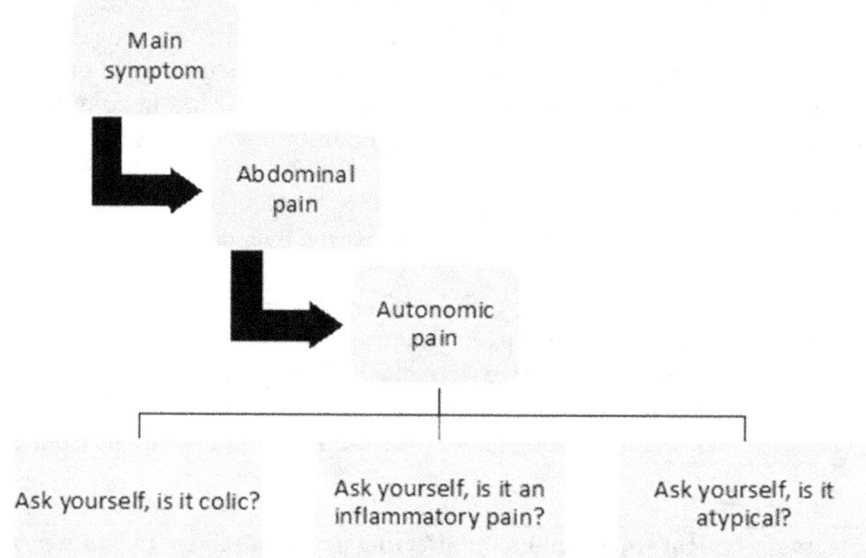

Patients who have difficulty describing their colic may be able to liken the pain to a "physiological colic" such as, "trapped wind" in the stomach, rectal filling with flatus or stool, a gastro-intestinal "upset", menstrual pain or the pain of a full bladder.

The pain of colic occurs when the wall of a tubular structure or a storage organ is acutely and intermittently excessively stretched during a wave of peristalsis. It indicates that luminal contents cannot be moved due to obstruction, "structural colic", or when peristalsis is disordered and uncoordinated, "neurologic colic". Regular waves of colic are likely to arise from a tubular peristalsing structure, such as the small intestine or the ureter. Irregular, occasional sporadic attacks of mild to moderate colic are likely to arise from a minimally peristalsing tube, such as the oesophagus, appendix, Fallopian tube or bile duct or a "storage" organ, such as the stomach, gall bladder or urinary bladder. For example:

- Retrosternal colic from oesophageal spasm ("nutcracker oesophagus").
- Upper abdominal colic from a mucocele of the gallbladder.
- Lower abdominal colic from sigmoid diverticular disease.
- Supra-pubic colic from chronic bladder outflow obstruction.

When the pain is characteristic of colic the location will indicate the likely tissues, organs or part of the body affected, reducing the list of possible diagnoses (Figure 57).

Figure 57: Line diagrams illustrating the possible location of the abnormality and differential diagnosis when the patient has abdominal colic.

Stomach. For example, gastric outlet obstruction, a gastric volvulus, or acute gastric dilation

Proximal small bowel. For example, proximal small bowel obstruction or Crohn's disease

Gall bladder and biliary tract. For example, biliary colic

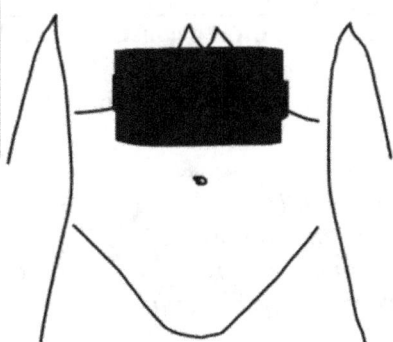

The small bowel. For example, obstruction, adhesions, volvulus, localized ischaemia or Crohns

The ascending and proximal two thirds of the transverse colon. For example, obstruction, localized ischamia or colitis

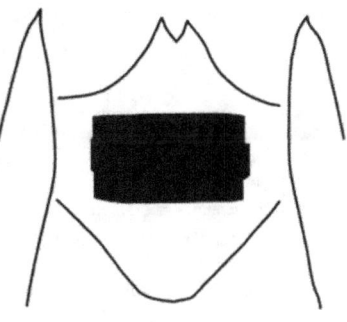

The large bowel. For example, large bowel obstruction, IBS, diverticular disease

The bladder. For example, a UTI, urinary retention

The Fallopian tubes. For example, an ectopic pregnancy

The uterus. For example, pregnancy, endometriosis

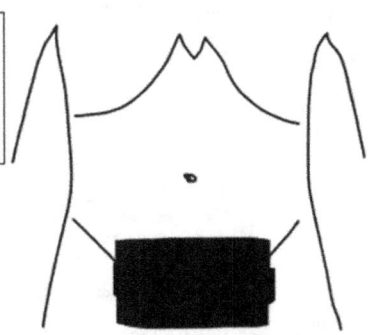

Figure 58: Line diagram illustrating the possible location of the abnormality and differential diagnosis when the patient has flank coli.

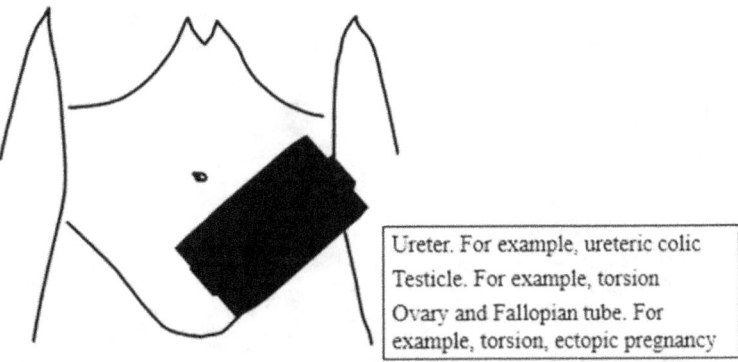

Ureter. For example, ureteric colic

Testicle. For example, torsion

Ovary and Fallopian tube. For example, torsion, ectopic pregnancy

When autonomic pain comes on gradually and is constant, aggravated by pressure, by moving or using the affected part, it is likely to be caused by inflammation. At rest the pain is of mild or moderate severity but it can be severe when moving or using the affected part. As a consequence, patients prefer to lie still, to rest and not use the affected part.

279

Inflammatory pain is a constant pain that is aggravated by moving or using the affected part

The questions to ask to confirm the pain is an inflammatory pain include:

Is the pain constant?
Do you prefer to lie still?
Does moving make the pain worse?
Does the pain feel more severe when you walk, laugh or cough?
Are you pain free when you lie still?

Inflammatory pain, as its name suggests, is caused by deep-seated inflammation and so is imprecisely localized. Consequently, the location of the abnormality is uncertain and the differential diagnosis long unless more localizing information is known, such as associated symptoms or the signs on examination (Figure 59).

Figure 59: Line diagrams illustrating the possible location of the abnormality and differential diagnosis when the inflammatory pain is in the abdomen.

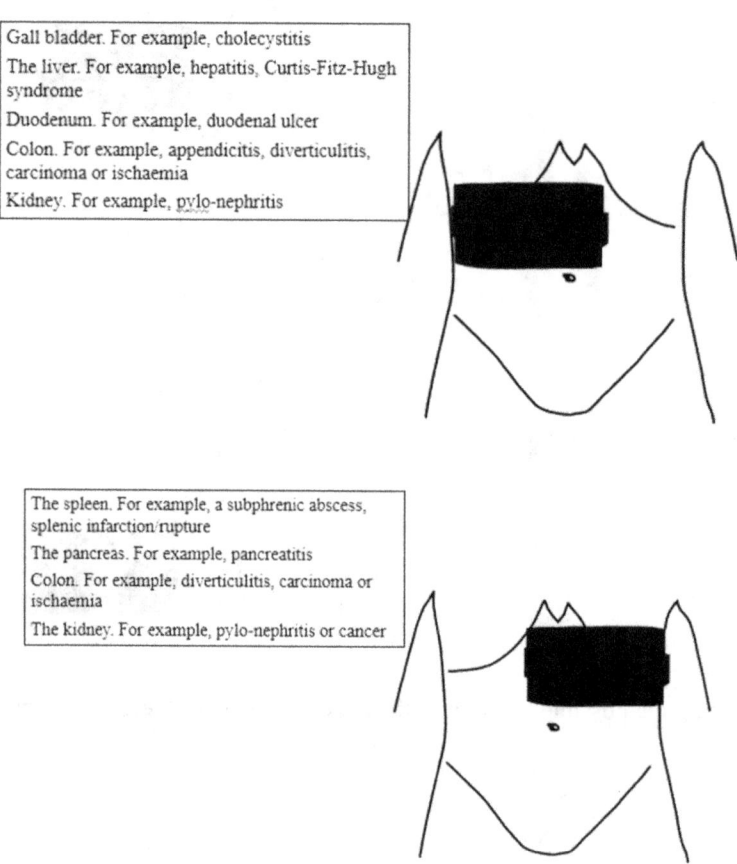

Gall bladder. For example, cholecystitis

The liver. For example, hepatitis, Curtis-Fitz-Hugh syndrome

Duodenum. For example, duodenal ulcer

Colon. For example, appendicitis, diverticulitis, carcinoma or ischaemia

Kidney. For example, pylo-nephritis

The spleen. For example, a subphrenic abscess, splenic infarction/rupture

The pancreas. For example, pancreatitis

Colon. For example, diverticulitis, carcinoma or ischaemia

The kidney. For example, pylo-nephritis or cancer

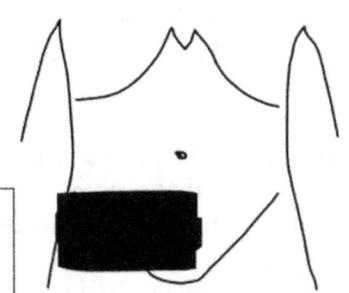

The terminal ileum. For example, Crohn's disease or Yersinia enterocolitica

The appendix. For example, acute appendicitis,

The caecum or ascending colon. For example, diverticulitis, colitis or cancer,

The ovary and Fallopian tube. For example, salpingo-oophoritis, ovarian torsion or haemorrhage into an ovarian cyst

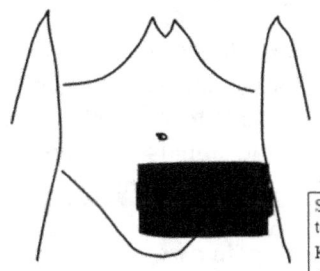

Sigmoid colon. For example, diverticulitis, colitis, a torted appendix epiploicua, carcinoma

Kidney. For example, pyelonephritis

Ovary. For example, salpingo-oophoritis, ruptured ovarian cyst or a tumour

Uterus. For example, an involuting fibroid, cancer or endometriosis

When the patient's description is not typical of inflammation or colic it is "atypical". It is important to ask questions to determine whether there is a mixed picture, a change caused by a secondary problem or a complication, whether the pain is caused by an abnormality affecting a solid organ or mass or by an uncommon problem, such as a metabolic problem or an autonomic neuropathy.

- When there is a mixed picture of a dull deep-seated inflammatory autonomic pain and a sharp superficial "somatic" pain, it is likely a deep-seated inflammation affecting the deep tissues, organs or structures is also affecting the somatically innervated parietal peritoneum or pleura. For example, acute appendicitis, acute cholecystitis or a diverticulitis.
- When there are features of both colic and inflammation, it may be because there has been a change caused by a secondary problem or a complication. Learning about a change in the symptoms will signpost the problem:
  - When the symptoms at the outset are typical of colic and then symptoms of inflammation developed later, the inflammation is likely to be a complication of colic, such as when acute cholecystitis complicates biliary colic, intestinal perforation complicates small bowel obstruction or intestinal ischaemia complicates a volvulus.
  - When the symptoms at the start were typical of inflammation and episodes of colic develop later, the colic is likely to be a complication or secondary problem. For example, mid-gut colic caused by a localized small bowel ileus secondary to nearby inflammation, such as acute appendicitis, or fore-gut colic caused by a duodenal ileus secondary to nearby inflammation, such as acute pancreatitis.
- When the abdominal pain is a constant atypical deep-seated mild discomfort, heaviness or ache aggravated by direct pressure, such as from tight clothes, but not by moving, it may be from a solid viscus or a large mass. Patients tend to prefer to lie in a certain position, such as on one side or another, similar to the effect of posture on the discomfort felt from a gravid uterus. The location of the pain will indicate the likely nearby organ affected. The differential diagnosis includes a structural type of problem, such as hepato- or spleno-megaly or a large cyst, inflammation, such as hepatitis, a circulatory problem, such as ischaemia, or cancer.
Solid organ pain, such as from the liver, spleen, pancreas, ovary or kidney or pain from a mass usually occurs when the enclosing capsule is being stretched by internal swelling, or the suspensory ligaments are stretched by the additional weight. If the organ or mass is tender and the pain is aggravated by using the affected part of the body, the pain is likely to be from an inflammatory problem, such as hepatitis or pancreatitis, or from or a circulatory problem, such as splenic infarction or mesenteric ischaemia.

- When a pain is highly atypical and widespread it may be caused by an unusual diagnosis. For example:
  - A peripheral neurological abnormality, such as autonomic neuropathy, MS, central prolapsed intervertebral disc or a tumour.
  - A central neurological abnormality affecting the spinal cord, the brain stem or the brain. The pain may be caused by a structural problem, such as an injury, spinal stenosis or a tumour, a circulatory problem, such as an infarction, a haemorrhage or an AV malformation, inflammation, such as arachnoiditis, or a neurological problem, such as reflex sympathetic dystrophy (complex regional pain syndrome), episodic pain syndrome or chronic fatigue syndrome.
  - Inflammation. For example, endometriosis, infection, such as TB, syphilis, EBV or HIV, or non-infective inflammation, such as SLE or coeliac disease.
  - A structural abnormality. For example, adhesions.
  - Cancer. For example, ovarian cancer.
  - A metabolic abnormality. For example, lead poisoning, hypercalcaemia, thyrotoxicosis or porphyria.

These are usually only considered when other diagnoses are excluded or on the basis of investigation results.

When the autonomic pain is a constant deep-seated pain affecting an area covering several adjacent dermatomes in the neck or trunk, away from a viscus, it is likely to be secondary to a problem affecting a viscus, i.e., "referred autonomic pain". Referred autonomic pain occurs when autonomic signals from an internal viscus are misinterpreted by the brain as being from equivalent somatic nerve root(s) that enter the spinal cord at the same level.

A constant widespread atypical deep-seated trunk pain away from a viscus is likely to be
"referred autonomic pain"

Referred pain is unaffected by pressure or using the part of the body at the site of the pain but is aggravated by using the abnormal part of the body and relieved when the abnormal part is rested. It is likely specific questions will be indicated to distinguish between a pain from an abnormality at the location of the pain and a referred pain. For example:

- When an atypical pain is felt in the neck and shoulder it may be referred from the diaphragm. For example, from a lower lobe pneumonia or a sub-phrenic abscess. The pain signals pass via the phrenic nerve and enter the spinal cord together with somatic sensory roots from C3,4,5. The brain maps the signals to the equivalent dermatomes. The pain is aggravated by breathing or coughing rather than moving the neck or shoulder. To help decide between a pain caused by a neck and shoulder problem and referred diaphragmatic pain questions to ask could include:

Does the pain feel like you have a problem with your neck or shoulder?
Is the pain brought on by moving the neck?
Does looking up, down or to the side, affect the pain?
Is it worse in some positions?
Is it worse when you take a deep breath or cough?

- When an atypical ache is felt in the left shoulder and upper arm it may be referred from the heart, such as ischaemic heart disease. The pain is signalled via the vagus and cardiac sympathetic plexuses to the inferior cervical ganglia and enters the spinal cord with upper thoracic roots T1-4. The brain maps the signals to the equivalent dermatomes. The shoulder pain is aggravated by walking up a hill and relieved by resting but not affected by moving the shoulder or neck. To help decide between a shoulder pain caused by a shoulder problem and referred cardiac pain questions to ask could include:

Does the pain feel like you have a problem with your shoulder?
Can you comb or wash your hair without pain?
Is the pain brought on by exercise and relieved by rest?
Is it worse when you move your arm?

The differential diagnosis when shoulder pain is caused by a shoulder abnormality or when it is referred from the chest.

Differential diagnosis of shoulder pain caused by a shoulder abnormality	Differential diagnosis of shoulder pain referred from a chest abnormality
Arthritis of the gleno-humeral or acromio-clavicular joint	Acute coronary syndrome
Rotator cuff tear	Myocarditis
Labral tear	Cardiac tamponade
Capsulitis	Pericarditis
Sub-acromial impingement	Diaphragmatic irritation
Sub-acromial bursitis	
Shoulder instability	
Tendinitis	

- When an atypical pain is felt in the lower thoracic back it is likely to be referred from an upper abdominal retroperitoneal organ. When it is central it is likely to be from the pancreas or aorta, when it is on the right, it is likely to be from the gallbladder and when on the left from the spleen. The pain signals pass via the coeliac axis and enter the spinal cord together with somatic sensory roots from T11 and 12. Referred pancreatic pain is likely to be aggravated by eating. To help decide between a back pain and referred pancreatic pain questions to ask could include:

Does the pain feel like you have a problem with your back?
Is the pain brought on by moving the back?
Does twisting or bending affect the pain?
Is it worse in some positions?
Is it worse when you eat a meal?

- When an atypical pain is felt in the sacrum and buttocks it may be referred from an abnormality affecting hindgut structures in the pelvis. The pain signals are carried via the pelvic parasympathetic afferents and enter the spinal cord with roots S2-4. The brain maps the signals to the equivalent dermatomes. It is important to distinguish between pain referred from the back and pain referred from the pelvis. When it is from the back, such as from a prolapsed intervertebral disc, it is on one side only and tends to be related to a back injury or aggravated by moving the back. When it is from the pelvis it tends to affect both sides, is unaffected by moving the back but, when it is from the rectum, the buttock pain is aggravated by stool or wind and relieved by defaecation. To help decide between a back pain and referred pelvic pain questions to ask could include:

Does it feel like you have a problem with your back?
Is the pain brought on by bending or twisting the back?
Is it worse in some positions?
Is it worse when you want to go to the toilet or passing wind?
Does it get better after going to the toilet or passing wind?

Ask yourself, how can information about the character of the pain, aggravating and relieving factors inform management?

When the character indicates a likely diagnosis, this informs management, such as investigations to confirm the diagnosis, determine a cause, or treatment. For example:

- A sharp unilateral chest pain, aggravated by inspiration, likely to be pleurisy is often investigated with a CXR to formulate a diagnosis or determine a cause.
- If ureteric colic is suspected an USS, intravenous urogram (IVU) or CT scan may be indicated to confirm the diagnosis and determine a cause.
- If biliary colic is suspected, LFTs and an USS are indicated to confirm the diagnosis and determine a cause.
- When the symptoms are typical for acute urinary retention, catheterization is indicated.
- If acute pancreatitis is suspected, a serum amylase is indicated to confirm the diagnosis.
- When the symptoms are classical for acute appendicitis an operation may be indicated.
- When retrosternal chest pain is likely to be from the oesophagus, an OGD may be indicated to confirm the diagnosis, assess severity and exclude a complication. For some patients, such as when there is diagnostic uncertainty, 24-hour oesophageal pH and manometry is indicated.

When the character indicates the likely location of the abnormality causing the problem, investigations are indicated to confirm the location and determine a likely diagnosis. For example:

- When groin pain is likely to be from the hip, an Xray is indicated to confirm the likely location of the abnormality.
- Central, mid-gut, colic, likely to be from small bowel obstruction is often investigated with a CT scan, to confirm the likely location of the abnormality and determine the diagnosis.
- When shoulder and upper arm symptoms are typical of angina, an ECG and serial troponin measurement are indicated to confirm the likely location of the abnormality. An angiogram may be indicated to determine the cause.
- When there is pain in the region of the tip of the scapula, likely to be referred from the gallbladder, an USS of the gallbladder is indicated to confirm the likely location of the abnormality and determine the diagnosis.

When the character indicates the likely type of problem, initial management will usually include investigations to confirm the type of problem and determine a likely diagnosis. For example:

- A deep-seated structural problem, causing, for example, colic, is usually investigated with an imaging investigation, such as an USS or CT scan.
- When inflammation is suspected, blood tests, such as a WBC and a CRP, are indicated to confirm the type of problem and assess the severity.
- When infection is suspected a representative tissue sample should be sent for microscopy, culture and serology to formulate a diagnosis.
- When auto-immune inflammation is suspected blood should be sent for measurement of auto-antibodies to confirm the type of problem and indicate a likely diagnosis. If there is a visible abnormality, a biopsy may be indicated. Imaging investigations, such as a joint Xray, may be indicated when deep-seated inflammation is suspected.
- When ischaemia is likely, a Doppler USS or angiogram is usually indicated to confirm the type of problem, the diagnosis and assess severity.
- When an acute inflammatory pain affects the great toe, measurement of a serum urate is indicated to confirm gout, a metabolic abnormality.

Aggravating and relieving factors may inform the advice given to patients, such as what to avoid doing. Information about the character may influence the priority of investigations or treatment.

Ask yourself, how can the information about the character of the pain, aggravating and relieving factors inform the examination?

When an examination is indicated, the character, aggravating and relieving factors may indicate the signs to look for. For example:

- An 80-year-old female may say "The ache in my knee when I walk up and down stairs has now become so bad that I have to sleep downstairs." The location and character of the pain would indicate a somatic pain likely to be caused by both a structural and inflammatory type of problem, such as degenerative arthritis affecting the knee. There are likely to be signs of a swollen, deformed, tender knee with a limited range of movement and crepitus.
- A 25-year-old patient may say "I have had a really uncomfortable headache for several days." The location and character of the pain would indicate a neurological type of problem affecting the brain, such as a tension headache or migraine. Signs are unlikely.
- A 50-year-old female may say "My abdominal cramps have got so bad over the last few months that, when they occur, I have to lie down and curl up into a ball." The location and character of the pain would indicate an autonomic pain; a colic. The colic is likely to be caused by a structural type of problem affecting the small bowel, such as adhesions or a hernia, or a neurological type of problem, such as IBS. The examination should include looking for signs of a hernia or abdominal scar, tympanic abdominal distension and tenderness and active bowel sounds or a mass.
- A 65-year-old man may say "I suddenly developed a very uncomfortable tightness or ache in my left shoulder and upper arm this morning." The location and character of the pain would indicate a referred autonomic pain caused by a circulatory type of problem affecting the heart. On examination, the heart may be enlarged or there may be a murmur to hear.
- When a patient presents with left sided chest pain following symptoms that suggest a viral illness, pericarditis is likely. Auscultation over the heart while the patient leans forward may reveal a rubbing or squeaking pericardial friction rub. Pulmonary signs are absent unless the patient has heart failure.
- When a patient presents with symptoms of chest pain likely to be caused by pleurisy, shallow fast breathing and pain aggravated when the patient takes a deep breath, a friction rub, and signs of a fever support the diagnosis. Reduced air entry, crepitations (crackles) and vocal fremitus on auscultation and dullness to percussion in a part of the lung field is indicative of consolidation likely to be caused by bacterial infection.
- When a patient presents with neuralgia the signs to look for on examination include altered sensation in the area affected and Tinel's test may be positive. There may be localized weakness or loss of tendon reflexes if the nerve is a mixed motor and sensory nerve.

Aggravating and relieving factors should be confirmed during the examination. For example:

- To confirm pain is increased on moving an inflamed joint.
- To confirm there is tenderness on palpating the abdomen.

It is important the symptoms and signs are consistent. In other words, the information should be considered together.

When the patient says they "feel ill", ask questions to learn and understand what the patient means, and aggravating and relieving factors

Feeling well embraces a state of physical and mental well-being. It is a state of mind measured against a subjective norm: how we feel most of the time is the baseline against which wellness/illness is measured. Feeling well does not mean the absence of disease; we may have an ongoing medical condition or various minor ailments but still feel relatively well. We may feel well because we feel good about ourselves despite having a medical condition or we may feel ill because of a social concern, such as an interpersonal conflict, despite being physically well.

Most of us expect to feel well and take being well for granted, because we spend most of our time feeling well. Unfortunately, we can become ill very quickly. We know it is normal to have day-to-day "ups and downs" and it is not unusual for us to have days when we feel ill or "under the weather". However, we usually know when it is different. Feeling ill is a non-specific or generic alarm signal that something is wrong with either the body or the mind. It is clinically significant when it is different, persistent, recurrent or more severe than would normally be expected.

Feeling ill means different things to different people and is often difficult to describe. When the information about the character, aggravating and relieving factors of their illness is likely to inform formulating a diagnosis, help determine the likely location of the abnormality causing the problem or the type of problem, management or the signs to look for when examining the patient, questions should be asked to understand what the patient means when they say they "feel ill". The patient's description of their problem may indicate the initial questions to ask. For example:

- A 50-year-old female may say "I've not felt well for many weeks. Everything seems too much. It has got so bad recently that I don't even want to go out and have stopped meeting friends." The initial questions to ask could include:

What do you mean when you say, you feel ill?
In what way do you feel ill?
Tell me about your illness?
How would you describe your illness?
Can you tell me more about why you feel ill?
What first made you think you were ill?
What do you mean when you say "everything seems too much"?

When the patient has difficulty describing their illness it may be helpful to compare it with an "every day" condition. For example:

Does the illness feel like [a viral illness/a fever/overwork]?
Do you feel very depressed?

When a patient describes the character of their illness it is important to decide between a non-specific symptom and a symptom associated with the underlying problem and part of a diagnostic pattern. Vague symptoms, such as feeling tired and listless, preferring to lie still and rest, finding even simple activities such as conversation or walking to be an effort, a loss of appetite, food seems tasteless and uninteresting and a low mood, apathy and impaired concentration that develop during the course of an illness are likely to be non-specific symptoms, felt as part of the "character" of the illness. Symptoms that precede or start at the same time as the illness, or that arise during the course of the illness but are emphasized or highlighted or are "red flag" symptoms are likely to be an associated symptom. Such symptoms may include, feeling depressed, fatigue, weakness, anorexia, weight loss, confusion, impaired memory or generalised aches and pains. It is important to learn about the timing of onset of such symptoms and to listen carefully to the patient's description, because they may indicate a possible diagnosis, help determine the location of the abnormality and the type of problem causing the illness and may indicate the signs to look for or inform management.

If the patient describes a number of symptoms present for a few days or more, it may be appropriate to ask what aggravates or relieves each symptom. The questions to ask could include:

What makes the [symptom] worse?
What do you avoid doing because it makes the [symptom] worse?
What makes the [symptom] better?
What do you do when you have the [symptom]?

When learning about the character of their illness:

Ask yourself, what is the likely diagnosis?

The character of their illness per se is unlikely to be diagnostic, whereas the associated symptoms may indicate a diagnostic pattern. For example:
- Feeling ill, in which the patient emphasizes a feeling of persistent sadness, low mood, apathy and loss of interest, poor concentration, low self-esteem, feeling worthless or hopeless or with suicidal thoughts, indicates depression.
- Feeling ill with odd, irrational thoughts (delusions) indicates schizophrenia.
- A patient who suddenly feels ill and appears slightly confused, disorientated or unsteady, may have had a "minor" stroke or "petit mal" seizure.

- Feeling ill associated with episodes of feeling hot and sweating followed by feeling cold, shaking all over and looking grey is likely to be caused by septicaemia.
- A patient who has been feeling ill and lethargic for several days, with generalized myalgia and arthralgia is likely to have a viral infection.
- A patient who initially felt slightly breathless, with a wheeze and a cough before feeling ill, is likely to have a chest infection.
- A patient who feels ill with chest discomfort or heaviness, sweating and breathlessness, may have had an AMI.
- A patient who has been feeling tired and increasingly run down for many weeks, globally weak and breathless on exertion may be anaemic.
- A patient who has been feeling ill with anorexia and increasing weight loss without a fever may have cancer.
- A patient who has been feeling ill, losing weight unexpectedly and has polyuria and polydipsia may have DM.
- Feeling ill, numbness or tingling in the fingers and toes or around the mouth, or noticing uncontrolled movements (tremor or fasciculation) may be caused by hypocalcaemia.

When a patient feels ill, aggravating and relieving factors may objectify the severity of an illness or influence management, but infrequently will help make a diagnosis: they are diagnostically more useful in patients presenting with a functional abnormality, or pain.

Ask yourself, what is the likely location of the abnormality causing the illness, the type of problem or the cause?

The character, aggravating and relieving factors may help discriminate between a primary brain abnormality and feeling ill secondary to a problem elsewhere and indicate the likely type of problem. This will signpost additional questions to ask and reduce the list of possible causes.

When the patient seems to be less alert, apathetic, less responsive to the environment or to stimulation, with poor concentration, or to have slow, disorganised or illogical thought processes, or be depressed, expressing negative thoughts, a feeling of helplessness, or isolation, they may have a primary brain abnormality. When a primary brain abnormality is suspected, it is likely to be caused by a neurological problem, a circulatory (vascular) or structural problem, cancer, or inflammation (usually infection).

The differential diagnosis of a neurological problem causing a person to feel ill, includes:

- Depression.
- Bipolar disorders.
- Schizophrenia.
- Autism.
- Personality or challenging behavioural disorders, such as anxiety, paranoia, panic attacks, obsessive-compulsive, body dysmorphic disorder, or eating problems.
- Disorders of sensory processing, such as chronic pain syndromes, phantom pains, irritable bowel syndrome, or fibromyalgia.
- Parkinson's disease.
- Seizures.

When a neurological problem is suspected, it may be appropriate to ask specific questions such as:

Has your mood changed?
What do you think about?
Do you behave differently?
Can you concentrate as well as you used to?
Have you had unusual or strange thoughts or feelings?
Have you noticed a tremor?
Have you had any fits, feints or funny turns?

Family members or friends may be able to give additional information.

Have you noticed a change in the way they behave?

Have you noticed anything different about their behaviour?

Patients who feel ill with a headache or have localizing neurological symptoms or signs, such as cranial nerve abnormalities (usually visual or auditory), or peripheral motor or sensory abnormalities, are likely to have a circulatory (vascular) problem, such as an embolus, carotid artery stenosis, thrombosis, or an aneurysm, or a structural primary brain problem, such as a tumour or cancer, or inflammation, usually infection.

If there is a suspicion the illness may be caused by a structural or circulatory type of problem, the questions to ask may include:

Have you had any unusual headaches?
Have you had any fits, feints or funny turns?
Have you had any blackouts?
Do you feel unsteady on your feet?
Have you had any visual disturbances, such as blurred vision, flashing lights or blindness in one or both eyes?
Have you had any funny feelings, such as tingling, in your hands or feet?
Have you felt weak, or numb on one side, or in one part of your body?

If there is a suspicion the illness may be caused by inflammation, the questions to ask may include:

Have you been confused or found it difficult to think clearly?
Have you felt tired and listless?
Have you had a headache?
Have you had any neck or back pain or stiffness?
Have you had a fever?
Do you find light uncomfortable?

Most patients feel ill secondary to an abnormality elsewhere causing a systemic inflammatory response, such as a UTI or an auto-immune condition, a metabolic problem, such as renal failure, or from cancer.

Systemic inflammation is usually caused by an infection and is associated with a fever and localizing symptoms or signs. It may be appropriate to ask:

Do you have a fever?
Does it feel like flu?
Do you feel breathless?
Do you have a cough?
Do you have to pass water more often? Does it sting when you pass water?
Have you any back or abdominal pain?

Some patients feel ill because of non-infective inflammation and do not get a fever. If auto-immune inflammation is suspected, it may be appropriate to ask:

Have you had a rash?
Do your muscles and joints hurt?

Fatigue and lethargy, feeling depressed or irritable, an impaired ability to concentrate and being forgetful, sleeping poorly and headaches associated with paraesthesia, palpitations, muscle weakness, twitches and cramps, anorexia, nausea and sickness or a loss of libido may be caused by a metabolic abnormality. The differential diagnosis of a metabolic problem includes:

- Deranged acid-base balance.
- Internal water and salt imbalance (particularly sodium, potassium, hydrogen, calcium, magnesium and phosphate ions).
- Abnormal nutrient supply (particularly glucose and amino acids).
- Deranged waste management; particularly bile salts or nitrogenous wastes.

Frequently, a metabolic problem is only considered when the results of investigations are abnormal.

When anorexia and unexpected weight loss are included in the description of their illness, cancer should be considered. Cancers, such as metastatic cancer, leukaemia or lymphoma may make patients feel unwell because they cause inflammation and a catabolic metabolism. Some cancers may affect the metabolism by increasing hormone resistance, as part of a paraneoplastic syndrome, or through effects on regulatory mechanisms. If the patient does not mention a change in weight, it may be appropriate to ask:

Have you been losing weight?

Less commonly, feeling unwell is secondary to a circulatory problem causing cerebral hypo-perfusion and hypoxia. The differential diagnosis of cerebral hypo-perfusion includes:

- Recurrent micro-emboli.
- Systemic hypotension caused by hypovolaemia or heart failure.
- Anaemia or respiratory failure.

Ask yourself, what is the likely location of the abnormality causing the illness, the type of problem or the cause?

When the patient is systemically ill, the examination takes priority. The initial focus is on assessing the severity of their illness and then on conducting a systematic examination in the hope of finding an abnormal sign.

- When a primary brain problem is suspected, it is important to examine the patient for neurological signs, if only to exclude them.
- When systemic inflammation is suspected, examine the patient for signs of a fever including, sweating, looking flushed, a pyrexia ($>38°C$) or hypothermia ($<35°C$), tachycardia with a bounding pulse, hypotension (systolic BP<101mmHg), tachypnoea (RR>21/min) with shallow mouth breathing ("panting"), or a slow (<8/minute) weak and shallow respiratory rate.

When the patient is unable to give meaningful description of their problem or believable answers to questions, a systematic examination may be indicated to look for an abnormal sign. In the confused patient, the initial focus will be on looking for signs of sepsis, when the patient has a mental illness, it is likely to be on a neurological examination.

For some patients presenting feeling ill, the signs may be diagnostic. For example:

- Signs of weight loss, lymphadenopathy, hepatomegaly, a pleural effusion or ascites in a patient with cancer.
- Unilateral facial, arm and leg weakness, hyper-reflexia and upgoing planters and a lateral visual field deficiency following a stoke.
- A tremor, muscle fasciculation, paraesthesia, scratch marks, coarse hair, brittle nails and dry skin, Chvostek and Trousseau's signs in a patient with hypocalcaemia.

Ask yourself, how can the information about the character, aggravating and relieving factors inform management

When the character indicates a likely diagnosis, treatment may be started. For example:

- When the working diagnosis is depression, treatment with anti-depressants may be indicated.
- When the patient is ill and there is a fever, likely to be caused by septicaemia, anti-microbial treatment may be indicated.

However, usually investigations are indicated to confirm or exclude a diagnosis, the location of the abnormality, the likely type of problem or the cause. Occasionally, "standard" blood tests indicate the likely location of the abnormality. For example:

- When the thyroid function is abnormal.
- When the urea and creatinine are abnormal.

- When the WBC is very abnormal.

Tests are also indicated to confirm the likely type of problem. For example:

- Measuring the WBC count and CRP to diagnose inflammation (Appendix 2).
- Measuring the serum creatinine and electrolytes to diagnosis a metabolic problem (Appendix 2).

Usually, more specific investigations are indicated, such as a CXR, a CT scan, or microbiological tests, such as of a urine sample.

Frequently, when a patient presents feeling ill, the blood is likely to be abnormal. Usually, a "standard" set of investigations are requested to screen for an abnormality, in addition to tests to confirm or exclude a diagnosis, such as a problem affecting the kidneys or liver, or to determine the type of abnormality, such as inflammation or a metabolic problem. Blood tests are likely to include (Appendix 2):

- A full blood count.
- Measurement of serum blood glucose.
- Serum electrolyte measurement.
- Measurement of serum urea and creatinine.
- LFTs.
- Measurement of serum calcium, magnesium and phosphate.

Aggravating and relieving factors may inform the advice given to patients, such as what to avoid doing.

When the patient describes a symptom of deranged function, ask questions to learn and understand what deranged function means to the patient, and aggravating and relieving factors

Symptoms of deranged function tell us about how parts of our body are working. They may be "normal", everyday symptoms, such as when we are tired and weak with myalgia after exercise, when we feel sick and bloated after eating too much or when we feel breathless after exercise. Symptoms that are unusual, excessive, unexplained, abnormal, atypical, unexpectedly persistent or recurrent tell us that something is wrong with a part of our body. Symptoms of deranged function include:

- Poor concentration, impaired memory, depression or confusion, fits, feints or funny spells.
- Problems with the senses, hearing, eyesight, taste, smell, balance, touch or coordination.
- Fatigue and weakness. A reduced range of movement.
- Anorexia, dysphagia, nausea, vomiting, weight loss, bloating, bleeding or a change in bowel habit.
- A cough, wheeze or breathlessness.
- Passing too much or too little urine or a slow urine stream.
- Excessive mucus, or pus or blood in the sputum, urine, stool, from the nose, ear, per-rectum or per-vagina.

It may be appropriate to ask questions to understand what they mean: i.e., to learn the "character" of the deranged function, when the information is likely to help formulate a diagnosis, determine the location of the abnormality or the type of problem or to inform the examination or management. For example:

- When a patient presents with vomiting, it may be appropriate to ask about the nature and volume of vomitus.

Do you feel sick?
What did it [the vomitus] look like?
How much did you bring up?
Was it clear and frothy, green or dark brown/black?
Was there any blood in it?

It may be appropriate to ask questions about specific aggravating or relieving factors. For example:

What makes you vomit?
Is there anything you can do to make it better?
What makes your sickness worse?
Do you feel sick after eating a meal?
Can you eat a small meal/drink without feeling sick?

- When a patient presents with diarrhoea, they may mean a change in bowel frequency, consistency, stool colour, such as melaena or steatorrhea, blood or mucus or faecal incontinence or urgency. It may be appropriate to ask:

What do you mean by diarrhoea?
What is the consistency?
What colour is the stool?
Is there any blood or mucus in it?
Do you have accidents or need to rush to the toilet?

It may be appropriate to ask questions about aggravating or relieving factors. For example:

When do you get diarrhoea?
Does it occur after meals?
Do you also get diarrhoea at night?
What do you do to prevent it?
Is it worse when you are stressed?
Have you limited what you do?

- When a patient presents with a cough they may mean a productive cough, a dry cough, a morning cough or a seasonal cough. It may be appropriate to ask:

Do you have a dry cough?
What do you cough up?
When do you get a cough?

When the cough is productive, it may be appropriate to ask:

What does the sputum look like?
Is it green, yellow or white?
Is it ever blood stained?

It may be appropriate to ask questions about aggravating or relieving factors.

What makes your cough worse?
Does lying down make it worse?
Is it better or worse when you get home/go to work?

- When a patient presents with breathlessness they may mean an increased respiratory rate, a change in the depth of breathing, an abnormal pattern of breathing, increased work of breathing or a wheeze. The questions to ask to understand what they mean include:

What do you mean when you say you feel breathless?
Describe your breathlessness?
What is the breathlessness like?

If the patient has difficulty describing their breathlessness it may be helpful to ask closed questions. For example:

Has your breathing rate changed [increased]?

Are you breathing more deeply than normal?
Do you feel you need to take deep breaths?
Is breathing more difficult?
Do you feel a tightness affecting your breathing?

It may be appropriate to ask questions about specific aggravating or relieving factors. For example:

What makes your breathlessness worse?
What do you do to relieve your breathlessness?
Do you get very breathless when anxious or frightened?
Can you walk to the shops?
Can you walk upstairs?
Is the breathlessness worse when you walk quickly or up a hill?
Is the breathlessness relieved by rest? Does lying down make the breathlessness worse Do you wake up at night feeling breathless?
Does sleeping in a chair help the pain?

When learning about the character, aggravating and relieving factors:

Ask yourself, what is the likely diagnosis?

A description of the character, aggravating and relieving factors when considered together with other information may indicate a diagnostic pattern. For example:

- Hyperventilation or panting that occurs when anxious or frightened is likely to be over-breathing. When tachypnoea starts suddenly and is persistent it may be caused by a PE, and when it is associated with a fever, by an infection. Hyperventilation or panting and sweet-smelling breath or a smell of ammonia noticed by others, could be caused by metabolic acidosis.
- Feeling breathless when lying down (orthopnoea), or suddenly waking up at night feeling very breathless (paroxysmal nocturnal dyspnoea) indicates heart failure as a cause of the breathlessness.
- Loud snoring at night and periods of apnoea, followed by loud deep breathing is characteristic of sleep apnoea. It is normally noticed by a sleeping partner. It is a form of obstructed breathing. Patients feel tired all the time and readily fall asleep during the day.
- A sequence of regular deep inspirations followed by apnoea is characteristic of Blot's respiration indicating raised intracranial pressure.
- Progressively faster and deeper breathing followed by apnoea is characteristic of Cheyne-Stokes's breathing in heart failure.
- In an elderly man a slow urine stream, with hesitancy and terminal dribbling indicates an enlarged prostate.
- Pale, bulky and very offensive stools, that are difficult to flush away, is characteristic of steatorrhea, likely to be caused by chronic pancreatitis.
- A purulent perianal spotting is likely to be from an anal fistula.

When the diagnosis is uncertain or the list of possible diagnoses long:

Ask yourself, what is the likely location of the abnormality, the type of problem and the cause?

It is obviously inappropriate to ask the patient the "location" of a symptom such as breathlessness or a change in bowel habit. Nevertheless, the patient's description of their problem may indicate the likely "location" of the abnormality. For example:

- Bright red bleeding indicates an abnormality nearby. For example,
  o Rectal bleeding indicates an anal or low rectal structural abnormality, such as haemorrhoids or an anal ulcer or a rectal abnormality, such as a polyp, a cancer or inflammation.
  o Frank haemoptysis indicates an upper airway abnormality, such as a bronchial cancer.
  o Frank haematuria indicates a bladder abnormality, such as TCC or a calculus.

- o Haemospermia indicates a prostatic abnormality, such as prostatitis.
- o Menorrhagia indicates a uterine structural abnormality, such as fibroids or inflammation, such as endometriosis or infection.
- Pus or a purulent discharge indicates an abnormality nearby. For example:
  - o Purulent sputum usually indicates an airway inflammatory abnormality, such as bronchitis, or pneumonia.
  - o A purulent vaginal discharge indicates vaginal inflammation, such as candida infection or bacterial overgrowth.
  - o Mucus and blood passed per-rectum indicates rectal inflammation, proctitis, or a tumour, such as an adenoma or a cancer.
- When a patient presents with vomiting, the nature and volume of vomitus may indicate the location of an abnormality, such as an obstruction. For example:
  - o Vomiting undigested food or frothy white fluid, indicates distal oesophageal or gastric outlet "obstruction".
  - o Green vomit indicates bile staining caused by duodenal or jejunal "obstruction".
  - o Frequent large volumes of vomit indicate proximal small bowel "obstruction".
  - o Small volumes of vomit or the occasional large volume vomit indicate a more distal cause.
  - o "Coffee ground" or "faeculent" vomit is usually from an ileus or a distal bowel obstruction.
- When breathing feels and appears strenuous or difficult, and the patient puts a lot of work into moving air into and out of the lungs, it is likely to be a primary respiratory problem affecting the airways, such as asthma, or pulmonary compliance, such as interstitial lung disease.
- A very slow respiratory rate is likely to be secondary to drugs, such as opiates or a raised ICP. A very slow respiratory rate is never caused by a primary respiratory abnormality.
- When a patient presents with diarrhoea, and the stools are pale, bulky, difficult to flush away and the smell is very offensive it is likely to be steatorrhea. Steatorrhea may be caused by inflammatory conditions affecting the pancreas, such as pancreatic exocrine deficiency in chronic pancreatitis, auto-immune small intestinal inflammation caused by Crohn's disease or coeliac disease, bacterial overgrowth or giardiasis.

The character may indicate the type of problem causing the deranged function. For example:

- When a patient presents with tachypnoea at rest the likely type of problem is:
  - o An inflammatory problem affecting the airways and lungs such as bronchitis or pneumonia.
  - o A structural problem, such as cancer or pulmonary fibrosis.
  - o A circulatory problem, such as anaemia, heart failure or hypovolaemia.
- When a patient presents with frequent watery diarrhoea and urgency the likely type of problem is:
  - o An inflammatory problem affecting the colon, such as colitis.
  - o A structural problem, such as a diverticular stricture or cancer affecting the colon, causing overflow diarrhoea.
  - o A circulatory problem, such as mesenteric ischaemia.

Ask yourself, how can the information about the character, aggravating and relieving factors of their illness inform the examinations?

Usually, when a patient presents with deranged function an examination is indicated. The character, aggravating and relieving factors may indicate the signs to look for. For example:

- When a patient presents with a productive cough, the chest should be examined for signs such as, localized unilateral reduced air entry, crepitations, dullness on percussion or a pleural rub.
- When a patient presents with rectal bleeding, the perineum and rectum should be examined for a visible or palpable abnormality.
- When a patient presents with weakness, this should be confirmed and the site examined for signs of muscle wasting and the reflexes assessed. The examination should also exclude weakness elsewhere or other neurological signs, such as paraesthesia.

For some conditions, the signs may be diagnostic. For example:

- A pericardial rub indicating pericarditis causing the breathlessness.

- In a patient with diarrhoea, a multifocal rash affecting the skin of the scalp and elbows is likely to be dermatitis herpetiformis caused by coeliac disease.

In some patients, the examination is used to look for signs to exclude a diagnosis. For example:

- In a breathless patient, exclude signs of heart failure, such as a raised JVP, an enlarged heart or peripheral oedema.
- When a patient has had a stroke, exclude signs of an embolic circulatory abnormality, such as a carotid bruit, an arrhythmia or a heart murmur.

Ask yourself, how can the information about the character, aggravating and relieving factors inform management

The character, aggravating and relieving factors may indicate the investigations to be requested, such as to assess severity or screen for an abnormality, and treatment to be started. For example:

- When tachypnoea is likely to be caused by a PE, measurement of oxygen saturation, an ABG (Text box?) and an ECG are indicated, oxygen and anticoagulation should be started, while awaiting a CT angiogram or VQ scan to confirm the diagnosis.
- When tachypnoea is associated with sweet-smelling breath or a smell of ammonia noticed by others, the blood glucose should be measured urgently. In addition, a standard set of blood tests should be requested.
- When loud snoring at night is characteristic of sleep apnoea, sleep monitoring may be indicated.
- In an elderly man a slow urine stream, with hesitancy and terminal dribbling is often investigated with a micturating cystogram to confirm bladder outflow obstruction.

Investigations are often indicated to confirm or exclude the likely location of an abnormality or the type of problem. For example:

- Pale, bulky and very offensive stools characteristic of steatorrhea, may be investigated with a faecal fat or a prosperol test, to confirm the type of problem. A CT scan or ERCP may be indicated to confirm the pancreas is the location of the abnormality.
- When there is purulent perianal spotting likely to be from an anal fistula an MRI may be indicated to define the anatomy prior to surgery.
- When the symptoms are typical of heart failure as a cause of the breathlessness an ECG and echocardiogram may be indicated to confirm the location of the abnormality.
- In an elderly man with bladder outflow obstruction a trans rectal USS and PSA may be indicated to determine the type of problem.

Frequently, when a patient presents with deranged function, the blood is likely to be abnormal. Usually, a "standard" set of investigations are requested to screen for an abnormality in addition to tests to confirm or exclude a diagnosis. Blood tests (appendix 2) are likely to include:

- A full blood count.
- Measurement of serum blood glucose.
- Serum electrolyte measurement.
- Measurement of serum urea and creatinine.
- LFTs.
- Measurement of serum calcium, magnesium and phosphate.

Often, specific investigations are indicated, such as measurement of oxygen saturation, an ABG (Appendix 2).and pulmonary function tests to investigate breathlessness or a colonoscopy to investigate a change in bowel habit.

Aggravating and relieving factors may inform the advice given to patients, such as what to avoid doing. Information about the character may influence the priority of investigations or treatment.

Ask questions to learn about the Location of the Problem and Use the available information to determine the likely Location of the Abnormality causing the problem

The aims of learning about the location of the problem are to formulate a diagnosis, to plan management and determine the signs to look for on examination. When the diagnosis is uncertain the aims are to determine the location of the abnormality causing the problem, the likely type of problem and the cause.

When patients first describe their problem, they usually describe the location, such as when they describe a "head"-ache, a "groin" lump or a weak "leg", or a location is inferred. For example:

- Symptoms of breathlessness suggest a problem affecting the chest.
- Dysphagia suggests an abnormality affecting the oesophagus.
- Palpitations suggest an abnormality affecting the heart.
- Forgetfulness suggests an abnormality affecting the brain.
- Weakness suggests an abnormality affecting the muscles.

When it is appropriate to identify the location of the problem and it is not mentioned it may be appropriate to ask:

Where do you get [the symptom]?

When a patient is in pain, it is important to try to be as precise as possible about the location of the problem as this is likely to indicate the abnormal tissue, organ or part of the body. When the patient describes or indicates the location of the problem it is understandably imprecise when the patient is sitting in a chair wearing clothes or in bed, and covered. Patients are more precise when identifying the location of a superficial problem or when their problem is in the limbs, but tend to be less precise for deep seated problems affecting the trunk.

It may be appropriate to ask:

Where exactly do you get [the pain]?
Is it in your [site] or [site]?

The gestures the patient uses may help. For example:
- If the patient points with a finger or shows you the part affected, the problem is likely to be localized. There may be a visible or palpable abnormality at the site indicated.
- When a patient indicates the area with a gesture, such as rubbing a knee or a part of the abdomen, clenching a fist over the chest, or moving the hand up and down the sternum it is likely to be from an internal or deep-seated abnormality.

The patient can usually distinguish pain felt in the head from the face and neck, the shoulder from the chest or the lower abdomen from the leg. For example:

- A "headache" can usually be distinguished from facial pain, such as toothache, otitis externa or temporomandibular joint pain or from neck pain, such as torticollis, a sub-luxed cervical facet joint or cervical nerve entrapment.
- A lower abdominal pain, such as acute appendicitis, ureteric colic or salpingo-oophoritis can usually be distinguished from upper thigh pain, caused by hip arthritis, upper lumbar spinal nerve entrapment or adductor tendinitis.

However, the patient may find it difficult to distinguish between lower chest and upper abdominal pain and between lower abdominal and pelvic pain because the viscera are innervated by autonomic nerves and the pain is poorly localized.

It is not unusual to ask about the location of the problem on at least 3 separate occasions during the consultation:

1. At the start, when the patient is asked to describe their problem.
2. When learning the details of the patient's symptoms.
3. When examining the patient.

When learning about the location of the problem:

Ask yourself, what is the likely diagnosis?

The headline information and the location of the problem may indicate a likely diagnosis based on probabilities. For example:

- An acute onset of right lower quadrant pain in a young man may be caused by acute appendicitis.
- A chronic knee pain in a middle aged or elderly patient is likely to be caused by osteoarthritis.
- A painful great toe may be caused by gout or an ingrowing toenail.
- Painful rectal bleeding on defaecation is likely to be caused by an anal fissure.
- A summer wheeze is likely to be caused by "hay-fever".

This will inform the questions to ask or signs to look for.
When learning about the location of the problem.

Ask yourself, what is the likely location of the abnormality?

The headline information and the location of the problem will usually indicate the location of the abnormality. For example:

- When pain, stiffness or a reduced range of movement affects one limb joint the abnormality is likely to be in the knee joint, such as osteoarthritis.
- A retrosternal burning chest pain is likely to be from an inflamed oesophagus, such as reflux oesophagitis.
- A persistently dry mouth indicates a problem affecting all the salivary glands, and is therefore likely to be caused by auto-immune inflammation from Sjogren's syndrome.
- Lower left-sided chest pain brought on by exertion and relieved by rest is likely to be caused by a cardiac circulatory problem, such as atherosclerotic ischaemic heart disease.

However, when there is uncertainty, ask questions to determine whether it is a primary problem at the site or secondary to an abnormality elsewhere, whether it is superficial or deep-seated, what tissue, gland, organ or structure is abnormal and whether it is a solitary problem or part of a multifocal or widespread problem.

Some problems can be caused by an abnormality at the site of the problem or be secondary to an abnormality elsewhere. For example:

- When a patient presents with small mass in the side of the neck likely to be an enlarged jugulo-digastric lymph node, it can be a primary abnormality, such as a lymphoma, or secondary to an abnormality in the face, mouth, head or neck, such as a dental abscess, or be part of a multi-focal disease, such as lymphoma.
- Collapse, without losing consciousness, may be caused by a primary brain abnormality, such as a seizure, or be secondary to a problem elsewhere, such as haemorrhage from a ruptured intra-abdominal aneurysm or a ruptured ectopic pregnancy.
- Breathlessness may be caused by a primary pulmonary abnormality or could be secondary to an abnormality elsewhere, such as heart failure, renal failure, thyrotoxicosis or a UTI.
- Palpitations could be caused by a primary cardiac conduction abnormality or be secondary to a metabolic abnormality, such as thyrotoxicosis or hyperkalaemia.
- Left sided shoulder and upper arm pain may be caused by a primary shoulder abnormality or be secondary to an abnormality affecting the neck or heart.
- Midline back pain may be caused by a primary musculo-skeletal abnormality nearby or be secondary to a retroperitoneal abnormality. For example:
  - A deep-seated mid-thoracic central back pain is likely to arise from a mediastinal abnormality, such as pericarditis, a thoracic aneurysm or lymphoma.
  - A deep-seated lower thoracic central back pain is likely to arise from an upper abdominal retroperitoneal abnormality, such as acute pancreatitis or pancreatic cancer.

- A deep-seated upper lumber central back pain is likely to arise from an abnormality affecting the abdominal retroperitoneum, such as an expanding abdominal aortic aneurysm, retroperitoneal haemorrhage, acute pancreatitis or para-aortic lymphadenopathy.
- A deep-seated sacral or perineal pain is likely to arise from an abnormality affecting a pelvic organ, such as proctalgia, proctitis, constipation or cancer.

In general, the abnormality is at the site of the main symptom:

- When the problem starts suddenly or acutely.
- When there is a visible or palpable abnormality at the site.
- When there are no associated symptoms.
- When the associated symptoms support the location of the problem being the location of the abnormality. For example, when the patient presents with:
  - An acute onset of breathlessness associated with a cough producing purulent sputum, is likely to be caused by an airway abnormality, such as bronchitis.
  - Pus or bright red blood indicate an abnormality nearby. For example:
    - Coughing up purulent sputum or frank haemoptysis, indicates a pulmonary abnormality.
    - A purulent vaginal discharge indicates a vaginal or uterine abnormality.
    - Frank haematuria or rectal bleeding indicates a bladder or rectal abnormality.
  - Frequent watery diarrhoea associated with blood and mucus is likely to be caused by a colonic abnormality; usually inflammation, such as UC or Crohn's disease.
  - Upper abdominal colic associated with vomiting is likely to be caused by a proximal small bowel abnormality, such as an obstruction.
  - Lower abdominal colic associated with constipation and abdominal distension is likely to be caused by a distal large bowel abnormality, such as obstruction, slow transit constipation or IBS.
  - Abdominal pain localized to the right lower quadrant associated with anorexia, nausea, bloating, diarrhoea or dysuria and a fever is likely to be an abnormality affecting the appendix, caecum, terminal ileum or right Fallopian tube and ovary, such as acute appendicitis, salpingo-oophoritis, Yersinia enterocolitica or Crohn's disease.
  - Left lower quadrant abdominal pain and tenderness associated with a change in bowel habit and a fever is likely to be caused by acute diverticulitis.
- When a precipitating factor supports the location of the problem being the location of the abnormality. For example:
  - Acute tachypnoea and a wheeze when in a room with an animal, such as a cat, and relieved when outside, is likely to be caused by an abnormality affecting the airways, such as a hypersensitivity reaction.
  - When eating bread causes diarrhoea and bloating, the abnormality is likely to affect the bowel, such as coeliac disease.
- When the character, aggravating and relieving factors indicate the location of the problem is the location of the abnormality. For example:
  - A sharp localized pain is likely to be caused by an abnormality in the skin or the sub-cutaneous tissues at the site indicated.
  - Neuralgia precisely localized to one spot is likely to be from a subcutaneous structural problem, such as a neuroma.
  - Upper abdominal colic aggravated by eating is likely to be caused by an abnormality that affects the foregut.
  - When a superficial shoulder pain is aggravated by moving the shoulder, such as to comb the hair it is likely to be caused by an abnormality that affects the shoulder.
- When the problem affects some locations. For example:
  - Problems affecting the face, cervical spine or a limb joint are likely to be caused by an abnormality at the site of the problem.
- Abdominal inflammatory pain or colic is likely to be from an underlying organ or tissue For example, midline trunk pain is likely to arise from a viscus that was embryologically midline.
  - Midline or "retrosternal" chest pain indicates an abnormality affecting:
    - The oesophagus, such as reflux oesophagitis or oesophageal spasm ("nutcracker" oesophagus).
    - The heart, such as ACS.
    - The mediastinum, such as lymphadenopathy.

- Midline upper abdominal pain, at the level of T6-9 dermatomes, is likely to be from the embryological foregut structures, including:
  - The stomach and duodenum. For example, gastritis, a peptic ulcer or gastric outlet obstruction.
  - The pancreas. For example, pancreatitis or cancer.
  - The biliary tract. For example, biliary colic, cholecystitis, choledocholithiasis or cholangitis.
- Midline mid abdominal pain, at the level of T9-11 dermatomes, is likely to be from the embryological midgut structures, including:
  - The jejunum and ileum. For example, infection, a Meckel's diverticulum, Crohn's disease, ischaemia or obstruction.
  - The caecum, appendix, ascending and proximal two thirds of the transverse colon. For example, appendicitis, diverticulitis, large bowel obstruction or colitis.
- Midline lower abdominal pain, at the level of T11-12 and L1 dermatomes, is likely to be from the embryological hindgut and pelvic structures, including:
  - Left side of the colon. For example, diverticular disease, colitis or cancer.
  - A pelvic abnormality. For example, acute retention of urine, endometriosis, an involuting uterine fibroid, a pyometrium or endometrial cancer.

In general, the problem is likely to be caused by an abnormality elsewhere:

- When the associated symptoms relate to a site elsewhere. For example:
  - Left shoulder and upper arm pain, associated with breathlessness, is likely to be referred from the heart, such as angina.
  - Lower thoracic back pain, associated with steatorrhea and weight loss is likely to be referred from the pancreas.
- When a precipitating factor indicates a site elsewhere. For example:
  - A neuralgia pain spreading down the back of the leg after lifting and moving heavy boxes is likely to be caused by an abnormality that affects the spine.
  - A dull aching shoulder pain aggravated by deep inspiration, coughing or sneezing is likely to be referred from the diaphragm.
- When the character is atypical for the site and aggravating and relieving factors are consistent with a site elsewhere. For example:
  - A dull ache or heaviness in the left shoulder and upper arm, aggravated by walking up stairs and relieved by sitting down and relieved by rest is likely to be referred from the heart, such as angina.
  - A constant dull ache in the lower thoracic back, unaffected by twisting, turning, bending or lifting but aggravated by eating is likely to be referred from the pancreas.
- When the pain or symptoms of deranged function are multifocal or widespread, they are usually secondary to an abnormality elsewhere. For example:
  - Widespread lower leg pain is likely to be secondary to an abnormality affecting the femoral artery, such as superficial femoral artery stenosis or the back, such as a prolapsed intervertebral disc.
  - Multi-focal myalgia or weakness is likely to be secondary to auto-immune inflammation, such as polymyalgia.
  - Weakness affecting one side of the body is likely to be secondary to a neurological abnormality, such as a stroke.

All available information about the problem should be used to determine the location of the abnormality causing the problem, i.e., the likely tissue, organ or part of the body affected. A knowledge or checklist of nearby structures will indicate the likely site of the abnormality. For example:

- Midline trunk pain is likely to arise from a viscus that was embryologically midline.
  - Midline or "retrosternal" visceral chest pain indicates an abnormality affecting:
    - The oesophagus, such as reflux oesophagitis or oesophageal spasm ("nutcracker" oesophagus).
    - The heart, such as ACS.
    - The mediastinum, such as lymphadenopathy.
  - Midline upper abdominal pain, at the level of T6-9 dermatomes, is likely to be from the embryological foregut structures:
    - The stomach and duodenum. For example, gastritis, a peptic ulcer or gastric outlet obstruction.

- The pancreas. For example, pancreatitis or cancer.
- The biliary tract. For example, biliary colic, cholecystitis, choledocholithiasis or cholangitis.
  o Midline mid abdominal pain, at the level of T9-11 dermatomes, is likely to be from the embryological midgut structures:
    - The jejunum and ileum. For example, infection, a Meckel's diverticulum, Crohn's disease, ischaemia or obstruction.
    - The caecum, appendix, ascending and proximal two thirds of the transverse colon. For example, appendicitis, diverticulitis, large bowel obstruction or colitis.
  o Midline lower abdominal pain, at the level of T11-12 and L1 dermatomes, is likely to be from the embryological hindgut and pelvic structures:
    - Left side of the colon. For example, diverticular disease, colitis or cancer.
    - A pelvic abnormality. For example, acute retention of urine, endometriosis, an involuting uterine fibroid, a pyometrium or endometrial cancer.

When there is uncertainty about the location of the abnormality, additional questions should be asked because this will limit the list of possible diagnoses. For example:

Does the pain feel deep inside?
Is the pain felt on the surface?

When the problem is a pain or a deranged function, or the differential diagnosis includes a diagnosis that can be solitary, multifocal or widespread, it is important to distinguish between a solitary localized problem, a multifocal problem, and a widespread or global problem. It may be appropriate to ask:

Is this the only site affected?
Have you noticed any problems elsewhere?
Are there any similar problems elsewhere?
Is this the only place you have [the problem]?
Are there any other parts affected?

When the symptoms of deranged function or pain are widespread or multi-focal, ask about the extent of the problem. The questions to ask could include:

Tell me all the sites affected.
How big an area is affected?

Ask yourself, how does the location inform the likely type of problem and the cause?

Some types of problem are more likely in some parts of the body. For example, when a patient presents with abdominal colic it is likely to be a structural problem or when a patient presents with an acutely painful leg it is likely to be a circulatory problem. This will indicate the questions to ask or the signs to look for to determine the type of problem.

The more precisely the location of the abnormality can be localized, the more likely the type of problem and the cause can be determined. For example:

- When the main presenting problem is breathlessness:
  o Caused by an abnormality affecting the airways compromising alveolar ventilation, it is likely to be an inflammatory problem, such as laryngitis, bronchitis or broncho-constriction, a structural problem, such as consolidation or a circulatory problem, such as pulmonary oedema.
  o When an abnormality affects gas transfer between alveolar air and the blood, it is likely to be a structural problem, such as pulmonary fibrosis or a circulatory problem, such as pulmonary oedema.
  o When an abnormality affects the blood, it is likely to be a circulatory problem, such as anaemia or a metabolic problem, such as acidosis or carbon monoxide poisoning.
  o When an abnormality affects pulmonary perfusion, it is likely to be a circulatory problem, such as a PE or heart failure.

- o When an abnormality increases oxygen demand, it is likely to be an inflammatory problem, such as sepsis or a metabolic problem, such as thyrotoxicosis.
  - o When an abnormality affects the regulation of ventilation, it is likely to be a neurological problem, such as from medications or a raised ICP.
- When the main presenting problem is a headache:
  - o Caused by a primary brain problem, it is likely to be a neurological problem, such as a tension headache, migraine, a mental health condition, such as depression, a structural problem, such as dementia, tumours, hydrocephalus or an intra-cranial abscess, a circulatory problem, such as an arterio-venous malformation, an aneurysm or a sub-dural or extra-dural haemorrhage, cancer or inflammation, such as encephalitis or meningitis.
  - o When the headache is secondary to an abnormality elsewhere, it is likely to be an inflammatory problem, such as an infection or auto-immune disease, a circulatory problem, such as hypovolaemia, anaemia or heart failure, or a metabolic abnormality, such as renal failure.

Table to show the relationship between the location of the pain and the type of problem.

			Location		
Type of presenting problem	Joint	Limb	Face	Chest	Abdomen
Inflammation	Likely	Likely	Likely	Likely	Likely
Structural abnormality	Likely	Unlikely	Unlikely	Likely	Likely
Cancer	Unlikely	Unlikely	Likely	Likely	Likely
Circulatory	Unlikely	Likely	Unlikely	Likely	Unlikely
Metabolic	Unlikely	Unlikely	Unlikely	Unlikely	Unlikely
Neurological	Unlikely	Likely	Likely	Unlikely	Unlikely

When the pain or symptoms of deranged function are multifocal or affect a wide area, the problem is likely to be mediated by an inflammatory, metabolic or neurological type of problem. For example:

- Pain affecting multiple joints and muscles indicates a multifocal abnormality affecting different tissues and is likely to be caused by a systemic inflammatory condition, such as rheumatoid arthritis, dermatomyositis, polymyositis, SLE or poly-myalgia rheumatica, or a metabolic problem, such as gout or porphyria.
- Global weakness may be caused by inflammation, such as Guillain-Barré syndrome.
- A widespread constant atypical generalised abdominal and bone pain may indicate a metabolic problem, such as hypercalcaemia.
- Widespread or multifocal persistent atypical pains affecting a limb or different parts of the body is likely to be caused by a peripheral neurological abnormality, such as poly-neuritis or poly-radiculopathy.

The location of the abnormality together with information about the onset may indicate the likely type of problem. For example:

- Peritonitis starting suddenly is likely to be caused by a non-infective inflammatory problem, such as acute pancreatitis or a perforated peptic ulcer, or a circulatory problem, such as mesenteric ischaemia. Peritonitis that starts gradually, increasing over several hours or a couple of days indicates infection, such as acute appendicitis or diverticulitis. When it is chronic it may be caused by infective inflammation, such as from an abscess or a walled off perforation, "auto-immune" inflammation, such as Crohn's disease or ischaemic bowel.

- Acute onset multifocal joint pain, widespread muscle aches, and a fever are likely to be caused by a viral infection, whereas chronic pains without a fever are likely to be caused by an auto-immune inflammation.

Frequently the location of the abnormality together with information about the associated symptoms indicate the likely type of problem. For example:

- Abdominal colic associated with anorexia, nausea, vomiting, abdominal distension and constipation indicate an intestinal obstruction, a structural problem.
- Jaundice associated with dark urine, pale stools and urticaria indicates bile duct obstruction, a structural problem.
- A headache associated with photophobia, neck and back pain and a non-blanching rash indicates meningitis, an infective inflammatory problem.
- Feeling unwell, associated with polyurea, polydipsia and weight loss indicating DM, a metabolic problem.
- Feeling unwell associated with numbness or tingling in the fingers and toes or around the mouth, muscle cramps, a tremor or muscle twitching indicate hypocalcaemia, a metabolic problem.
- Excessive urine output or oliguria associated with frothy urine, breathlessness, hiccups, peripheral oedema, constipation and pruritis, may indicate renal failure, a metabolic problem.

Occasionally, the location of the abnormality together with a precipitating factor indicates the likely type of problem. For example:

- When breathlessness, a cough and a wheeze are brought on by an allergen, such as pollen, it is likely to be a hypersensitivity reaction.
- When dysphagia develops after a foreign body, it is likely to be a structural problem.
- When jaundice develops after a paracetamol overdose it is likely to be a metabolic problem.

The character, aggravating and relieving factors together with the location of the abnormality may indicate the likely type of problem. For example:

- A constant abdominal pain, aggravated by moving and relieved by rest is likely to be caused by inflammation.
- Intermittent episodes of pain and an inability to get comfortable are likely to be caused by colic, a structural problem or IBS, a neurological problem.
- Feeling unwell, with persistent sadness, low mood, apathy and loss of interest, aggravated by anxiety or stress indicate depression, a neurological problem.
- Breathlessness characterised by shallow fast breathing and pain aggravated when the patient takes a deep breath, indicate pleurisy, an inflammatory problem.

When there is uncertainty about the type of problem, additional questions should be asked because this will limit the list of possible diagnoses.
When learning about the location of the problem:

Ask yourself, how does the location inform management?

Frequently, investigations are indicated to confirm the location of the abnormality (Appendix 2). For example:

- When the patient feels ill and the location of the abnormality is uncertain, blood tests may indicate a likely location of the abnormality. For example:
  o A full blood count may reveal anaemia.
  o Measurement of serum blood glucose may confirm DM.
  o Measurement of serum electrolyte urea and creatinine may identify a renal abnormality.
  o Measurement of LFTs may identify a liver abnormality.
  o Measurement of serum calcium, magnesium and phosphate may indicate an endocrine abnormality.
- When there is a change in bowel habit, investigation with a colonoscopy or a CT scan may be indicated to determine the location of the abnormality.

- An USS may be indicated to identify the location of the abnormality when the patient presents with an upper abdominal pain, whereas a CT scan may be indicated to investigate a lower abdominal pain.
- A Dopplar USS or angiogram may identify the location of the abnormality when the patient presents with claudication.

The location of the abnormality may influence the choice of treatment. For example:

- A skin cancer on the back of the hand may be excised with a primary closure, whereas a skin cancer on the face may need plastic surgery to cover the excision defect.
- An infection in a foot of a patient with DM may need intravenous antimicrobial medication, whereas upper limb cellulitis may be treated with oral antimicrobial medication.

The location may influence the priority of a management option. For example:

- Chest pain is likely to be considered a higher priority than limb pain.
- Bacterial meningitis is a medical emergency that should be treated with antibiotics urgently whereas a UTI in a healthy person can be treated routinely.

When learning about the location of the problem:

Ask yourself, how does the location inform the signs to look for?

In general, the location of the problem and the likely location of the abnormality causing the problem indicate the sites to be examined and the method to use. For example:

- When there is a visible or palpable abnormality the examination of the site is likely to be diagnostic.
- When there is a problem likely to affect the brain, such as migraine or depression, there are unlikely to be any local signs so examining the head is not indicated. However, there may be associated signs, such as cranial or peripheral neurological signs to look for.
- When there is a problem affecting the heart auscultation is likely to be the most useful method.

The examination can assess the extent of the problem. For example, when the patient presents with neuralgia:

- To determine whether neuralgia is precisely localized.
- To determine whether neuralgia is in the distribution of a named sensory nerve, such as trigeminal neuralgia, ilio-hypogastric nerve entrapment following a hernia operation, or meralgia paraesthetica.
- To determine whether neuralgia affects a dermatome, such as sciatica or shingles caused by Herpes zoster infection.
- To look for an associated motor weakness affecting a nearby group of muscles, indicating the abnormality affects a mixed motor and sensory nerve, such as when the median nerve is entrapped at the wrist in carpal tunnel syndrome or a central disc prolapse.

The examination may also be undertaken to look for associated signs. For example:

- All patients with symptoms indicating a primary brain problem should be carefully examined for neurological signs, including sensory, motor or tendon reflex abnormalities and for signs of a raised ICP. These changes are subtle, and should be carefully looked for.
- To examine for signs of heart failure when a patient presents with atypical shoulder pain.

The examination can determine the likely location of the abnormality. For example:

- When there is a visible or palpable abnormality.
- When a patient has an ischaemic limb, the signs on examination may indicate the likely location of the stricture or occlusion.

- When a patient has neuralgia in the distribution of a named sensory nerve there may be a structural or inflammatory abnormality affecting the sensory nerve axon proximal to the location of the pain.
- When neuralgia affects a dermatome, it is likely to be from a structural abnormality affecting a spinal nerve root. This may be confirmed by examining the spine.

Use Available Information and Ask Additional Questions to Determine the Type of Problem and the Likely Cause

When the diagnosis is uncertain, determining the likely type of problem and cause, together with the likely location of the abnormality, will indicate a descriptive diagnosis or a list of possible diagnoses, inform management and the signs to look for when examining the patient.

The patient's main symptom and the location of the abnormality will often indicate the likely type of problem. For example:

- When a patient presents with chest pain the likely type of problem is either:
  o An inflammatory problem, such as pleurisy, pericarditis, reflux oesophagitis or a ruptured oesophagus.
  o A circulatory problem, such as angina, acute myocardial infarction, aortic dissection or an aortic aneurysm.
- When a patient presents with breathlessness the likely type of problem is:
  o An inflammatory problem affecting the airways and lungs, such as laryngitis, bronchitis or pneumonia.
  o A structural problem, such as bronchospasm, COPD, cancer, or pulmonary fibrosis.
  o A circulatory problem, such as anaemia, heart failure or hypovolaemia.
- When a patient presents feeling ill, the likely types of problem include:
  o A neurological problem, such as depression, anxiety or ME.
  o An inflammatory problem, such as a viral infection, a chest infection, a UTI or an auto-immune disease.
  o A metabolic problem such as DM, liver failure or renal failure.

This will indicate the likely type of problem and can be used to inform additional questions to ask.

Ask yourself, is it an inflammatory type of problem and how should it be managed?

Inflammation is a high priority problem that should be considered in all patients, and particularly in patients who are immuno-compromised. Superficial inflammation is usually associated with a visible or palpable abnormality, whereas, deep-seated inflammation usually presents with symptoms of deranged function, pain or feeling ill. The pain or symptoms of deranged function are usually mild when the patient rests the inflamed part but are increased when it is used or moved. There may be an associated systemic inflammatory response causing the patient to feel ill, hot and sweaty with non-specific associated symptoms, such as a headache, anorexia, tiredness and listlessness, general weakness, myalgia or arthralgia. When there are symptoms of inflammation, the descriptive diagnosis often includes the location of the abnormality with a post-fix "- itis". For example, cellul-itis, ulcerative col-itis, osteoarthr-itis, cholecyst-itis, or hip arthr-itis. However, inflammation is not a diagnosis; it is the immune response to many problems. Inflammation becomes a definitive diagnosis when the underlying cause is identified (Figure 60).

The different causes of inflammation include:

- A chest infection or pneumonia is inflammation of the lung, likely to be caused by a bacterium. When the infecting organism, such as pneumococcus or haemophilus is identified it is a definitive diagnosis.
- Appendicitis is inflammation of the appendix, likely to be caused by infection complicating an obstructing faecolith.
- Dermatomyositis is auto-inflammation affecting the skin and muscles.
- Oesophagitis is inflammation of the oesophagus likely to be caused by chemical irritation from reflux of gastric fluid.
- Osteoarthritis is inflammation of the joint likely to be caused by senescent degeneration, repetitive trauma or an injury.
- Thrombophlebitis is inflammation of a vein likely to be caused by intra-venous thrombosis.

Figure 60: Illustrating the different causes of inflammation.

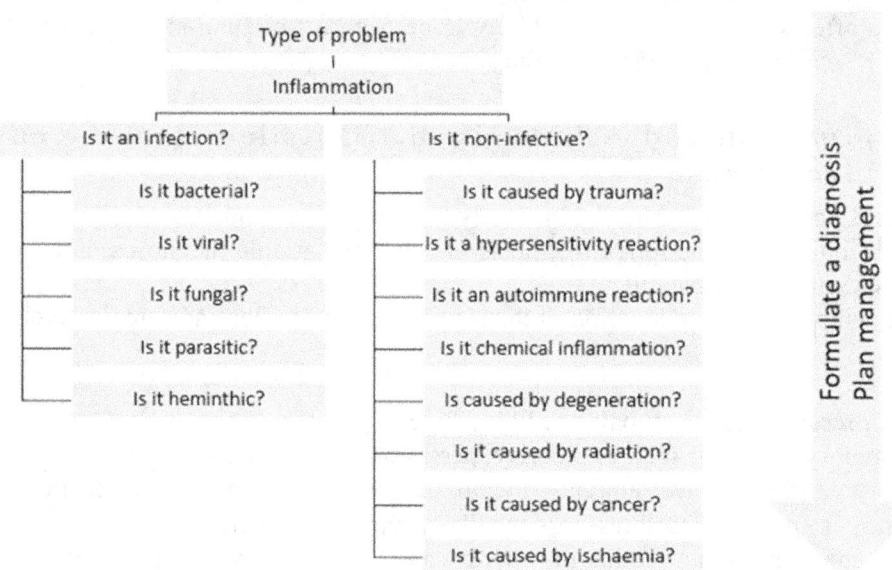

Information about the person and the person as a patient may include a risk factor suggesting a likely cause for the inflammation. For example:

- In the elderly, infection, degenerative or circulatory inflammation are more likely.
- Repetitive manual work is a risk factor for osteoarthritis.
- A low fibre diet is a risk factor for diverticular disease and diverticulitis.
- Smoking, DM and elevated blood lipids are risk factors for ischaemia.
- Known gallstone disease is a risk factor for cholecystitis.
- Previous allergic reactions are a risk factor for other allergies.
- An immuno-compromised patient is at increased risk of infection.
- A known auto-immune condition is a risk factor for another auto-immune condition.
- A previously treated cancer may recur.

Information about the person and the person as a patient may exclude a likely cause for the inflammation. For example:

- An absence of previous radiotherapy excludes this as a cause.
- In a young patient ischaemia is unlikely.

Information about a precipitating factor may indicate a likely cause for the inflammation. For example:

- Inflammation associated with a recent penetrating injury is likely to be caused by a bacterial infection.
- Elbow pain brought on by playing tennis may be lateral epicondylitis.
- Breathlessness and wheezing when in the company of a cat is likely to be a hypersensitivity reaction.
- Vomiting and diarrhoea occurring within hours of eating out at a restaurant is likely to be caused by gastroenteritis.
- Breathlessness and pleuritic chest pain following a long journey is likely to be from a PE.
- Diarrhoea following recent pelvic radiotherapy may be proctitis.

Information about the onset, duration or severity may indicate a likely cause for the inflammation. In general, an acute onset over several hours or days of constant but progressively deteriorating symptoms is likely to be caused by infection. Infection is more common in parts of the body at the interface with the environment, such as the respiratory, gastro-intestinal or urinary tract than in the soft-tissues, solid organs, bones or joints unless there has been a recent injury. There is usually pain, tenderness, swelling and symptoms of deranged function of the affected part of the body. The symptoms are aggravated by actively or passively using or moving the affected part. Feeling hot and sweaty, with anorexia, tiredness and generalised weakness, thirst and a dry mouth indicate a fever, likely to be caused by an infection. Rigors, an altered mental state with impaired conscious level, confusion, irritability, hallucinations and convulsions would indicate septicaemia, a medical emergency. The pattern of symptoms may indicate the likely cause of the infection. This should then be used to inform the signs to look for and management. For example:

- When there are symptoms of a fever, the signs to look for would include, sweating, looking flushed, pyrexia (>38 °C) or hypothermia (<35 °C), tachycardia with a bounding pulse, hypotension (systolic BP<101mmHg), tachypnoea (21/min) with shallow mouth breathing ("panting"), or a slow (<8/min) weak and shallow respiratory rate. If dehydrated the patient may be peripherally cold but centrally hot, the pulse fast but weak and difficult to palpate, with a low volume and concentrated urine with a low volume output. When the cause is uncertain, possible sites should be carefully examined for localizing signs. The WBC count and CRP should be measured to confirm an inflammatory response and cultures sent for microscopy, culture and serology to make a diagnosis.

- A constant headache that develops or increases over hours or a few days and is associated with drowsiness, impaired concentration, an impaired or fluctuating conscious state, confusion, a change in personality or behaviour, agitation or disturbed speech or hearing and a fever developing over several days, in the absence of symptoms of a problem elsewhere is characteristic of encephalitis. Associated neck stiffness and pain, aggravated by moving the head, and photophobia, are characteristic of meningitis. Patients prefer to lie down in a dark room and not be disturbed. On examination, signs of a fever and neurological signs, such as weakness, should be looked for. If meningitis is suspected, the neck should be examined for pain on flexing the neck and there may be a rash. If a bacterial infection is suspected, antimicrobial medication should be started and, in addition to blood tests, a CT scan and a lumbar puncture may be indicated to make a diagnosis.

- Urinary frequency, urgency and dysuria increasing over several days is likely to be caused by a UTI. The abdomen and loins should be examined for deep-seated tenderness. If a UTI is likely urine should be sent for microscopy, culture and serology to make a diagnosis and guide treatment.

- A gradual onset over a few hours of breathlessness associated with a productive cough and a fever is characteristic of a chest infection. There may be associated pleuritic chest pain. Signs of a fever and an increased respiratory rate are likely. Dullness to percussion and reduced air entry and crepitations (crackles) in part of the lung support the diagnosis of a chest infection. A rubbing, grating, crunching or squeaking sound is characteristic of a pleural friction rub. The absence of a rub does not exclude pleurisy. If a chest infection is likely sputum should be sent for microscopy, culture and serology and a CXR to confirm the diagnosis and treatment with antimicrobial medications may be indicated.

- Pain and localised tenderness in a joint that gradually increases over several hours or a couple of days may be from an infection. Rest does not relieve the pain and any movement, active or passive, causes severe pain. There may be an associated swelling and fever. On examination the joint or affected area is swollen, tender and warm. The joint is held partially flexed and not moved by the patient. Even gentle passive movement causes severe pain. If infection is suspected, in addition to blood tests to assess the severity of the inflammation a knee joint aspiration for microbiological assessment may be indicated to make a diagnosis prior to starting antimicrobial medication.

- A constant abdominal pain, increasing over several hours or days, is likely to be caused by intra-abdominal infection. At rest the pain may be absent or mild but it is aggravated by moving or using the affected part, when it can be severe. As a consequence, patients prefer to lie still, to rest and not use the affected part. When the inflammation is localized, the location indicates the likely location of the abnormality. When the pain affects the whole abdomen, the site where the pain started is likely to be the location of the abnormality. Associated symptoms of anorexia, abdominal distension, nausea and constipation indicate the inflammation is adjacent to or involving the bowel causing a localized ileus. Jaundice would indicate liver involvement. The abdomen is likely to be tender and there may be guarding. There may be a fullness or an ill-defined tender mass or, when it affects an organ, tender organomegaly. The area of maximal tenderness indicates the likely location of the abnormality. If infection is suspected, antimicrobial medication should be started, blood tests sent to confirm and assess the severity of the inflammation and to screen for deranged homeostasis, and an USS or CT scan ordered to formulate a diagnosis.

- A constant deep-seated right sub-costal aching pain, discomfort or heaviness aggravated by direct pressure is likely to be arising from the liver or gall-bladder. If there is associated jaundice, there may be dark urine and pale stools. If there is a deep-seated right sub-costal tender mass to feel it may be a diffuse mass, indicating hepatomegaly or more localised, indicating an enlarged gall bladder. In addition to blood tests to measure the

WBC count and CRP to assess the severity of the inflammatory response, blood should be sent to screen for deranged homeostasis and to assess liver function. Blood cultures or viral hepatitis antibody tests may be indicated. Imaging with an USS or CT scan may be indicated to formulate a diagnosis.

Viral and bacterial infections usually present with symptoms and signs of acute inflammation but some infections, such as endocarditis, osteomyelitis, an abscess, HIV, TB, Brucellosis, Coxiella burnetti (Q fever), Rickettsia, fungal, helminthic or parasitic infections are atypical and may present with chronic or relapsing symptoms. Information about the person and the person as a patient may indicate the patient is at increased risk of an atypical infection.

Some atypical infections present with a characteristic pattern of symptoms. For example:

- A generalized itchy rash, diarrhoea and weight loss, drowsiness, impaired concentration, an impaired or fluctuating conscious state, confusion, a change in personality or behaviour, agitation or disturbed speech or hearing, and with tender cervical, axillary or groin swellings may be caused by HIV infection. Risk factors include drug taking and sharing needles or sexual behaviour. The signs to look for include a red/purple rash and swellings compatible with lymphadenopathy. Blood should be tested for HIV antibodies.
- TB can occur anywhere and mimic many different conditions. High-risk groups include previous travel to, or living in, an endemic area, ongoing HIV infection or an immuno-compromised patient. Investigations may include a CXR, CT scan or sending a specimen for microbiological analysis to formulate a diagnosis.
- A rash, abdominal discomfort, weight loss and diarrhoea may be caused by Actinomycosis infection. There has usually been a previous contaminated injury, or the patient is vulnerable to infection, such as following cancer chemotherapy or radiotherapy treatment. The signs to look for include red or purple patches of skin discolouration, sub-cutaneous skin swelling with sinuses. Investigations may include a CT scan or a biopsy for microbiological assessment to confirm the diagnosis.
- Chronic localized abdominal inflammatory pain and an intermittent fever and rigors may be caused by an abscess or a walled off perforation. When the patient has had a recent abdominal operation, this may be a complication. Antimicrobial medication should be started, blood tests sent to help assess the severity of the inflammation and to screen for deranged homeostasis, and a CT scan ordered to formulate a diagnosis.
- Chronic joint, abdominal and eye pain, bloody diarrhoea, feeling ill, fatigue, significant weight loss and impaired vision may be caused by Trophymera whipplei infection (Whipple's disease) when the patient has lived in an endemic area or is immunocompromised. An OGD and duodenal biopsy for microbiology, culture and serology may be indicated to confirm the diagnosis.

Symptoms of inflammation are not always caused by an infection. Non-infective inflammation may be caused by degeneration, a hypersensitivity reaction, an autoimmune disease, injury, including "chemical" injury, ischaemia, previous radiation exposure or cancer. In general, a sudden onset of pain or symptoms of deranged function or chronic symptoms, with intermittent relapse and remission, affecting the sub-cutaneous soft tissues, bones or joints and be multi-focal, without a fever are more likely to be caused by non-infective inflammation than infection. Information about the person and the patient may indicate a likely cause or exclude some causes, such as whether injury or radiotherapy induced inflammation are likely.

The prevalence of degenerative inflammation increases as we get older. It should be considered when a patient presents with chronic, progressive, persistent or relapsing pain and/or symptoms of deranged function over many months or years that are aggravated by active use and helped but not completely relieved by rest. Patients do not usually get a fever or feel unwell. Symptoms tend to affect the joints, the colon or the lungs. There may be a characteristic pattern of symptoms. For example:

- A progressively reduced range of movement in a joint over many months or years, or impaired ability to use a joint, such as when walking or climbing stairs, associated with joint discomfort and swelling indicate degenerative inflammation. Pain is aggravated by use, such as at the end of the day, and is reduced when rested. There is never a fever. On examination the joint is swollen and tender with a reduced range of movement. When joint degeneration is chronic there are structural changes, such as Heberden's nodes, loss of leg length or genu valgus/varus and there may be crepitus on moving the joint. The WBC count and CRP should be measured to exclude a systemic inflammatory response. Investigations with an X-ray may be indicated to confirm the diagnosis and assess severity and initial treatment is aimed at alleviating symptoms.
- Recurrent episodes of a variable bowel habit associated with lower abdominal discomfort and fullness, particularly before defaecation over many months or years may be caused by diverticula disease. On

examination, the left lower quadrant of the abdomen may be mildly tender and a thickening or fullness palpable. A CT scan or a barium enema may be indicated to confirm the diagnosis. Initial treatment is aimed at alleviating symptoms.

- Increasing breathlessness and a productive cough over many months or years may be caused by COPD or emphysema. On examination, the chest may be barrel shaped and there may be clubbing and cyanosis. There are coarse crepitations on auscultation. A CXR may be indicated to exclude other conditions and pulmonary function tests to confirm the diagnosis.

When the inflammation is *unlikely* to be caused by an infection or degeneration it may be caused by a hypersensitivity reaction or auto-immune inflammation.

An acute generalised pruritic erythematous rash, associated with breathlessness and a wheeze is characteristic of a hypersensitivity reaction. Seasonal symptoms are likely to be caused by a pollen allergen, whereas intermittent symptoms may be caused by exposure to an environmental allergen, such as dust or insect bites, or dietary, such as a nut allergy. Patients usually know what has precipitated the reaction, but sometimes patch testing is indicated. Avoiding the allergen, antihistamines and a salbutamol or steroid inhaler may be indicated.

A delayed-type hypersensitivity reaction may occur several hours or even days after exposure. There may be a characteristic pattern of symptoms. For example:

- Abdominal colic, bloating, sickness or a change in bowel habit and weight loss, may be caused by a dietary allergen, such as gluten.
- Widespread blistering pustules in the skin and mucosae or liver damage may be caused by toxic epidermal necrolysis (Stevens-Johnson syndrome) following paracetamol ingestion.

Stopping or avoiding the allergen is indicated.

Chronic recurrent or relapsing pain, symptoms of deranged function, feeling unwell, tired and listless may be caused by auto-immune inflammation, a type of hypersensitivity reaction. Symptoms are often widespread or multi-focal affecting the skin, soft tissues or joints. A fever is usually absent. There may be a characteristic pattern of symptoms. For example:

- A multi-focal ache affecting joints and muscles, aggravated by using the affected parts and associated with feeling ill and tenderness, for many weeks, with periods when it is more severe, is characteristic of auto-immune inflammation. A fever is unusual. On examination, the skin should be inspected for skin lesions, such as purpura, and the painful sites examined for signs of swelling, reduced power and range of movement. They may be warm and tender to touch. The distribution of the inflammation and the signs may be diagnostic. The pattern of symptoms indicates the signs to seek on examination and informs management. For example:

  o A violet or dusky red rash is characteristic of dermatomyositis.
  o Tender red nodules are characteristic of erythema nodosum.
  o Weakness and myalgia or joint stiffness, swelling and arthralgia in polymyalgia.

  The WBC count and CRP should be measured to confirm an inflammatory response and blood should be tested for a range of auto-antibodies to formulate a diagnosis.

- A gradual onset of mild to moderate sharp lower left chest pain radiating to the back and shoulders associated with breathlessness may be caused by pericarditis. Patients may feel ill with a mild fever. Most patients are likely to have had a recent viral infection or have an associated condition, such as rheumatoid arthritis. On examination, auscultation of the left side of the chest, particularly on leaning forward, may reveal a rubbing or squeaking sound in time with each heartbeat, particularly on leaning forward, characteristic of a pericardial friction rub. The WBC count and CRP should be measured to confirm inflammation, viral antibodies measured and an ECG and an ECHO cardiogram indicated to confirm the diagnosis, exclude an effusion and assess heart function.
- Increasing breathlessness, progressing over many months and associated with a dry cough and fatigue, myalgia and arthralgia is characteristic of pulmonary fibrosis: a chronic non-infective pulmonary inflammatory type of problem. The signs to look for include widespread crepitations, clubbing, and multifocal tender muscles. Sputum should be sent for microscopy, culture and serology to exclude an infection and a CT scan and pulmonary function tests may be indicated to confirm the diagnosis and to assess severity.

- Persistent or recurrent episodes of diarrhoea for several weeks associated with blood and mucous is likely to be caused by auto-immune inflammation, such as a dietary allergen, UC or Crohn's disease. The abdomen may be mildly generally tender. Stool should be sent for microscopy, culture and serology to exclude an infection, a WBC count and CRP should be measured and a faecal calprotectin and a colonoscopy may be indicated to confirm the diagnosis and to assess severity.
- Increasing jaundice and feeling ill, with upper abdominal discomfort a skin rash and joint pains may be caused by auto-immune hepatitis. On examination a tender right, sub-costal mass, consistent with hepatomegaly may be palpable. There may be a rash and ascites. Blood tests are indicated to confirm the diagnosis, exclude anaemia or other causes of hepatocellular damage and to assess the severity of liver inflammation and damage and a liver USS to exclude biliary tract obstruction, a common cause of jaundice.
- Recurrent episodes of urinary frequency, urgency and dysuria over many months without a fever and associated with pelvic pain and dyspareunia indicate interstitial cystitis. On examination, there may be suprapubic tenderness. Urine should be sent for microscopy, culture and serology to exclude a UTI. A cystoscopy may be indicated to confirm the diagnosis.

Occasionally, inflammation is caused by caustic liquid in the wrong place ("chemical" inflammation). It may affect the skin, the lungs, the oesophagus, the mediastinum, the peritoneal cavity or the retro-peritoneum. Most patients present with a sudden onset of severe pain. The pain is initially constant but usually reduces after a few hours. It is worse when moving or using the affected part and relieved by rest. Loss of function of the affected part of the body quickly follows. A fever is absent unless infection supervenes. There may be a characteristic pattern of symptoms.

- A retrosternal burning pain, "heartburn", is characteristic of reflux oesophagitis. Reflux may be precipitated by swallowing certain foods, when stressed or lying flat and may be associated with waterbrash, halitosis, a wheeze, cough or recurrent chest infection due to aspiration. A fever is absent.
- Episodes of severe retrosternal chest pain may be caused by oesophageal spasm, a type of colic (a "nutcracker" or a "corkscrew" oesophagus) often precipitated by gastro-oesophageal reflux. Unlike ACS, oesophageal spasm is short lasting and is not brought on by exercise or associated with breathlessness. Oesophageal spasm occurs when there is a strong and non-propulsive smooth muscle contraction in the oesophagus. It is one of several oesophageal motility disorders, including achalasia and diffuse oesophageal spasm.
  There are no relevant signs on examination. When the symptoms are characteristic of reflux oesophagitis, patients can be reassured and treatment started to alleviate symptoms and reduce the risk of future complications. An OGD and 24-hour oesophageal pH and manometry may be indicated.
- A sudden onset of severe retrosternal chest pain, brought on by severe retching or vomiting, aggravated by movement, including breathing or coughing, that improves over a few hours to become a mild or moderate pain could be caused by "chemical" inflammation from a ruptured oesophagus (Boerhaave's syndrome). The signs to look for include crepitus, reduced air entry and dullness to percussion of the lung bases. Signs of a fever are likely. The WBC and CRP should be measured to diagnose and assess the severity of the inflammation and an emergency CT scan is usually indicated to confirm the diagnosis.
- A sudden onset of severe abdominal inflammatory pain that then improves over a few hours to become a mild or moderate pain could be caused by "chemical" inflammation. There is usually an associated ileus, causing anorexia, abdominal distension, nausea and constipation. There may be a fever. The location at the start indicates the likely cause. For example:
  o If the peritonitis follows a period of constant upper abdominal pain or "indigestion" it may have been caused by a perforated peptic ulcer.
  o If previously the patient had episodes of upper abdominal colic, gallstone pancreatitis is likely.
  o Back pain indicates a retroperitoneal "chemical" inflammation, such as from pancreatitis or a posterior duodenal ulcer.
  On palpation, the abdomen is initially very tender, with guarding. The area of maximal tenderness may indicate the likely location of the abnormality. Blood tests to diagnose and assess the severity of anaemia and inflammation and to measure serum amylase are indicated. An USS and CT scan are usually indicated to confirm the diagnosis.

In some patients, the clinical features indicate an inflammatory type of problem but the problem is caused by another type of problem. For example:

- Cancer may cause inflammation, such as when it is ischaemic.
- Ischaemia may cause inflammation, such as when infection supervenes.
- A structural problem may perforate causing inflammation.

When the type of problem is uncertain:

Ask yourself, is a circulatory type of problem likely and how should it be managed?

A circulatory problem is more likely in older patients and those with risk factors, such as smoking, DM, obesity, abnormal blood lipids or a family history of cardiovascular disease who present with recurrent or chronic mild pain or a sudden onset of severe persistent pain, or with symptoms of deranged function, such as weakness or breathlessness. The symptoms are aggravated by active movement or use of the affected part of the body and relieved by rest because increased metabolic activity increases the demands on the local circulation. For example, when limb circulation is compromised and blood flow cannot increase to meet increased demand, calf pain is increased, whereas passive movement is pain free. Feeling ill may be caused by a systemic circulatory problem, such as anaemia or heart failure. As with other circulatory problems, the symptoms are aggravated by activity and relieved by rest and the pattern of associated symptoms is characteristic. Occasionally, a visible or palpable abnormality is caused by a circulatory problem. For example, petechial haemorrhages in thrombocytopaenia, a "strawberry" naevus or a glomus tumour. The signs are usually pathognomonic.

When determining whether or not a pain is a circulatory problem, it should be remembered that ischaemia only causes pain when the sensory nerves are functioning. This may occur during the process of tissue death, when the tissue is re-perfused or at the margin between dead and living tissue. When the nerves are dead, pain is no longer felt. For example, a "mummified" finger or dead bowel are painless. Therefore, if the pain is severe the tissues are still ischaemic but not dead. A reduction in pain intensity may be caused by reperfusion and healing or progression to gangrene giving a false sense of reassurance. When a dead viscus perforates and infection supervenes, or at the margins of ischaemic tissues, a systemic inflammatory response develops and there is pain typical of inflammation.

A characteristic pattern of symptoms may indicate a circulatory type of problem. For example:

- A sudden onset of an atypical headache, with or without a blackout or unilateral weakness, may be caused by a sub-arachnoid haemorrhage or a stroke. There may be associated neurological symptoms, such as amaurosis fugax, lateral visual field deficiency (hemianopia), slurred speech, and unilateral facial, arm and leg weakness (hemiparesis). When they occur, the neurological symptoms are usually the dominant presenting symptoms but, in some patients, the neurological symptoms partially or completely resolve. When a circulatory type of problem is suspected, signs of a circulatory problem should be sought, such as a weak pulse, an arrythmia, a bruit or a heart murmur in addition to an examination of the neurological system to look for signs of paraesthesia, weakness or abnormal reflexes. Any patient suspected of having a "vascular headache" should have a CT head to confirm the diagnosis, determine the cause and assess severity.

- A progressive change in personality, loss of short-term memory and the ability to concentrate over many months may be caused by multi-infarct dementia. There may be previous or ongoing circulatory problems elsewhere, an arrythmia, a weak or absent carotid pulse, a bruit or a heart murmur. Blood tests to screen for a metabolic abnormality, and a CT scan may be indicated to confirm the diagnosis, exclude other diagnoses and distinguish it from other causes of dementia.

- Chronically feeling tired, run down, lethargic, globally weak and breathless on exertion may be caused by anaemia. If anaemia is suspected it is important to ask if there has been any blood loss. The signs to look for include, pallor, tachycardia, hypotension and tachypnoea. A FBC and ferritin may be indicated to confirm the diagnosis and assess severity.

- Feeling light headed or dizzy with a headache, particularly when lying or bending down, coughing or sneezing, stressed or anxious, may indicate severe hypertension. If it is associated with weight gain and swollen ankles and feet it is characteristic of fluid retention and proteinuria from renal failure. The blood pressure will be very high and there may be a renal artery bruit. Urgent antihypertensive treatment and an ECG is indicated.

- A sudden onset of a deep-seated central or left sided chest pain or an atypical left shoulder and upper arm pain is characteristic of ACS. The pain may be felt as a discomfort, heaviness, a crushing pain or a tight band across the chest. Recurrent pains, brought on by exercise or stress and relieved by resting are likely to be angina, whereas a persistent pain, not relieved by rest, may be an AMI. Associated breathlessness, palpitations or swollen ankles support a circulatory type of problem. On examination, signs are unlikely but there may be hypertension, an arrhythmia, a raised JVP, basal crepitations and pitting oedema. Any patient presenting with chest pain suspected of having ACS should have an urgent ECG performed and, if the pain has been felt within the last few hours, blood tests sent for serum troponin levels to confirm the diagnosis.

- A gradual increase in breathlessness on exertion or when lying flat (orthopnoea) is typically caused by heart failure. The patient may wake up at night feeling very breathless (paroxysmal nocturnal dyspnoea) and have to sit up to recover. Usually there is associated nocturia and weight gain due to water retention. On examination there may be dependent oedema, a raised JVP, an enlarged heart and bilateral basal crepitations or dullness to percussion. Diuretic treatment is indicated and an ECG and echocardiogram may be indicated to confirm the diagnosis and assess severity.

- A sudden onset of severe unremitting generalised abdominal visceral pain can be caused by ischaemic bowel. The pain remains severe from the onset. Ischaemia is not associated with a fever unless a complication develops. There may be bloodstained diarrhoea. On palpation of the abdomen there is mild tenderness and no guarding unless infection or perforation has supervened. It is important to distinguish ischaemia from infection or chemical inflammation. Classically, acute ischaemic pain is "out of proportion to the signs". Mesenteric ischaemia is an indication for a CT angiogram to confirm the diagnosis. Chronic or recurrent generalised mild or moderate abdominal inflammatory pains present for many weeks or months may be caused by chronic ischaemia. The pain may be present all the time, day and night or only when eating. Patients avoid eating so dramatic weight loss is a common feature. Diarrhoea is also a frequent symptom. On palpation of the abdomen there may be mild tenderness.

- A sudden onset of breathlessness associated with chest pain on deep inspiration is likely to be caused by a PE. There may be an associated DVT. Signs of a fever or chest signs, with the exception of tachypnoea, are unlikely. There may be a pleural rub. A PE is should be managed as a medical emergency and, while awaiting the results of investigations, such as a CT scan to confirm the diagnosis, anticoagulation should be started.

- A sudden onset of constant aching pain and tenderness in the calf made worse on passive dorsi-flexing of the foot is likely to be caused by a DVT. The patient minimizes weight bearing on the affected side. When a DVT is suspected, the signs to look for are a swollen lower limb, muscle tenderness and increased calf pain on dorsiflexing the foot. When a DVT is suspected blood should be tested for the presence of D-dimer and a Doppler USS performed to confirm the diagnosis. It is likely anticoagulation will be indicated.

  A constant chronic severe "bursting" limb pain, aggravated by and limiting walking and associated with the limb becoming swollen and appearing blue is typical of extensive deep venous thrombosis; "phlegmasia caerulea dolens". The limb is swollen and cyanosed. Peripheral veins may be prominent. There may be tenderness on deep palpation. A Doppler USS or venogram may be indicated to confirm the diagnosis.

- Progressive unilateral calf and lower limb weakness and fatigue, associated with an ache or deep-seated discomfort, brought on by walking is characteristic of claudication. Most patients will have noticed the distance they can walk has reduced over many months and if they walk faster or up a gradient the distance they can walk is reduced. Resting relieves the claudication after a few minutes. When the pain has deteriorated to become a severe constant limb pain that wakes the patient from sleep at night and is relieved by sitting upright ("rest pain") the limb is critically ischaemic.

  The limb looks pale and feels cold distally. When the symptoms are longstanding, paradoxically, parts of the more proximal limb, such as around the knee may feel warm because of superficial collaterals. The venous refill is very slow ("guttering") and capillary refill time slow. The distal arterial pulses are absent. Buerger's test is positive. An FBC is indicated to exclude anaemia, an ECG to screen for heart disease and a Doppler USS or angiogram is indicated to confirm the diagnosis and identify the location of the abnormality.

- A sudden onset of constant severe lower limb pain and paralysis is likely to be caused by an occluding femoral artery embolus or acute thrombosis. Associated symptoms include weakness or a limp and, in some patients, peripheral paraesthesia or numbness. An USS or angiogram may be indicated to confirm the diagnosis.

- An acute onset of progressively more severe pain in a group of limb muscles is characteristic of compartment syndrome. The pain is increased if the muscles in the part affected are actively used or passively stretched and the pain is least when rested and the adjacent joints are in a position to minimise muscle stretch. Compartment syndrome may follow trauma, such as a long bone fracture or a crush injury, or reperfusion following arterial occlusion.

  When compartment syndrome is suspected, the overlying skin appears stretched and pale due to swelling, distal pulses may be weak or absent, there is muscle tenderness and increased pain on stretching the muscle. There may be numbness (paraesthesia) distally. Blood tests, including creatine kinase, ABGs and urine testing

310

for myoglobin are indicated to assess severity and to screen for deranged homeostasis and the compartment pressures should be measured urgently.

Table showing the clinical features that distinguish abdominal ischaemia from infection or chemical inflammation.

Type of inflammation	Infection	Ischaemia	"chemical"
Age	Any	Elderly	Any
Risk factors	Immuno-compromised	Lifestyle, Cardiovascular disease	Lifestyle, medications
Onset and duration	Gradual over several days	Usually sudden, may be chronic	Usually sudden
Severity	Starts mild but increases over a few days	Starts severe and stays severe. "Pain out of proportion to signs"	Starts severe but improves slowly
Location	Starts localized, may become generalised	Usually localized but may appear generalised	Starts localized to quickly become generalised peritonitis
Character	Initially, aching but may become sharp	Aching	Burning, sharp
Aggravating factors	Movement	Use of the affected organ	Movement
Relieving factors	Rest	Rest	Rest
Fever	Fever	No	No
Tenderness	Severe with guarding	Minimal	Initially severe with guarding, but later minimal

Determining the problem is a circulatory problem together with the location of the abnormality will indicate a descriptive diagnosis. For example:

- Meno-rrhagia.
- Haemat-emesis.
- Ischaemic heart disease.
- Renal infarction.
- Brachial embolus.
- A popliteal aneurysm.
- A DVT.
- An-aemia.

Determining the problem is a circulatory type of problem is not a diagnosis. It is then necessary to determine the likely cause. Information about previous or ongoing medical conditions may suggest a likely cause. For example:

- A previous heart attack may suggest widespread or multi-focal peripheral vascular disease.
- A previous stroke or TIA may indicate a cardiac source for emboli.
- A known circulatory problem, such as anaemia or angina may have recurred.
- Risk factors, such as family medical history of significant cardio-vascular disease, smoking or hyperlipidaemia may increase the likelihood of peripheral vascular disease.

If the pattern of symptoms is not diagnostic, a checklist of abnormalities associated with the location of the abnormality may indicate a list of possible diagnoses, which can be used to inform additional questions to ask or the signs to look for (Appendix 1).

When the underlying cause is identified it becomes a definitive diagnosis. For example:

- IHD caused by coronary artery atherosclerosis.
- Renal infarction caused by an embolus from renal artery atherosclerosis.
- A brachial embolus caused by an embolus from left atrial thrombus in a patient with AF caused by IHD.
- A popliteal aneurysm caused by atherosclerosis.
- A DVT caused by venous stasis during a long journey.

Usually management includes investigations, such as blood tests, an ECG, a Doppler USS, an echo cardiogram, a CT scan or angiogram to confirm or exclude a likely diagnosis.

When the type of problem is uncertain:

Ask yourself, is a structural type of problem likely and how should it be managed?

A structural problem should be considered in any patient who presents with a visible or palpable abnormality, an acute onset of colic, recurrent or chronic mild pain affecting a part of the body, and symptoms of deranged function, such as a reduced range of movement, vomiting or breathlessness. Use of the affected part may aggravate the symptoms or be prevented. When a joint is affected, both active and passive movement is painful. A fever is absent. Structural problems do not usually cause a patient to present feeling ill unless a complication or secondary problem arises. A structural problem should be considered in older patients or in patients with risk factors, such as previous injury or occupation.

A characteristic pattern of symptoms may indicate a structural type of problem and a likely cause. For example:

- Acute onset of abdominal colic is likely to be caused by a structural problem. The location of the colic and the associated symptoms will indicate the likely diagnosis. For example:
  o Mid-gut colic associated with anorexia, nausea, vomiting, bloating and constipation are characteristic of small bowel obstruction caused by adhesions, a hernia or cancer. The signs to look for include a distended tympanic abdomen with active bowel sounds. A visible or palpable tender irreducible hernia, a surgical scar or an intra-abdominal mass indicate a likely cause.
  o Lower abdominal colic and absolute constipation is characteristic of large bowel obstruction, usually caused by a diverticular stricture or cancer. The signs to look for include a distended tympanic abdomen and a rectal or left lower quadrant mass to feel.

  Blood tests are indicated to screen for abnormal homeostasis, anaemia and inflammation and a CT scan may be indicated to confirm or exclude a likely diagnosis and inform management.
- A persistent mild to moderately severe atypical headache, present day and night, that has been present for more than a few weeks may be caused by a structural type of problem. The associated symptoms, aggravating and relieving factors will indicate the likely diagnosis. For example:
  o When the headache is accompanied by a slowly progressive change in behaviour and a deterioration in short-term memory it may be caused by dementia.
  o When the headache wakes the patient from sleep or occurs in the morning and is worse when coughing, sneezing or bending down, it indicates a raised ICP which may be caused by an intracranial structural abnormality. The patient may feel ill, with lethargy, fatigue, drowsiness and a change in personality or behaviour, visual disturbance and pulsatile tinnitus. If a raised ICP is suspected, the patient's optic discs should be examined for papilloedema. If there is hypertension, a widened pulse pressure and bradycardia ("Cushing's triad"), an irregular breathing pattern or periods of rapid breathing followed by absent breathing for a time (Blot's respiration) the patient may have severe ICP and should be managed as a medical emergency.
  o When the headache is accompanied by seizures, characterised by vigorous tonic-clonic movements at one extreme ("grand mal") or a momentary loss of awareness ("petit mal") at the other, or focal neurological symptoms, such as weakness or paraesthesia, it may be caused by an intracranial structural abnormality.

The neurological system should be examined for focal neurological signs, such as weakness, paraesthesia, hyper-reflexia and a positive Babinski reflex. Blood tests are indicated to exclude a metabolic abnormality and a CT scan may be indicated to formulate a diagnosis and inform management.

Determining the problem is a structural problem together with the location of the abnormality will indicate a descriptive diagnosis. For example, obstructive jaundice, small bowel obstruction, a goitre, COPD, acute retention of urine, or ureteric colic. However, a structural problem becomes a definitive diagnosis only when the underlying cause is identified. For example:

- Choledocho-lithiasis causing obstructive jaundice.
- Adhesional small bowel obstruction.
- COPD caused by chronic smoking.
- Acute retention of urine caused by benign prostatic hypertrophy.
- Ureteric colic caused by an oxalate calculus.

Information about the person and the patient may indicate a likely diagnosis. For example:

- When the patient presents with colic:
  o A previous laparotomy indicates adhesions are likely to be the cause.
  o Previous episodes of diverticulitis indicate large bowel colic may be a relapse.
  o When previous investigations have shown renal or gall stones.
- When the patient presents with a headache:
  o The risk of dementia increases with age and in some families. Other risk factors include occupations or hobbies, such as playing football or being a boxer, and atherosclerosis or micro-emboli.
  o When the patient is prone to falls, a head injury may be the cause of a sub-dural haematoma.
  o Brain metastases are possible if there has been previous treatment for cancer.
  o A brain abscess is possible if the patient is being treated for a chronic infection, such as infective endocarditis.

If the pattern of symptoms is not diagnostic, the onset, associated symptoms and location of the problem may indicate a likely diagnosis based on probabilities. For example:

- Jaundice associated with itching, dark urine, pale stools and urticaria indicates bile duct obstruction. The absence of pain increases the likelihood it is caused by cancer.
  On examination the liver is likely to be mildly tender and may be enlarged. Blood tests to assess liver function and a hepato-biliary USS are indicated to confirm the diagnosis.
- When a patient presents with symptoms of small bowel obstruction:
  o An acute onset is usually caused by a hernia, adhesions or a volvulus.
  o Symptoms that develop over many days or weeks or are recurrent are more likely to be caused by adhesions, a Crohn's stricture or cancer.
  On examination the abdomen is likely to be distended and tympanic. Bowel sounds may be active. Blood tests to screen for deranged homeostasis, anaemia and inflammation and a CT scan or an MRI may be indicated to confirm or exclude a likely diagnosis.
- When a patient presents with symptoms of oesophageal obstruction.
  o A sudden onset while eating, associated with inability to swallow saliva, is likely to be caused by an obstructing foreign body.
  o Symptoms that develop and progress over several weeks indicate a malignant stricture.
  o Symptoms that develop over many months or years are likely to be from a benign stricture or pharyngeal pouch.
  Signs are unlikely unless cancer is suspected when there may be an abdominal mass or signs of metastatic spread, such as a Virchow's node. An OGD or barium swallow may be indicated to make the diagnosis and inform management.
- Feeling full after eating, associated with vomiting undigested food, anorexia, nausea and weight loss, indicates gastric outlet obstruction.

- o Previous abdominal or back pain over many months and a succession splash indicates gastric outlet obstruction caused by a peptic ulcer or stricture.
  - o Progression over several weeks with profound weight loss indicates gastric cancer.
    The examination is unlikely to reveal any signs unless cancer is suspected when there may be an abdominal mass or signs of metastatic spread. Blood tests to screen for deranged homeostasis and anaemia and an urgent OGD or CT scan may be indicated to confirm or exclude a likely diagnosis.
- Breathlessness associated with a wheeze or stridor indicates turbulent air flow caused by airway obstruction.
  - o An acute onset is likely to be caused by exposure to an allergen.
  - o Recurrent episodes are likely to be caused by asthma.
  - o Persistent and progressive symptoms over a few weeks may be caused by cancer.
  - o Chronic symptoms may be caused by bronchitis.
    A wheeze is likely to be audible and the lung fields should be examined for consolidation. A CXR or a CT scan may be indicated.
- A poor urinary stream or passing small volumes of urine associated with hesitancy and terminal dribbling, in the absence of dysuria, indicate bladder outflow obstruction.
  A dull suprapubic mass, likely to be a palpable bladder, supports the diagnosis of chronic urinary retention and an enlarged prostate may be palpable on rectal examination. Blood tests to assess renal function and to measure the PSA to screen for prostate cancer and the FBC for anaemia, an USS to assess the urinary tract and urodynamic studies to assess the severity of the obstruction may be indicated.

In some patients, the clinical features indicate a structural type of problem but the problem is caused by another type of problem. For example:

- Cancer will frequently cause obstruction.
- Intestinal ischaemia may cause bowel obstruction.
- A neurological problem may obstruct function. For example, achalasia or a localized ileus.
- Inflammation may obstruct function. For example, a duodenal ileus in acute pancreatitis.

When the type of problem is uncertain:

Ask yourself, is cancer likely and how should it be managed?

Cancer is highlighted as a separate type of problem because it may have recognizable clinical features and is a high priority diagnosis that should be deliberately considered. Information about the person and the patient may indicate cancer is more likely. For example:

- The elderly.
- When a patient has previously been treated for cancer or are receiving treatment for cancer.
- Patients who smoke are at increased risk of many cancers.
- Patients with a genetic risk, such as FAP, HNPCC, or BRAC.
- Patients with chronic inflammatory conditions, such as chronic ulcers, Barrett's oesophagus, chronic atrophic gastritis, chronic pancreatitis, calcified cholecystitis or chronic inflammatory bowel disease are at increased risk of cancer.
- Repeated or chronic sun exposure increases the risk of developing skin cancer.

In general, cancer should be considered in all patients with constant and deteriorating symptoms over several weeks or months or when there is a characteristic pattern of symptoms: "red flag" symptoms, including:

- When a patient presents with a palpable mass.
- Unexplained weight loss of >5% over <6 months.
- Haemoptysis in a patient >40 years of age.
- An unexplained change in bowel habit in a patient >60 years of age.
- Rectal bleeding and a change in bowel habit in a patient >50 years of age.
- Painless visible haematuria in a >45-year-old.

Cancer may present as another type of problem. For example:

- Feeling increasingly or persistently non-specifically unwell, tired, lethargic, breathless and pale over many weeks may be caused by iron deficiency anaemia. The positive predictive value of anaemia for oesophageal, gastric, renal and bladder cancer is about 1% and for colo-rectal cancer about 6%.
- A constant and unremitting deep seated pain present day and night for several weeks or more may be bone pain caused by a metastasis from breast, bronchus, prostate, kidney or thyroid cancer or by a primary malignant tumour, such as an osteosarcoma.
- A persistent mild to moderately severe atypical headache, present day and night, that has been present for more than a few weeks, could be caused by intra-cranial cancer causing increased intracranial pressure due to either growth in a confined space or by obstructing the CSF circulation.
- Dysphagia, abdominal colic or a change in the bowel habit may be caused by bowel cancer.
- Painless jaundice associated with itching, dark urine, pale stools, urticaria, and weight loss, may be caused by pancreatic or biliary cancer
- An inflammatory problem, such as dermatomyositis or pyoderma gangrenosa may be caused by cancer.
- A metabolic problem may be caused by cancer. For example:
  o Cancer may affect body metabolism directly by autonomously releasing hormones (paraneoplastic syndromes), such as Cushing's syndrome, insulinoma, gastro-intestinal stromal tumours (carcinoid) or prolactinoma.
  o Cancer may affect body metabolism indirectly by causing hormone resistance or through effects on endocrine regulatory mechanisms.
  o A complication of cancer may include chronic renal failure or jaundice.
- An embolus causing peripheral ischaemia may be a tumour embolus.
- Cancer may cause neurological syndromes, such as Eaton-Lambert myasthenic syndrome or encephalomyelitis.

When there are symptoms of cancer the descriptive diagnosis usually includes the location of the cancer. For example:

- Carcinomatosis peritonei.
- Cervical carcinoma in-situ.
- Lung cancer.
- Breast cancer.
- Malignant pleural effusion.

However, cancer is a definitive diagnosis only when the location of the primary and the cell type or genetic mutations are identified. When the location of the primary is uncertain consider lung, breast (in females), prostate (males), bowel, kidney, oesophagus, pancreas or stomach.

If cancer is suspected the signs to look for on examination include, weight loss and in particular a loss of muscle mass (sarcopaenia), a palpable mass including lymphadenopathy, pulmonary consolidation or a pleural effusion, jaundice, hepatomegaly or ascites. Investigations, such as blood tests, a CT scan or endoscopy are indicated to confirm or exclude a likely primary and inform management.

When the type of problem is uncertain:

Ask yourself, is a neurological type of problem likely and how should it be managed?

The neurological system regulates the activities of many different parts of the body and may be the cause of feeling ill, an atypical pain, symptoms of deranged function or occasionally a visible or palpable abnormality. In general, a neurological type of problem should be considered when the patient presents with recurrent, persistent or atypical pains, such as headaches or paraesthesia, deranged function, such as an unexplained change in behaviour or affect, problems with the special senses of hearing, eyesight, taste, smell, balance, touch, coordination or balance, abnormal peripheral pains or sensation, weakness, uncontrolled movements, a seizure or a tremor. There may be a characteristic pattern of symptoms. For example:

- More than 90% of headaches are caused by a neurological type of problem. When a patient presents with an atypical headache:
  - o Recurrent severe, frequently disabling, pulsating headaches that develop over minutes are characteristic of a migraine. They can be brought on by triggers, such as cheese or red wine.
  - o A severe atypical headache associated with nausea, photophobia or phonophobia is likely to be migraine. Patients often need to lie down in a dark quiet room until the headache passes.
  - o Recurrent severe headaches that develop over minutes in the region of one eye and are associated with lacrimation and nasal congestion, are characteristic of cluster headaches. Patients often need to lie down in a dark quiet room until the headache passes.
  - o A headache that is associated with a change in mood, behaviour or personality may be caused by a mental health problem, such as depression, personality or bipolar disorders or schizophrenia.

  There are unlikely to be any signs on examination but the neurological system should be examined to exclude signs. Blood tests may be indicated to exclude metabolic or inflammatory problems and a CT scan to exclude a structural or circulatory cause or cancer.

- When a patient presents with persistent or recurrent abnormal behaviour, such as poor concentration, impaired memory, depression or confusion, odd or irrational thoughts or hallucinations a neurological problem should be considered. For example:
  - o Persistent sadness, low mood, apathy and loss of interest, poor concentration, low self-esteem, feeling worthless, hopeless and suicidal, disturbed sleep and lethargy indicate depression is likely.
  - o Hallucinations, odd or irrational thoughts (delusions) suggesting schizophrenia.
  - o Phobia's, anxiety, paranoia, panic attacks, obsessive-compulsive, body dysmorphic disorder or eating problems may indicate a personality disorder.

  There are unlikely to be any signs on examination. Investigations, such as blood tests to exclude a metabolic problem and a CT scan to exclude a structural problem may be indicated.

- When a superficial "pain" feels atypical and is very different from that normally felt in the affected area a neurological problem should be considered. For example, paraesthesia, dysesthesia, hyperaesthesia or allodynia. Typically, the sensory abnormality is precisely localized to one spot or is felt in the distribution of a cranial nerve, a named cutaneous nerve, or a dermatome. It may be aggravated by movements or postures that stretch or pinch the nerve along its course. There may be an associated weakness if a mixed motor and sensory nerve is affected.

- When a patient presents with weakness a neurological problem should be considered. There may be an associated sensory abnormality, such as paraesthesia.
  - o Localized weakness affecting a muscle or muscle group innervated by a named nerve or nerve root, with or without associated sensory abnormality indicates a neurological problem affecting a peripheral nerve.
  - o Regional weakness. For example, paraplegia, indicates a spinal neurological problem or unilateral weakness a motor cortex problem.
  - o The differential diagnosis of a global weakness includes ME, Guillain-Barré syndrome, motor neurone disease or multiple sclerosis. A global weakness that gets worse with repetitive use, is characteristic of myasthenia gravis.

  The examination should confirm the weakness, assess the severity and the distribution of the weakness. Sensation, the reflexes and the cranial nerves should all be assessed. A CT or MRI scan may be indicated to formulate a diagnosis or exclude diagnoses, such as structural or circulatory abnormality.

- When a patient presents with a tremor, associated with reduced taste or smell, a flat facial expression, slow movements, poor balance and clumsiness Parkinson's disease is likely. On examination, the appearance of a "pill-rolling" tremor and unsteady coordination may distinguish Parkinson's disease from a cerebellar or "intention" tremor. Blood tests may be indicated to exclude a tremor caused by a metabolic problem, such as hyperthyroidism or hypercalcaemia.

- Intermittent dysphagia over many months or years, slowly becoming more persistent and severe may be caused by an oesophageal motility problem, such as achalasia or a pharyngeal pouch. Food takes longer and more effort to swallow. It may need to be "washed down" with liquids. The patient may not lose weight. The patient should be asked if they regurgitate undigested food or if anyone has commented on their bad breath. Episodes of severe retrosternal pain indicate oesophageal spasm. The examination is unlikely to reveal any signs. A barium swallow and/or an OGD is indicated to confirm the diagnosis.

- Recurrent attacks or chronic and persistent mild or moderately severe abdominal colic may indicate neurologic colic. There is likely to be symptoms of deranged function, such as bloating, anorexia, or a changeable bowel habit. The colic may be triggered by stress, the menstrual cycle, eating certain foods or follow recent abdominal or back trauma, including a recent operation. Frequently, it is a diagnosis of exclusion, but distinguishing a neurological abnormality from inflammation or a structural abnormality can be difficult. When the symptoms are classic for colic, it is rarely a neurological type of problem. The differential diagnosis of neurological abdominal colic includes:

  o Disordered peristalsis, from IBS or diverticular disease.
  o An autonomic abnormality, such as slow transit constipation, biliary dyskinesia or detruser sphincter dyskinesia.
  o Nearby intra-abdominal inflammation, such as small bowel colic from acute appendicitis or gastro-duodenal colic from acute pancreatitis.
  o A metabolic problem, such as renal failure or hypercalcaemia.
  o Recovery from an ileus, when the resumption of normal gut function and peristalsis is disordered, with different parts recovering at different times. For example, after an abdominal operation, following abdominal trauma, following a retroperitoneal bleed or inflammation, following resolution of a severe metabolic abnormality.
  Investigations, including blood test or a CT scan, may be indicated to exclude another diagnosis.

- Autonomic neurological problems (autonomic neuropathy) usually present with symptoms of deranged function. Autonomic neuropathy is usually only considered when the symptoms are atypical or non-specific, other types of problems have been excluded or in high-risk patients, such as patients with DM. Autonomic neurological problems are typically persistent and chronic. When advanced they have characteristic features. For example:
  o Recurrent episodes of dizziness and fainting when standing, exercising or entering a hot environment is characteristic of postural hypotension. It may cause collapse, a blackout or even a seizure.
  o In a diabetic taking insulin, the inability to recognize hypoglycaemia is characteristic of autonomic neuropathy.
  o Sweating too much or too little.
  o Feeling full while eating a meal and uncomfortable for a long time after eating, associated with anorexia, upper abdominal bloating and nausea may be caused by gastroparesis.
  o Longstanding and progressive constipation may be caused by slow transit constipation. Patients may not open their bowels for several weeks. It is usually associated with increasing abdominal discomfort, bloating, nausea and anorexia and occasional colic.
  o Difficulty driving at night or blurred vision when driving into tunnels or being dazzled when exposed to bright lights, is characteristic of a slow pupil reaction.
  o Lack of awareness of needing to pass urine, dribbling small volumes of urine or difficulty starting to urinate, incomplete emptying yet feeling full or repeated urinary tract infections are characteristic of chronic urinary retention from a neuropathic bladder.
  o Erectile dysfunction or failure to ejaculate in men or vaginal dryness and low libido in women are characteristic of autonomic neuropathy.
  Specialist investigations may be indicated.

In some patients, the clinical features indicate a neurological type of problem, but the problem is caused by another type of problem. For example:

- A primary brain abnormality may be caused by:
  o A structural problem, such as dementia, a benign tumour, hydrocephalus or an intra-cranial abscess.
  o A circulatory problem, such as an arterio-venous malformation, an aneurysm or a sub-dural or extra-dural haemorrhage.
  o Cancer.
  o Inflammation. For example, encephalitis or meningitis.
- A peripheral neurological abnormality may be caused by:
  o A structural problem: usually nerve entrapment. For example, sciatica from a prolapsed intervertebral disc, carpal tunnel syndrome, ileo-inguinal nerve entrapment following an open inguinal hernia repair or peroneal nerve compression from a plaster cast.
  o Cancer, usually malignant infiltration.
  o Inflammation. For example, Herpes zoster infection or neuritis.

When there are symptoms of a neurological problem the descriptive diagnosis may include the location of the abnormality or simply describe the problem. For example:

- Sciatica.
- Peripheral neuropathy.
- Depression.
- Schizophrenia.
- Mania.

Information about the person and the patient may indicate a likely diagnosis. For example:

- Previous operations, medical conditions, such as chickenpox or ongoing problems such as cancer, DM or an arrhythmia and medications, such as anti-coagulant medications may indicate a possible cause for abnormal peripheral sensation.
- Information about the patient may indicate a tremor is likely to be caused by alcohol, drugs or medications use or withdrawal.
- When a patient has autonomic neuropathy, it is usually a complication of comorbidity, such as a stroke, paraplegia, a head injury, ME, DM or chemotherapy.

A precipitating factor may indicate the likely cause of a neurological type of problem. For example:

- Recurrent acute mild to moderate headaches that are triggered by stress, grief, exercise, hormones or sex are likely to be "tension" headaches.
- Sciatica following twisting the back is likely to be caused by a structural problem.
- Wound paraesthesia following an operation is likely to be caused by damage to a nerve.
- Global weakness following a viral illness is likely to be caused by neuritis.

When the type of problem is uncertain:

Ask yourself, could it be caused by a metabolic problem and how should it be managed?

Metabolic problems disturb the body's homeostasis and affect cellular function, and nerve and muscle function in particular. A metabolic problem is usually only considered after excluding other types of problem or when the results of blood tests show an abnormality. A patient will usually present with symptoms of deranged function or feeling ill. Rarely do patient's present with a visible or palpable abnormality or pain.

In general, a metabolic problem should be considered when a patient presents with sub-acute or chronic non-specific symptoms such as a headache, confusion, forgetfulness or impaired concentration, lethargy, fatigue, depression or irritability, impaired memory, palpitations or loss of libido. Systemic symptoms of weakness, muscle spasms or cramps, or paraesthesia are likely to be multifocal or widespread. There may be uncontrolled movements, seizures, fasciculation or a tremor or symptoms of deranged gastro-intestinal function including, anorexia, nausea, vomiting and constipation and weight loss. There may be a characteristic pattern of symptoms. For example:

- Polyurea, polydipsia and weight loss indicating DM. When DM is suspected an urgent blood glucose level should be measured. The signs to look for include tachycardia, hypotension, peripherally cold and sweaty and loss of skin turgor, sweet smelling breath (due to ketones), breathlessness and evidence of weight loss. Laboured breathing ("Kussmaul" breathing) occurs in diabetic ketoacidosis.
- Feeling unwell, with constant atypical generalised abdominal and bone pain, associated with thirst, nausea, constipation, polyuria, palpitations and thin hair may indicate hypercalcaemia. The signs to look for include, thin hair, hypertension, an arrhythmia and a soft, non-tender abdomen. The causes of hypercalcaemia to consider include, hyper-parathyroidism, osteolytic bone metastases, multiple myeloma, paraneoplastic syndromes and chronic kidney failure.
- Feeling unwell and describing numbness or tingling in the fingers and toes (paraesthesia) or around the mouth, muscle cramps, a tremor or muscle twitching indicate hypocalcaemia. The signs to look for include, uncontrolled movements, such as a tremor and muscle fasciculation, paraesthesia, scratch marks, coarse hair, brittle nails and dry skin, Chvostek and Trousseau's signs.

If hypo- or hyper-calcaemia is suspected blood should be sent to the laboratory for calcium, electrolyte and acid-base measurement to confirm the diagnosis and assess severity.

- Agitation and irritability, poor concentration, hyper-activity, palpitations, weight loss, diarrhoea, twitching, a tremor and increased sweating, indicate thyrotoxicosis. The signs to look for include twitching, a tremor and increased sweating, a tachycardia, an arrythmia, hyper-reflexia, exophthalmos, lid lag and a goitre. The likely diagnosis includes Graves' disease or a toxic nodular goitre.
- Fatigue and weakness, depression, slow movements and thought processes, constipation, weight gain, dislike of the cold, hoarseness, dry skin and a puffy face are characteristic of hypothyroidism. The signs to look for include dry skin and a puffy face, loss of hair and thinned eyebrows, bradycardia, hypertension and a goitre. The likely diagnosis is Hashimoto's disease. Blood should be sent to the laboratory for measurement of serum TSH to confirm the diagnosis and assess severity.
- Severe fatigue and light headedness, nausea, vomiting and weight loss, myalgia and arthralgia, and dark skin (hyperpigmentation) is characteristic of Addison's disease. Apart from hyperpigmentation signs are unlikely. Blood should be sent to the laboratory for measurement of serum electrolytes, urea and creatinine, an FBC and serum cortisol and adrenocorticotrophic hormone to confirm the diagnosis.
- Persistent steatorrhea, characterised by pale, bulky and very smelly stools, that are difficult to flush down the toilet, for more than a few weeks is characteristic of pancreatic exocrine failure. The abdomen should be examined for tenderness but there may not be any signs to find. A faecal fat stool test or a prosperol test may confirm the diagnosis. A blood test should be performed to exclude DM because there may be an associated pancreatic endocrine failure. A CT scan of the pancreas may be indicated to formulate a diagnosis.
- Jaundice, dark urine and pale stools, a tendency to bruise easily and itching is characteristic of liver failure. The signs to look for include, yellow skin, sclera and palate, spider naevi, palmar erythema, malar flush, a liver flap, peripheral oedema, scratch marks, bruising, ascites, a tender liver, hepatomegaly, splenomegaly, and caput medusae. The differential diagnosis of jaundice includes, biliary obstruction, parenchymal liver disease, Gilbert's syndrome and drugs, such as chlorpromazine, carbamazepine, erythromycin, or rifampicin, haemolysis, ineffective erythropoiesis, blood transfusion or resorption of a haematoma. Blood should be sent to the laboratory for measurement of liver function tests, electrolytes, urea and creatinine and an FBC and a liver USS performed to confirm the diagnosis and assess severity.
- Change in urine output (too much or too little) and frothy urine, breathlessness, hiccups, peripheral oedema, constipation and pruritis, may indicate renal failure. The signs to look for include, pitting oedema in dependent areas, hypo- or hyper-tension and an arrhythmia. The differential diagnosis of renal failure includes:
  - o Urinary tract obstruction. For example, a TCC or BPH.
  - o Renal ischaemia. For example, emboli, renal artery stenosis or MSOF.
  - o Urinary tract infection. For example, pyelonephritis.
  - o Auto-immune inflammation. For example, glomerulonephritis.
  When renal failure is suspected blood should be sent to the laboratory for measurement of electrolytes, urea, creatinine and proteins and urine tested for proteinuria and osmolality to confirm the diagnosis.

Information about the person and the patient may indicate a likely diagnosis. For example:

- Previous thyroid surgery causing hypo-calcaemia from hypo-parathyroidism or hypothyroidism.
- Medications, such as anti-epileptic drugs, loop diuretics or bisphosphonates causing hypo-calcaemia. Medications, such as amiodarone, interferon or lithium causing thyrotoxicosis.
- An atypical diet.
- The environment, such as causing iodine deficiency.
- Malabsorption, from, for example Crohn's disease.
- Hypothyroidism may be caused by previous radiotherapy or some medications.

Frequently, metabolic problems are revealed by the results from relevant blood tests.

Use Available Information to Formulate a Diagnosis and to Inform Management and the Signs to Look For

In the absence of pathognomonic symptoms or a recognised diagnostic pattern a series of steps is followed to bridge the divide between the presenting problem and the diagnosis. For example:

Main presenting symptom:	Breathlessness
Information about the person	60-year-old retired male
Information about the patient:	Smokes 10 cigarettes per day and has done for 40 years Previously worked as a coal miner.
	Not immunocompromised. No Allergies
Associated symptoms:	An unproductive cough, and a wheeze. No haemoptysis or weight loss.
Onset and duration:	Increasing over several days.
Severity:	Resting at home, on sick leave from work. Increasing cough
Character, aggravating and relieving factors	Tachypnoea, increased on exercise, even walking up a flight of stairs. Prefers to rest.
Ask yourself, what is the likely location of the abnormality?	A primary problem affecting the lungs.
Ask yourself, what is the likely type of problem?	Infective inflammation
Ask yourself, what is the likely cause?	Streptococcal pneumonia on a background of COPD or pneumoconiosis
Diagnoses to exclude:	COPD, Cancer
Provisional management plan:	A CXR, sputum sent for MC&S and treatment with a penicillin. Pulmonary function tests when infection resolved
Signs to look for:	Tachypnoea, signs of consolidation or a pleural effusion, a wheeze. Signs of a fever. Signs of weight loss or lymphadenopathy.

Main presenting symptom:	Abdominal pain
Associated symptoms:	A fever. Anorexia, nausea and constipation
Onset and duration:	Suddenly, a few hours ago
Severity:	Severe
Character:	Constant pain aggravated by movement
Ask yourself, what is the likely location of the abnormality?	Uncertain: widespread inflammation throughout the peritoneal cavity
Ask yourself, what is the likely type of problem?	Infective or non-infective inflammation
Learn about the person:	50-year-old manual worker
Learn about the patient:	Takes regular NSAIDs for back pain
Ask yourself, what is the likely cause?	Chemical inflammation from a duodenal perforation
Diagnoses to exclude:	Acute pancreatitis, other causes of peritonitis
Provisional management plan:	Admit to hospital, blood tests, intravenous fluids, oxygen, broad spectrum antibiotics, CT abdomen
Signs to look for:	Widespread abdominal tenderness and guarding. Absent bowel sounds. A fever, tachycardia and hypotension.

Chapter 9
Learn and Understand Information
from the Examination

Abstract

The examination is an opportunity to gather additional information about the problem, the person and/or the patient. The headline information and the information learnt while talking to the patient determines whether an examination is indicated and informs the aims, focus and format of the examination. When a patient presents with a new problem, an examination is frequently indicated with the aims of formulating a diagnosis, understanding the problem, assessing severity and planning management. Occasionally, the aims of the examination include pro-actively screening for signs or to assess function. The same examination can meet different aims, different parts of the examination may be performed for the same aim and the aims can change during the examination.

When a patient presents with a new problem or to review an existing problem, the examination usually starts by examining the site of the problem, and, if different, the site of the abnormality. When a patient presents with a visible or palpable abnormality, the findings then inform the questions to ask. In all patients, the local signs indicate whether or not it is appropriate to examine for associated or systemic signs, what signs to look for, what additional questions to ask and inform management. In some patients, such as when the aim of the examination is to exclude a diagnosis or assess the severity of a problem, the focus may be on looking for associated or systemic signs. Occasionally, such as when the patient is unable to describe their problem or the diagnosis is unclear, a systematic examination is indicated in the hope of finding a sign.

Signs that are pro-actively sought are more likely to be identified and their absence is more likely to exclude them. When there is an abnormality on examination, look for pathognomonic signs or a diagnostic pattern. If the diagnosis is uncertain or the differential diagnosis long, use the examination to determine the location of the abnormality causing the problem, the type of problem and the likely cause. Additional questions may need to be asked.

Relevant and appropriate information about the person, the patient, the problem and the examination findings should be linked and together used to determine the working diagnosis and plan management. When the symptoms and signs are consistent, the likelihood of a diagnosis is increased.

In conclusion, when indicated, a well conducted examination is an important part of the consultation, contributing to meeting the aims.

Introduction

It's not what you look at that matters; it's what you see.

Henry Thoreau (1817-1862)

For many patients the examination is an important part of the consultation and for some, such as those with a visible or palpable abnormality, it is the key to formulating a diagnosis and planning management. The context of the consultation and information learnt from talking to the patient will determine the aims of the examination, whether or not it is indicated and the focus and format of the examination.

Throughout the examination, the HCP should use their medical knowledge and a clinical method to ensure all relevant information is learnt, understood and interpreted to meet the aims. A well conducted, professionally undertaken examination gives the patient confidence that they are being looked after and reassures them that the HCP is competent and thorough and thereby helps build a working relationship with the patient. If the patient perceives an examination or a part of the examination to be unnecessary, inadequately or incompetently performed, inappropriately intrusive or caused them distress it may undermine the working relationship.

The aim of this chapter is to discuss how the examination can contribute to meeting the aims of the consultation.

Determine the Aims of the Examination

The examination should be undertaken with purpose and not as a ritual in the hope of finding something abnormal. The aims determine the focus and format of the examination. The aims are determined by the context, the patient and the information learnt from talking to the patient. Frequently, the examination is undertaken with the aims of formulating a diagnosis and planning management. For some patients, the aims are to understand the problem, to assess severity, functional performance, change or to screen for a secondary problem or a complication or to look for signs of another abnormality. Occasionally, the aim is to demonstrate something to the patient. At all times, the aims of the examination should be clear to the HCP and to the patient who is consenting to the examination. To summarize, examination aims may include:

- Information exchange:
  - To learn and understand available information.
  - To learn relevant signs.
  - As a baseline assessment.
  - To inform the patient.
  - To document relevant information.
- To formulate a diagnosis:
  - To confirm a diagnosis.
  - To make a diagnosis.
  - To exclude a diagnosis.
  - To determine the location of the abnormality causing the problem.
  - To determine the type of problem.
  - To determine the cause.
  - To screen for:
    - Another abnormality.
    - A secondary abnormality.
    - A complication.
- To help plan management:
  - Of the problem.
  - Of the symptoms.
  - Of the diagnosis
  - To assess:
    - The local problem.
    - The impact on the patient.
    - Future risk.
- To build on the working relationship.

The aims of the examination should contribute to meeting the aims of the consultation. That does not mean the aims are the same. For example, the aims of the consultation may be to formulate a diagnosis and plan management whereas the aims of the examination may be to exclude a diagnosis or assess the impact of the problem on the patient. The examination can be undertaken not only to meet several aims but also different parts of the examination may be performed for different aims and the aims can change during the examination.

Determine Whether an Examination Is Indicated

Most patients expect to be examined and, for many patients, an examination is indicated because it is likely to provide relevant additional information about the person, the patient or the problem, to meet the aims of the consultation. However, an examination is an intrusion into a patient's personal and private space and should only be undertaken if it is indicated and with the consent of the patient. Consent is dependent on trust. The patient trusts that the examination is appropriate and indicated and will be undertaken sensitively and respectfully with regard to the patient's dignity, thoughts and feelings. An examination may *not* be indicated when:

- The facilities or necessary equipment are inadequate or unavailable.
- Privacy is inadequate.
- A chaperone is needed but is unavailable.
- The examination is unlikely to be safely undertaken, such as when the patient is likely to be violent.
- Signs are not expected. For example, when a patient presents with a change in mood, behaviour or personality likely to be caused by a mental health problem, such as depression, personality or bipolar disorders or schizophrenia.

- The problem has resolved.
- The examination is soon to be done by someone else.
- The examination is unlikely to be helpful. For example, trying to palpate a kidney in a morbidly obese patient.
- A test is going to be performed that is more accurate than the examination.

When an examination is not possible, such as during a telephone consultation, a patient can describe their problem or, in some circumstances, send a photograph or video of the abnormality. This is usually a poor substitute for a proper examination and there is an increased risk of error.

An examination is contra-indicated when the patient refuses to be examined. Some patients, such as those who are very nervous, anxious or self-conscious may postpone being examined until a later date. Not examining the patient should be a deliberate decision and the reasons documented.

Decide When to Examine the Patient

The context of the consultation, the patient, the nature of the presenting problem and information learnt from learning about the problem determine when to examine the patient. When the HCP has not previously met the patient, when a patient is challenging or difficult or has a complex medical background the examination usually follows learning about the person and the person as a patient. This helps establish a working relationship and puts the problem in context, ensuring the patient is treated as a person with a problem. When a patient presents with a new problem, feeling ill, a new pain or symptoms of a deranged function, or as a follow up consultation to assess change, examining the patient usually follows learning about the problem. When the presenting problem is a visible or palpable abnormality, examining the problem is usually the initial focus of the consultation. Questions are asked to learn and understand about the problem while examining the patient or after. When the consultation follows an investigation, the results dictate when the examination should be undertaken. If the patient is new to the HCP, such as when they are seen following a screening investigation or following referral from another HCP, learning about the person and the patient usually also precedes learning about the problem and the examination.

Use the Headline Information and the Introductory Conversation to Inform the Examination

The headline information and introductory conversation not only inform the aims and the initial focus of the consultation but also, together with information about the person, the patient and the problem, informs the aims, focus, format and conduct of the examination. For example:

- When a patient presents with a new problem the aim of the examination is usually to formulate a diagnosis and plan management.
- When the patient presents with a new visible or palpable abnormality, the site of the problem is usually examined first and then questions are asked to learn more about the problem.
- When the patient is very ill, a systemic examination is indicated initially, with the aim of assessing the severity of the illness.
- If the patient is a child the conduct of the examination is different from that of an adult.

Use the context of the consultation to inform the examination

Patients arrive at a consultation via different referral routes and at different stages in the pathway of care. The information available and the aims of the consultation are different in different contexts and this may influence the aims, focus and format of the examination. For example:

- When a patient presents with a new problem and the aim is to formulate a diagnosis, the examination usually follows learning about the problem and the initial focus of the examination is on the location of the presenting problem.
- When the consultation follows an investigation, including a screening test, the examination usually follows sharing information with the patient and learning about the problem. The results of the investigation, together with the information learnt from talking to the patient, inform the aims, focus and format of the examination. For example:

- When a CXR demonstrates an asymptomatic pulmonary abnormality and the differential diagnosis includes cancer, the aims of the examination may be to screen for signs of metastatic spread. The initial focus of the examination is likely to be on the regional lymph nodes and liver to look for associated signs.
- When a screening mammogram has shown a breast abnormality the aims of the examination may be to assess "local" severity and to screen for signs of metastatic spread, to plan management. The initial focus of the examination is likely to be on the breasts to determine if there is a visible or palpable abnormality, such as a mass, nipple retraction or peau d'orange and then on the regional lymph nodes and liver to look for associated signs.
- When a screening USS has revealed an abdominal aortic aneurysm, the aims of the examination may be to assess the severity of the vascular disease and the patient's functional performance to inform management. The examination is likely to focus on the peripheral vascular system and the chest to look for associated signs.

- When the consultation is a follow up to assess change, such as to assess resolution of cellulitis following a course of antibiotics or the range of joint movement following physiotherapy, the initial focus is on the site of the problem.
- When the consultation follows referral from another HCP, the aims are determined by the referral and this is likely to influence the focus of the examination. For example:
  - When an anaesthetist sees a patient pre-operatively with the aim of assessing the patient for an anaesthetic, the focus of the examination is usually on the upper airway, the chest and the circulation.
  - When the consultation is with a physiotherapist with the aim of improving shoulder movement, the focus of the examination is likely to be on the shoulder.

Use demographic information to inform the examination

Demographic information, and age and gender in particular, may influence the conduct of the examination, the aims, the interpretation of the signs and the differential diagnosis. For example:

- The conduct of the examination of an infant is different from an adult
- In some patients, the examination may need to respect cultural differences.
- There are anatomic and physiologic differences between males and females.
- In the elderly, the aims of the examination may include an assessment of physical function or to assess biological age to help plan management.
- Many signs, such as visual acuity, power and the range of movement of a joint are influenced by age.
- Demographic information influences the differential diagnosis and this influences the signs to look for. For example:
  - A breast lump in a male is likely to be gynaecomastia. A breast lump in an adolescent female is likely to be a cyst or fibroadenoma. When a middle aged or elderly female presents with a breast lump, cancer is more likely.
  - When a young adult presents with a swollen stiff knee joint the differential diagnosis may include an auto-immune disease, such as rheumatoid or psoriatic arthritis. There may be early signs of inflamed joints elsewhere or a skin rash. In the elderly, it is more likely to be caused by osteoarthritis.
  - A young or middle-aged patient presenting with sudden onset of loin to groin pain is likely to have ureteric colic. In an elderly patient it is important to exclude a AAA.

Use first impressions to inform the examination

When talking to the patient and before examining the patient:

Ask yourself, are you at risk?

Before examining a patient, it is important to ensure you and your staff are safe. This is usually only a concern when examining an unpredictable, difficult or vulnerable patient.

Ask yourself, is the patient seriously ill, very distressed or agitated, in severe pain or very breathless?

When a patient is very ill, the focus and format should follow an emergency protocol. The examination usually starts with an assessment of the airway and breathing and then of the chest and cardiovascular system.

A patient who is very distressed or agitated may not be able to relax sufficiently for an examination. Talking to the patient to help them relax or postponing the examination may be indicated.

A patient who is in severe pain or very breathless may need treatment before they can be examined.

Ask yourself, does the patient have special needs?

When a patient has a special need, such as a physical or mental disability, learning about the person should precede the examination because this information may inform the conduct of the examination.

Use Information About the Person to Inform the Examination

Learning about the person usually precedes the examination. Occasionally, the information may influence whether or not an examination is indicated or contra-indicated and it may influence the conduct of the examination, the aims, focus or format of the examination. For example:

- An examination is contra-indicated when the patient refuses to be examined or is very nervous or anxious and manifestly unhappy about being examined.
- It may not be safe to examine a potentially violent patient.
- When it becomes apparent a patient is unable to hold a meaningful conversation, a systematic examination may be indicated in the hope a localizing sign will be identified.
- An examination may need to be conducted with extra sensitivity and empathy in some patients, such as children or vulnerable adults.
- The focus and format of the examination may be influenced by the patient's views and expectations or past experiences, or by a disability. This may preclude examining some parts of the body.

Occasionally, information about the person may indicate signs to look for or the interpretation of signs. For example:

- When a patient has a very sedentary lifestyle the aim of the examination may be to assess function to inform management or the interpretation of signs, such as the pulse rate or blood pressure.
- When a patient's home, work or lifestyle exposes them to a potential risk factor, such as air pollution, stress or an unusual diet the aims of the examination may include screening for associated signs.
- When it is suspected that a patient may be drinking excessive quantities of alcohol or taking drugs, or withdrawing from alcohol or drugs, the examination may include looking for relevant signs.
- Information about the person may influence an assessment of tenderness or power.

Use Information About the Patient to Inform the Examination

Learning about the person as a patient usually precedes the examination because the information may change the aims, focus or format of the examination and indicate signs to look for or the interpretation of signs. For example:

- The aim of the examination may be to assess the severity of an ongoing medical condition. For example:
  - When there is concern a patient drinks excessive quantities of alcohol or takes drugs or is withdrawing from alcohol overuse or taking drugs, the examination may focus on assessing the impact on the patient.
  - When a patient is taking anti-hypertensive medication, the examination may include measuring the blood pressure to assess severity or change.
  - When a patient has been treated for cancer, the examination may include looking for signs of recurrence or metastatic spread to assess severity.
- The examination may include an assessment of the severity of a risk factor, such as the extent of peripheral vascular disease.
- An ongoing or previous medical condition or its treatment may influence the interpretation of the examination findings. For example, paraplegia or opioids may mask tenderness.

- The aim of the examination may be to screen for a complication or problem secondary to a known medical condition or risk factor. For example:
  - When the patient has previously been treated for a stroke or a heart attack, the examination may include an examination of the cardio-vascular system to screen for an abnormality.
  - When a patient has a chronic condition, such as a varicose ulcer or Crohn's disease the examination may include screening for a complication, such as an SCC or an abscess.
  - When the patient's occupation or lifestyle exposes them to chemicals or heavy metals, such as lead, arsenic or thallium, the aim of the examination may be to screen for signs of toxicity.
  - When a patient eats an unusual diet, the aim of the examination may include screening for signs of nutritional deficiency.
- Medications may cause adverse effects. Occasionally, relevant signs should be sought during the examination to screen for an adverse reaction. For example:
  - Peripheral neuropathy from chemotherapy.
  - Anaemia from occult blood loss while taking anti-coagulants or NSAIDs.
  - Hypotension while taking anti-hypotensive medications.
- When the consultation is to discuss an invasive procedure in a patient with a complex medical background, the examination may include an assessment of performance and suitability for the procedure.

Use Information About the Problem to Inform the Examination

The patient's description is a springboard to examining the patient to learn and understand the problem. This information usually determines the aims and initial focus of the examination. For example, to look for signs or a pattern of signs to formulate a diagnosis, to assess the impact on the patient to plan management or to screen for a complication or secondary problem.

When the patient presents with a new visible or palpable abnormality the location of the abnormality as described by the patient is first examined. Asking questions to learn more about the problem, the person and the patient can be undertaken during or after the examination. Looking for associated or systemic signs may then be indicated (Figure 61).

Figure 61: A figure illustrating the focus and format of the examination when a patient presents with a visible or palpable abnormality

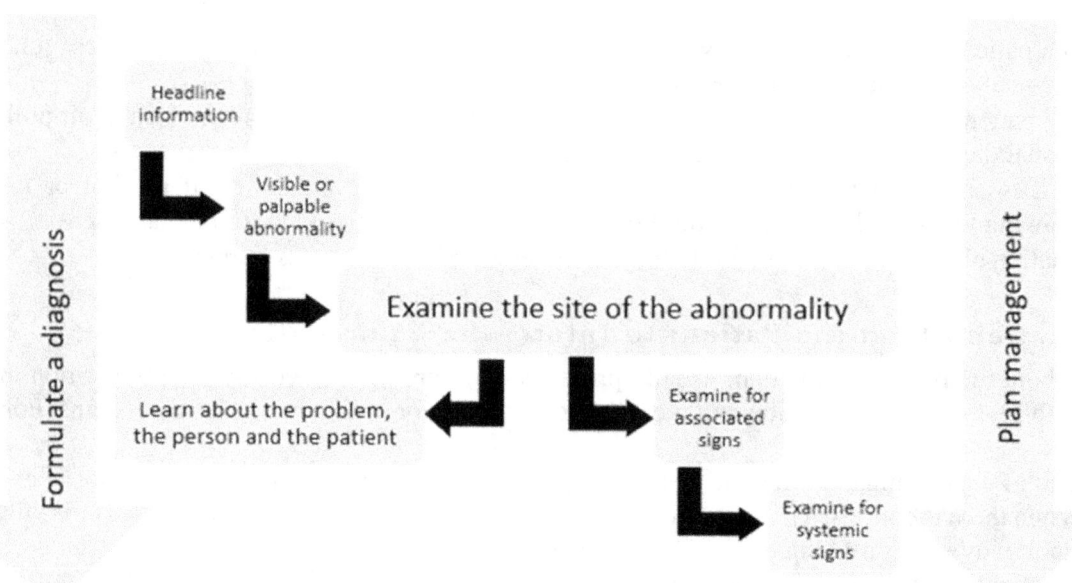

When the patient presents feeling ill, with pain or deranged function the examination is usually undertaken after talking to the patient and the information will inform the examination (Figure 62). Usually, the location of the abnormality is examined first. When information about the problem indicates the location of the abnormality is different from the location of the problem or the location has changed during the course of the illness it may be appropriate to examine both sites. For example:

- When a patient presents with shoulder pain likely to be angina, it may be appropriate to examine the shoulder first to exclude an abnormality and then the heart, the likely location of the abnormality.
- When a patient presents with back pain likely to be from the retroperitoneum, it may be appropriate to examine the back first to exclude an abnormality and then the abdomen, the likely location of the abnormality.
- When a patient presents with paraesthesia, the site of the paraesthesia should be examined first and then the nerve pathway examined to look for the location of the abnormality.
- When a patient first gets upper or central abdominal pain that moves to the right lower quadrant both sites should be examined.

Frequently, the examination will then focus on looking for associated or systemic signs. Information learnt about the person, the patient, the problem and from examining the site of the problem will determine the signs to look for.

Figure 62: A figure illustrating the focus and format of the consultation when a patient presents feeling ill, with pain or symptoms of deranged function.

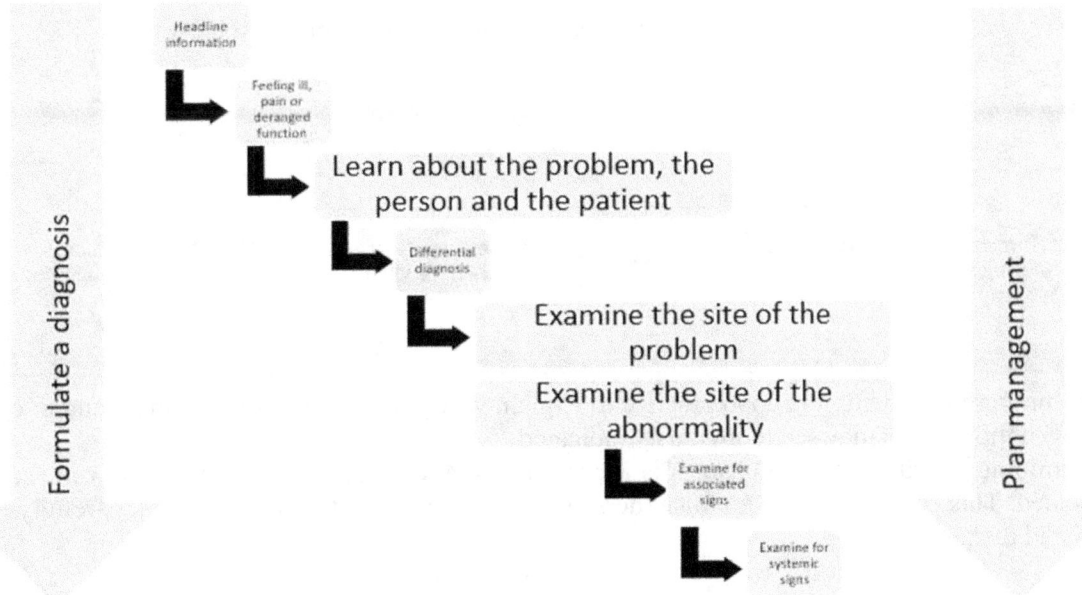

For some patients, the aim of the examination is to look for associated or systemic signs. For example:

- When a primary brain abnormality is likely, such as when the patient presents with a headache, an examination of the head is unlikely to be informative and the examination starts by looking for associated or systemic signs.
- To assess the impact on the patient.
- To screen for a complication or secondary problem.

Occasionally, a systematic examination is undertaken in the hope of finding an abnormal sign. For example:

- When the location of the abnormality causing the illness is uncertain, such as when the patient is unable to give a reliable description of their problem, a systematic examination may be indicated.
- When the patient is very ill, a systemic examination is usually undertaken early to assess the severity of their illness, request urgent investigations and initiate supportive treatment.

Examine the site of the problem

When the patient presents with a visible or palpable abnormality the site of the problem is examined early in the consultation, frequently before learning the details of the problem. When the patient presents with pain, symptoms of deranged function or feeling ill, and learning about the problem has preceded the examination, available information will indicate the site to examine and the signs to look for. For example:

- When a patient presents with palpitations and breathlessness and AF is suspected, palpate a named artery and auscultate the chest for an arrythmia.
- When a patient presents with pleuritic chest pain, the chest should be examined for a pleural rub and a likely cause, such as signs of consolidation.
- When a patient presents with intestinal colic, associated with nausea and vomiting, the abdomen should be examined for signs of previous surgery or a hernia, tenderness, a mass active, tympanic distension and bowel sounds.
- When a patient presents with neuralgia the signs to look for on examination include altered sensation in the area affected and Tinel's test may be positive. There may be localized weakness or loss of tendon reflexes if the nerve is a mixed motor and sensory nerve.

Examining the site of the problem is not always indicated. However, a decision not to examine the site of the problem should be a deliberate decision. The aims of examining the site of the problem are to formulate a diagnosis, assess local severity, determine the location of the abnormality, the type of problem, whether associated or systemic signs are likely, and to plan management (Figure 63).

Figure 63: Illustrating the aims of examining the site of the problem

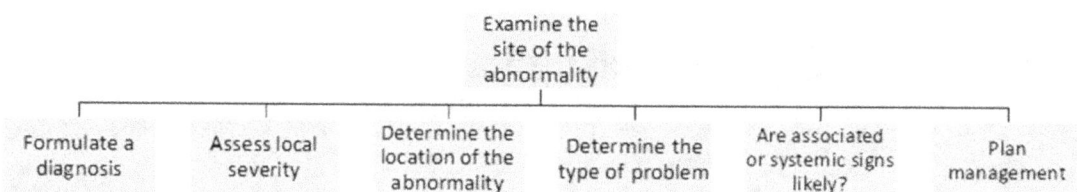

Before examining the patient, it is good practice to explain why you want to examine them and to check they give their consent even though this may seem obviously indicated.

Before examining the site of the problem, it is appropriate to ask the patient again to show you exactly where the problem is located. This ensures there is no misunderstanding. Before palpating the site, look carefully for any visible abnormalities and then ask:

Is it painful or tender?
Does it hurt?

If so:

Where is it most tender?

When the patient presents with a visible or palpable abnormality and the site is examined early in the consultation, questions should be asked to learn about the problem while examining the problem or afterwards. For example:

- A visible and palpable midline mass in the throat that moves on swallowing is likely to be a goitre. The patient should be asked about any symptoms of hyper- or hypo-thyroidism. For example:

Do you feel anxious or irritable?
Do you feel very tired and slow?
Have you noticed a tremor?
Have you been losing weight? Are you eating a lot more than normal yet losing weight?
Do you feel the cold or do you feel hot?
Have you had a change in bowel habit? Do you tend to have diarrhoea or be constipated?

The associated signs to look for include a dry skin, a puffy face and abdominal bloating. The hands should be examined for an associated tremor, the eyes for exophthalmos and lid lag and the pulse rate and rhythm measured.

There may be signs of increased sweating, weight loss, or hyper-reflexia. An USS and thyroid function tests are indicated.

When the patient is examined after learning about the problem, additional questions may be indicated. The signs determine the questions to ask and the aims of asking those questions. The aims may be to simply check information, to ensure all relevant information has been learnt and understood to confirm or exclude a diagnosis, to determine whether associated signs should be sought or to inform management.

While examining the site of the problem/abnormality, ask yourself:

What is the likely diagnosis or the differential diagnosis?

When the diagnosis is uncertain, ask yourself:

What is the location of the abnormality?
What is the type of problem?

Throughout the examination, ask yourself:

How severe is the problem?
What is the management plan?
What associated or systemic signs are likely?

While examining the site of the problem:

Ask yourself, what is the likely diagnosis or the differential diagnosis and how should it be managed?

When there is an abnormality, the signs may be diagnostic and this will inform management. For example:

- A spinal deformity with increased curvature and rigidity is characteristic of kypho-scoliosis. An Xray may be indicated to confirm the diagnosis, to assess severity and exclude other diagnoses such as a fracture or ankylosing spondylitis.
- Asymmetric facial features with unilateral mouth drooping, facial paralysis and loss of blinking are characteristic of Bell's (facial nerve) palsy. Antiviral treatment, analgesics, and steroids may be indicated.
- Kayser-Fleischer rings are characteristic of copper deposition in Wilson's disease. Blood tests are indicated to confirm the diagnosis and exclude secondary problems.
- Ptosis and miosis is characteristic of Horner's syndrome. Referral to an ophthalmologist may be indicated.
- A new onset of unexplained bronze skin pigmentation is characteristic of Addison's disease. Blood tests are indicated to confirm the diagnosis and screen for deranged homeostasis.
- Exophthalmos is characteristic of Graves' disease. Blood tests are indicated to confirm the diagnosis.
- A discoloured slightly raised skin tag on the back is likely to be actinic (solar) keratosis. If it is troublesome excision may be indicated.
- An expanding circle of erythema with a darker centre (a "bull's eye" rash) is characteristic of Lyme disease. Blood tests are indicated to confirm the diagnosis and antimicrobial treatment started.
- Café au lait patches and sub-cutaneous fusiform nodules are characteristic of neurofibromatosis. Genetic testing and a CT or MRI scan may be indicated.
- Exquisite superficial tenderness is characteristic of an abscess. Incision and drainage may be indicated.
- A sub-cutaneous firm, lower-midline swelling in the throat that moves up on swallowing is likely to be a multi-nodular goitre. An USS and thyroid function tests are indicated.
- A groin swelling palpable only on coughing is likely to be an inguinal hernia. A hernia repair may be indicated.
- A firm circumscribed non-tender mass with a punctum, arising from within the skin of the head or back is likely to be a sebaceous cyst. If it is troublesome excision may be indicated.
- A small peri-anal shallow nodule with a central pit is likely to be the external opening of an anal fistula. An MRI may be indicated to confirm the diagnosis.
- A pilonidal pit, with or without a surrounding firm swelling is likely to be a pilonidal sinus Referral to a surgeon for treatment may be indicated.

- Hard palmar chord like thickening and nodularity of the skin along the line of the flexor tendons to the ring finger and adjacent fingers, tending to produce a fixed flexion deformity, is characteristic of a Dupuytren's contracture. Referral to a hand surgeon for treatment may be indicated.
- A deep-seated pulsatile mass in the popliteal fossa is likely to be a popliteal aneurysm. A Doppler USS may be indicated to confirm the diagnosis.
- An early diastolic murmur is likely to be caused by aortic valve regurgitation. An echocardiogram may be indicated to confirm the diagnosis.
- A grating or crunching sound heard just before S1 and just after S2 is likely to be a pericardial friction rub caused by pericarditis. An ECG and echocardiogram may be indicated to confirm the diagnosis.
- Multiple scars or healing cuts on the arms or abdomen are likely to be from self-mutilation. A psychiatric opinion may be indicated.

When there are no pathognomonic signs, the pattern of local signs may indicate a short list of possible diagnoses. The differential diagnosis will inform management. For example:

- Patches of skin erythema, with flaking or cracking, usually affecting the limbs and face, are characteristic of eczema. The differential diagnosis may include psoriasis or a fungal infection. If a fungal infection is suspected, scrapings may be sent for microscopy and treatment with a topical antifungal cream indicated.
- A soft sub-cutaneous smooth, well-defined non-tender swelling may be a lipoma. The differential diagnosis will depend on the location but could include a sebaceous cyst, a neuroma/fibroma, a sarcoma or a lymph node. Excision may be indicated for treatment and to confirm the diagnosis.
- A small pearly pink/red shallow nodule with a central pit or ulcer on the face or back of the hands is likely to be a BCC. The differential diagnosis may include a sebaceous cyst or an SCC. Excision may be indicated for treatment and to confirm the diagnosis.
- A compressible non-tender groin swelling only visible or palpable when upright or while coughing may be a saphena varix or a hernia. An USS may be indicated.
- A firm non-tender well-demarcated intra-abdominal mass may be cancer. The differential diagnosis includes other tumours or cysts. If it is midline and arising from the pelvis it may be a gravid uterus, a full bladder or an ovarian mass. An USS may be indicated.
- A subcutaneous midline swelling in the throat that moves on protruding the tongue is likely to be a thyroglossal cyst. The differential diagnosis includes a submental lymph node or a thyroid goitre. An USS may be indicated.
- A multifocal itchy blistering rash affecting the skin of the scalp and elbows is characteristic of dermatitis herpetiformis caused by coeliac disease. The differential diagnosis of a blistering rashes includes an adverse reaction to a medication, pemphigus or pemphigoid. A review of the medications being taken and an anti-transglutamase antibody test is indicated. If pemphigus is suspected a skin biopsy for microscopy and immunohistochemistry may be indicated.
- The differential diagnosis of unexplained bruising may indicate a clotting abnormality, such as von Willebrand disease or haemophilia. Blood tests are indicated to measure the FBC and clotting and to formulate a diagnosis.
- Deformity and deviation of the fingers is characteristic of rheumatoid arthritis, but may be caused by arthritis or trauma. An Xray may be indicated.
- Exquisite tenderness in a joint is characteristic of gout or septic arthritis. Blood should be sent for a urate level and a joint aspirate sent for microbiological analysis. Antimicrobials should be started if septic arthritis is likely.

Occasionally, the signs are pathognomonic or fit a pattern indicating a likely diagnosis but, for many problems, the diagnosis is unclear. In which case, use the symptoms and signs together to determine the location of the abnormality, the type of problem and the likely cause (Figure 64). This may lead to a descriptive diagnosis or a list of possible diagnoses and inform management.

Figure 64: Illustrating the questions to ask yourself when examining the site of the problem

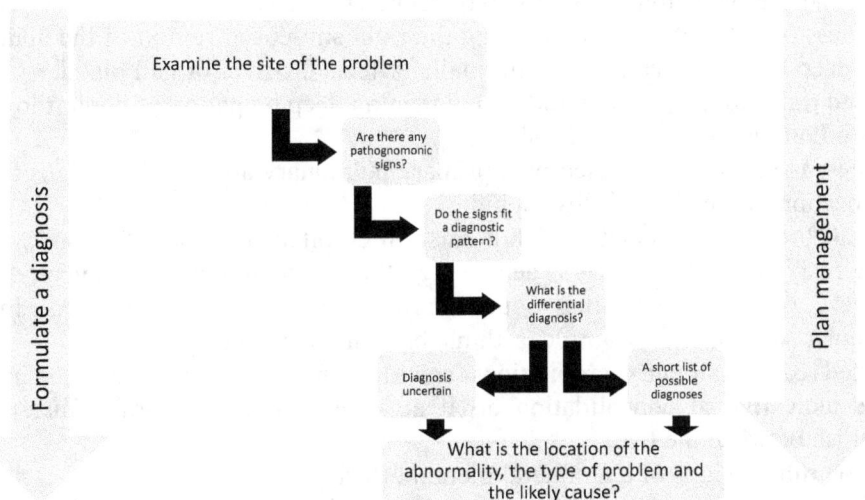

When the diagnosis is uncertain or the differential diagnosis long, while examining the site of the problem:

Ask yourself, what is the location of the abnormality and how should it be managed?

Often the symptoms or an examination of the site of the problem will indicate the likely location of the abnormality. However, when there is uncertainty, use the examination to determine whether it is a primary problem at the site or secondary to an abnormality elsewhere, whether it is superficial or deep-seated, what tissue, gland, organ or structure is abnormal and whether it is a solitary problem or part of a multifocal or widespread problem (Figure 65).

Figure 65 Illustrating a systematic method to determine the location of the abnormality causing the problem.

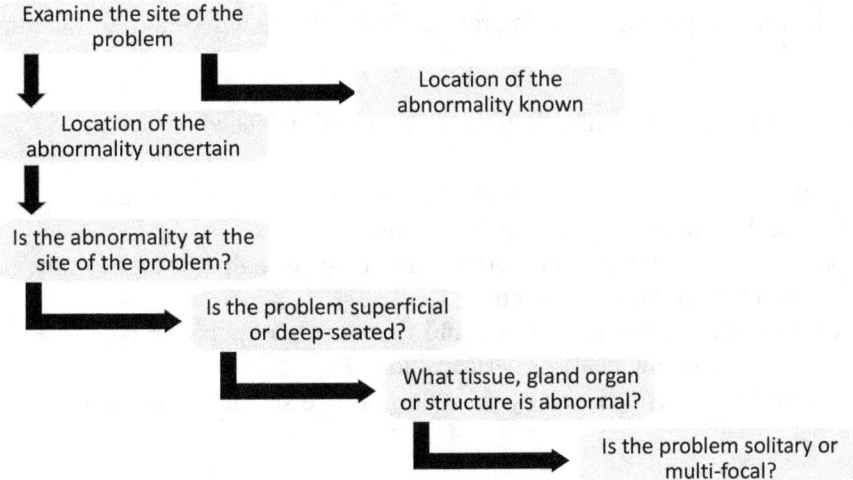

In general, the problem is likely to be caused by a primary abnormality at the site of the problem when:

- The symptoms indicate it is caused by a primary abnormality.
- There are signs at the site of the problem. For example:
  - A solitary visible or palpable abnormality, localized tenderness or a characteristic pattern of local signs. For example:
    - A midline mass in the throat that moves on swallowing is likely to be a goitre, whereas if it moves on protruding the tongue it is likely to be a thyroglossal cyst.
    - A right sub-costal mass that is more easily felt during deep inspiration is likely to be related to the liver.

- A left sub-costal mass that is more easily felt when the patient lies in the right lateral position is likely to be related to the spleen.
- A mass that can be balloted is likely to be related to the kidney.
- Tenderness or a "catch" when palpating the right sub-costal region of the abdomen when the patient takes a deep breath indicates the abnormality affects the liver or gall bladder, "Murphy's sign".
- Increased right lower quadrant abdominal pain on deep palpation of the left lower quadrant indicating nearby inflammation, "Rovsing's sign".
  - Breathlessness is likely to be caused by a primary pulmonary abnormality. Signs that confirm the chest is the likely location of the abnormality include:
    - Strenuous breathing associated with a harsh, high-pitched whistle, "stridor". This would indicate an upper airway obstruction, such as acute epiglottitis, a foreign body or cancer.
    - A wheeze (a coarse whistling sound during inspiration or expiration) indicating branchial or bronchiolar stenosis. For example, asthma, bronchitis or cancer.
    - Localized reduced air entry, crepitations (crackles) and dullness to percussion in a part of the lung field. This is indicative of consolidation or, if at a lung base, a pleural effusion. Vocal fremitus may distinguish between the two.
    - A friction rub, or signs of a unilateral pleural effusion.
      A CXR may be indicated to confirm the location of the abnormality and indicate a likely diagnosis. If cancer is suspected a CT scan may be indicated.
  - A change in bowel habit is likely to be caused by a primary abdominal abnormality. Signs that confirm the abdomen is the likely location of the abnormality include abdominal tenderness, with or without guarding, an abdominal mass or fullness, abdominal distension or active or absent bowel sounds. An US or CT scan may be indicated.
- The problem is typically caused by an abnormality at the site. This usually applies to localized superficial problems or problems affecting the limbs or face.
- The associated signs indicate a primary abnormality. For example:
  - When there is a suspicion of a midline throat mass, likely to be a goitre, associated signs of thyrotoxicosis or hypothyroidism would support a thyroid abnormality.
  - When a patient has breathlessness, associated chest signs would support a primary chest abnormality.
  - When a patient has a persistent unilateral headache, localized weakness or numbness would support a primary brain abnormality.

In general, the problem is likely to be secondary to an abnormality elsewhere when:

- The symptoms indicate the problem is secondary to an abnormality elsewhere.
- There are no signs at the site of the problem. For example:
  - When the pain is felt in the back, yet there are no visible or palpable signs in the back. The pain is likely to be referred from a retroperitoneal structure.
  - When the pain is felt in the left shoulder and there are no visible or palpable signs in the shoulder, it is likely to be referred from the heart or pericardium.
- The problem is known to be also caused by an abnormality elsewhere. For example:
  - Anaemia.
  - Neuralgia.
  - Ischaemic leg pain.
  - Back pain.
  - Shoulder pain.
- There are abnormal signs at another site. For example:
  - When the pain is felt in the back, yet there is abdominal tenderness or a mass. For example:
    - Lower thoracic back pain may be referred from acute pancreatitis or pancreatic cancer.
    - Lumber back pain may be referred from an expanding abdominal aortic aneurysm, pancreatitis, a retroperitoneal haematoma or from para-aortic lymphadenopathy.
  - When the pain is felt in the left shoulder yet there is a cardiac sign, such as a pan-systolic murmur.
- The associated signs indicate an abnormality elsewhere. For example:

- o When the patient presents with breathlessness likely to be secondary to heart failure, basal crepitations and bilateral basal dullness to percussion, associated with a laterally displaced heart apex beat, a raised JVP and pitting oedema in dependent areas would support the diagnosis.
- o When the patient presents with a change in the bowel habit likely to be secondary to thyrotoxicosis, an absence of abdominal signs and associated twitching, a tremor and increased sweating, a tachycardia, an arrythmia, hyper-reflexia, exophthalmos, lid lag and a goitre would support the diagnosis.
- o An umbilical mass is usually a hernia, a primary abnormality, but rarely it may be secondary to an abnormality elsewhere. If it is compressible rather than reducible, it may be secondary to ascites or divarication of the recti. If it is a firm and non-reducible, it may be a metastasis from an intra-abdominal malignancy. The rest of the abdomen should be examined to exclude a weakness in the linea alba, ascites, hepatomegaly or an intra-abdominal mass.
- The signs are multi-focal or widespread. For example:
- o When pain, tenderness or altered sensation extends over an area that corresponds to a named nerve, dermatome or extends widely affecting a large part of the body or multiple areas. For example:
  - Meralgia paraesthetica.
  - Trigeminal neuralgia.
  - Post-herpetic neuralgia.
  - Hyper-aesthesia in the region of the tip of the scapula (Boas' sign).
  - Unilateral loss of sensation from a stroke affecting the sensory cortex.
  - Chronic fatigue syndrome or fibromyalgia.
  - Episodic pain syndrome.
  - Reflex sympathetic dystrophy (complex regional pain syndrome).
- o A multi-focal joint deformity, swelling and pain is usually secondary to an autoimmune condition, such as rheumatoid arthritis or psoriasis.
- o A multi-focal rash is usually secondary to an autoimmune condition, such as eczema, psoriasis, polyarteritis nodosum, pemphigoid, pemphigus, epidermolysis or dermatitis herpetiformis.
- o Multi-focal unexplained bruising or petechiae is likely to be secondary to a clotting abnormality, such as von Willebrand disease, haemophilia or thrombocytopaenia.
- o Widespread bilateral muscle wasting is likely to be secondary to motor neurone disease.
- o When a patient presents with calf pain likely to be claudication, a cooler pale limb with absent peripheral pulses would support the diagnosis of a proximal arterial abnormality.

When the signs are multi-focal or widespread, examine each site or representative sites, to identify the local signs and determine a common link.

While examining the site of the abnormality it may be appropriate to ask questions to help determine whether it is a primary abnormality or secondary to an abnormality elsewhere. For example:

- When a patient presents with a marble sized non-tender mass in the left supraclavicular fossa it could be a primary lymphoma in a lymph node or secondary to an abnormality elsewhere. After examining the site, it would be appropriate to ask:

Have you recently had a sore throat or an infection affecting your mouth or face?
Have you noticed any lumps or abnormalities elsewhere?
Have you felt more breathless than normal?
Have you lost weight?

It would then be appropriate to examine the patient for associated signs, such as a mass or lymphadenopathy elsewhere, the chest for a pleural effusion and the breast, the abdomen or rectum to exclude hepatomegaly or a mass caused by a primary cancer.

- When a patient presents with a non-blanching purple patch it could be bruising from a direct blow or secondary to a clotting abnormality, such as von Willebrand disease. After examining the site, it would be appropriate to ask:

Do you know what caused the bruise?
Do you bruise easily?

When you cut yourself do you bleed for a long time?
Have you noticed any bleeding elsewhere, such as when you cough or go to the toilet?
Are your periods very heavy?
Have you had any problems with your joints?

The conjunctiva should be examined for pallor and the pulse measured to diagnose associated anaemia and the abdomen examined for a hepato- or spleno-megaly.

- When a patient is noted to be jaundice, it could be caused by a primary hepatocellular abnormality or be secondary to biliary disease or increased haemolysis. After examining the abdomen, it would be appropriate ask the patient:

Have you noticed a change in colour of your urine or stools?
Have you been itching?
Have you had any abdominal pain or discomfort?
Have you felt ill?
Have you felt very tired, weak and listless?
Have you had a fever, any shaking attacks or episodes of feeling alternately hot and cold?

The abdomen should also be examined for tenderness and a palpable mass likely to be arising from the liver or gallbladder. The temperature and pulse rate should be measured to exclude a fever and the conjunctiva inspected to screen for anaemia.

When there is a visible or palpable abnormality, determine the precise position in relation to the surface, superficial landmarks and named nearby anatomical structures, such as bone, a joint, a major artery or an organ. For example:

- When the patient presents with scrotal pain and, on examination, there is local tenderness, the precise location of the tenderness will distinguish between orchitis and epididymitis. Treatment with antimicrobials or sending a urine sample for MC&S to confirm the diagnosis and identify the pathogen may be indicated.
- When the patient presents with a mass in the scrotum, the precise location will distinguish between a testicular mass, such as cancer, an epididymal cyst or a hydrocoele. Imaging with an USS may be indicated to confirm the diagnosis.
- When the patient presents with groin pain, the precise location of the tenderness will distinguish between ileo-inguinal nerve entrapment, hip pain, lymphadenitis, adductor tendinitis, osteitis pubis, testicular torsion or epidymo-orchitis. Imaging with an USS of the groin and scrotum or an Xray of the hip or pelvis may be indicated to confirm or exclude a diagnosis.
- When the patient presents with a mass in the groin, the precise location will distinguish between an inguinal hernia, a femoral hernia, an undescended testicle, an encysted hydrocoele of the cord, a lipoma of the chord, a femoral lymph node, a saphena varix or a femoral artery aneurysm. Imaging with an USS may be indicated to confirm a diagnosis.
- When pain is in the elbow, the precise location of tenderness will inform the likely diagnosis.
  - Tenderness of the lateral epicondyle of the humerus is likely to be caused by lateral epicondylitis, "tennis elbow".
  - Tenderness of the medial epicondyle is likely to be caused by epicondylitis, "golfer's elbow".
  - Tenderness anteriorly over the biceps brachii tendon is likely to be caused by biceps tendinitis. Contracting the muscles against resistance should aggravate the pain.
  - Tenderness in a small area over the tip of the olecranon process is likely to be from olecranon bursitis.
  - Tenderness in the joint is likely to be from arthritis.

  Imaging with an MRI may be indicated to confirm the diagnosis or an Xray if arthritis is suspected and symptomatic treatment may be indicated.
- When pain is in the knee joint, the precise location of tenderness will inform the likely diagnosis.
  - A superficial tenderness lateral to the knee joint aggravated by stressing the knee medially is likely to be arising from a lateral ligament injury.
  - Tenderness, swelling, deformity and crepitus in the joint is likely to be from arthritis.
  - Pre-patellar tenderness is likely to be from pre-patellar bursitis.
  - Popliteal fossa or upper calf pain, tenderness and swelling may be from a popliteal, "Baker's" cyst.

- o Upper calf tenderness may be from a calf muscle injury or from a DVT.
  Imaging with an MRI of the knee may be indicated to determine the location of the abnormality and confirm the diagnosis, an Xray if arthritis is suspected or an USS if a Baker's cyst or DVT are suspected.
- When pain is in the heal, the precise location of tenderness will inform the likely diagnosis.
  - o A tender Achilles tendon is likely to be due to tendinitis.
  - o Tenderness between the tendon and the calcaneum indicates retrocalcaneal bursitis.
  - o Tenderness in the calcaneum is likely to be due to periostitis or a fracture.
    Imaging with an MRI scan to confirm the diagnosis and symptomatic treatment may be indicated.
- When the problem is arising from a deep-seated abnormality affecting the chest, abdomen, pelvis or back, an examination of the site will not localize the abnormality precisely. In which case, consider a checklist of nearby tissues, organs or parts of the body. This will indicate a list of possible diagnoses and inform management. For example:
  - o Midline or "retrosternal" chest pain could be arising from:
    - The oesophagus, such as reflux oesophagitis or oesophageal spasm ("nutcracker" oesophagus).
    - The heart, such as ACS.
    - The mediastinum, such as lymphadenopathy.
    An ECG is indicated to exclude ACS. An OGD or CT scan may be indicated to determine the location of the abnormality and formulate a diagnosis.
  - o A deep-seated upper mid-line mass could be arising from:
    - The stomach, such as cancer.
    - The pancreas, such as a pseudocyst.
    - The transverse colon, such as a cancer.
    - The liver, such as a liver cyst or cancer.
    A CT scan is indicated to determine the location of the abnormality and formulate a diagnosis.
  - o A deep-seated unilateral cervical mass could be arising from:
    - A salivary gland, such as a sub-mandibular gland tumour.
    - A lymph node, such as a lymphoma.
    - The carotid artery, such as a carotid body tumour.
    - The sterno-mastoid muscle, such as torticollis.
    An USS or CT scan may be indicated to determine the location of the abnormality and formulate a diagnosis.
  - o Knee tenderness could be arising from a tendon or ligament, such as following an injury, a bursa, such as bursitis, the bone, such as a stress fracture, or the joint itself, such as a meniscal injury.
    An MRI may be indicated to determine the location of the abnormality and formulate a diagnosis.

When an abnormality is separate from a named anatomical structure, it may be arising from the connective tissue. For example, a lipoma, neuroma, a haematoma, infection, fibroma, angioma or a sarcoma. This will then limit the differential diagnosis and inform management. When the location of the abnormality is uncertain, consider a checklist of tissues or organs nearby.

Usually, a patient will describe whether their problem is solitary, multifocal or is part of a widespread problem. However, some problems present as a solitary problem when they are in fact part of a multifocal or widespread problem. For example:

- A solitary neck, axillary or groin mass, likely to be lymphadenopathy, may be the first presentation of carcinomatosis.
- A soft subcutaneous lump likely to be a lipoma is often solitary but can be multifocal.
- A patient who presents with a groin swelling likely to be an inguinal hernia may have an asymptomatic hernia on the other side.
- When a patient presents with a breast lump, the contralateral breast should also be examined for asymptomatic bilateral breast disease.
- A skin lesion likely to be caused by sun exposure may be a multifocal problem.
- When the patient presents with a swollen salivary gland, the other salivary glands may also be enlarged.
- Thrombophlebitis is usually solitary but it may be multifocal. In which case, it may indicate an underlying malignancy.
- A painful swollen joint likely to be caused by arthritis may be a multifocal problem.
- When a patient presents with paraesthesia or numbness in the fingers of one hand, other digits may be affected.

- A swollen foot is usually part of a generally swollen limb and is likely to be a bilateral problem when the swelling is caused by heart failure or hypoproteinaemia. The rest of limb and the cardio-vascular system should be examined.
  - Aneurysmal or occlusive vascular disease is frequently caused by atherosclerosis which is usually a multifocal problem. The rest of the cardio-vascular system should be examined.
  - Raynaud's syndrome is usually a bilateral problem.
  - Intra-epithelial neoplasia may be multifocal or affect a wide area.
  - Arthritis usually affects multiple joints.
  - Hidradenitis often affects multiple sites.

When there is doubt, other sites should be examined. Asking additional questions may be indicated after examining the site of the abnormality to determine whether it is a solitary problem or part of a widespread or multi-focal problem. For example:

- When a patient, known to have DM, presents with numbness in one hand, it may be a localized problem, secondary to a nerve entrapment or part of a widespread problem, such as peripheral or autonomic neuropathy. After examining the patient, it would be appropriate ask:

Can you eat a large meal? Do you feel full quickly?
Are your bowels normal? Do you tend to be constipated?
Do you have difficulty controlling your urine?
Do you get an erection?

It would then be appropriate to examine the patient for associated signs of autonomic neuropathy, such as reduced vibration and light touch sensation elsewhere, orthostatic hypotension and a slow pupil reaction time.

The distribution of multi-focal or widespread signs may indicate the likely location of the abnormality and the possible diagnosis. For example:

- When weakness is widespread, affecting several different muscle groups the abnormality is likely to be central, in the spinal cord, such as paraplegia or in the brain, such as unilateral weakness following a stroke. When weakness is generalised, the abnormality may be central, in the spinal cord, such as motor neurone disease, or secondary to an auto-immune condition, such as rheumatoid arthritis, dermatomyositis, polymyositis, SLE or Guillain-Barré syndrome.
- When anaesthesia or paraesthesia affects a wide area, the abnormality is likely to be central: in the spinal cord, such as cauda equina syndrome or paraplegia, or in the brain, such as following a stroke. When anaesthesia or paraesthesia is multifocal, the abnormality is likely to be metabolic, such as chemotherapy induced peripheral neuropathy or polyneuritis.

When the type of problem is uncertain:

Ask yourself, what is the likely type of problem and how should it be managed?

When the diagnosis is uncertain, determining the likely type of problem and possible cause, together with the likely location of the abnormality, will indicate a likely descriptive diagnosis or a list of possible diagnoses. This can be used to inform the associated signs to look for or additional questions to ask with the aims of confirming or excluding a diagnosis and informing management. Information about the problem and the local signs will often indicate the likely type of problem. For example:

- A tachypnoea is likely to be caused by inflammation, such as an infection, or a structural type of problem, such as COPD, bronchiectasis, pneumothorax or pleural effusion. Occasionally it is caused by cancer.
- Most chest pains are caused by a circulatory problem, such as angina or an acute myocardial infarction, or inflammation, such as reflux oesophagitis, pericarditis or pleurisy.
- Abdominal tenderness is likely to be caused by intra-abdominal inflammation, such as cholecystitis, appendicitis, colitis or endometriosis. Rarely it is caused by a circulatory problem, such as ischaemic bowel.

- Abdominal distension is likely to be caused by a structural type of problem, such as intestinal obstruction, cancer, a neurological type of problem, such as IBS, slow transit constipation or autonomic neuropathy, or a metabolic problem, such as an ileus due to uraemia or ascites due to hypoproteinaemia.
- Feeling ill due to a primary brain abnormality is usually caused by a neurological type of problem, such as depression, and there are no signs to find on examination. Occasionally it is caused by inflammation, such as encephalitis, a structural problem, such as dementia, or a circulatory type of problem, such as a sub-dural haemorrhage when there may be associated signs on examination.
- Widespread or multifocal signs affecting the skin, such as a rash, joints, such as tenderness, a reduced range of movement or deformity, or muscles, such as tenderness or reduced power are likely to be caused by auto-immune inflammation. Occasionally, they are caused by a metabolic or neurological type of problem.
- Soft-tissue limb, superficial head and trunk tenderness is likely to be caused by, non-infective inflammation, such as myositis, a structural problem, following an injury, or occasionally by a neurological or a circulatory type of problem, such as ischaemia.
- Joint tenderness is likely to be caused by inflammation, such as osteoarthritis, or occasionally by a metabolic problem, such as gout.

When the type of problem and cause are uncertain:

Ask yourself, are there local signs of inflammation and how should it be managed?

The classical signs characteristic of superficial inflammation, are well known and include:

- Local warmth ("calor").
- Localized blanching erythema ("rubor").
- Local pain and tenderness ("dolor"), aggravated by active or passive movement.
- A tender swelling ("tumour").
- Loss of function.

Superficial signs of inflammation and the location will indicate a likely diagnosis. For example, cellul-itis, furuncul-itis, paronychia, or a breast, pilonidal, peri-anal or a vulval, "Bartholin's", abscess.
The signs indicating deep seated inflammation include:

- Local warmth and erythema are not usually apparent when the inflammation is deep-seated. Nevertheless, they should be looked for. For example:
  o Warmth and erythema of a joint is characteristic of septic arthritis.
  o Warmth and erythema over a tender groin mass may be caused by a strangulating viscus in a hernia or an infected lymph node.
  o Warmth and erythema in part of the breast is characteristic of mastitis or a breast abscess. Occasionally, it may be caused by an "inflammatory cancer".
- Pain and tenderness aggravated by active or passive movement of nearby structures. For example:
  o Joint pain and tenderness increased on active or passive movement of the joint indicates joint inflammation. When any movement is severely painful it may be septic arthritis or gout.
  o Upper abdominal tenderness indicates deep-seated inflammation, such as from cholecystitis or hepatitis. The tenderness is likely to be aggravated by deep inspiration while palpating under the liver (Murphy's sign).
- A tender swelling ("tumour"), ill-defined fullness or firmness. For example:
  o A circumscribed very tender swelling is characteristic of an abscess.
  o A right sub-costal tender swelling may be due to hepatitis, severe cholecystitis, an empyema of the gallbladder or a local perforation.
  o Tender non-fluctuant joint swelling may be caused by synovial inflammation. When it is fluctuant, the swelling is likely to be caused by intra-articular fluid, usually secondary to inflammation.
  o Tender non-fluctuant muscle swelling may be caused by myositis.
  o Muscle spasm when the site is palpated indicates nearby inflammation. In the abdomen, this is felt as guarding.

When there is local inflammation, there may also be systemic inflammation. Systemic inflammation should be considered in any patient who presents feeling ill with nonspecific symptoms such as fatigue, poor concentration, global weakness and a change in weight. When there are symptoms of systemic inflammation or local signs of inflammation, the patient should be examined for associated signs of a fever. Signs of a fever include sweating, looking flushed, a pyrexia >38°C, tachycardia with a bounding pulse and tachypnoea >21/min with shallow mouth breathing ("panting"). Signs of a fever are likely to be caused by infective inflammation. If the patient appears ill, peripherally cold and sweaty but centrally hot, the pulse fast but weak and difficult to palpate, the patient hypotensive with a systolic BP<101mmHg and passing a low volume of concentrated urine, septicaemia is likely. When septicaemia is suspected intravenous antibiotics should by started and the patient managed as a medical emergency.

Inflammation is the immune response to a variety of problems; it is not a diagnosis. Inflammation may be caused by infection or a non-infective cause, such as degeneration, a hypersensitivity reaction, an auto-immune disease, an injury, including "chemical" injury, ischaemia, atherosclerosis and thrombosis, previous radiation exposure or cancer. The onset, symptoms and the location of the problem, together with information about the person and the patient may indicate a likely cause or exclude some causes.

When the classical signs of inflammation arise acutely and are localized, they are usually caused by a superficial infection. The likely infecting organism is based on probabilities and awaits the results of microbiological tests. However, some signs are indicative. For example:

- The presence of blistering or wheals indicates a Staphylococcal infection; "bullous impetigo". When a Staphylococcal infection is likely treatment with antibiotics is usually indicated.
- Blistering or vesicles in a dermatomal distribution is likely to be caused by herpes zoster infection; "shingles". If diagnosed early, treatment with an antiviral medication may be indicated.
- Patches of itchy slightly raised and scaly blanching erythema affecting the groin or perianal skin or under the breasts or skin folds is characteristic of a fungal infection. When a fungal infection is likely scrapings may be taken for microbiological examination and treatment started with a topical anti-fungal cream.
- Pitting, scarring, skin thickening, erythema or small abscesses in the groin, pilonidal or perineal regions, armpits or below the breasts is characteristic of hidradenitis. When hidradenitis is likely, treatment with antibiotics or surgery may be indicated.
- Pitting, scarring, skin thickening, erythema or small abscesses in the cheeks is characteristic of acne. When acne is likely treatment with antibiotics is usually indicated.
- Small painless sores or ulcers affecting the genitals, peri-anally or the mouth are characteristic of syphilis. When syphilis is suspected blood tests to measure syphilis VDRL (Venereal disease research laboratory) antibody are indicated to confirm the diagnosis.

Occasionally, although the signs are classical for a superficial infection, the cause is non-infective. However, usually the location and the pattern of local signs are characteristic. For example:

- When acute superficial inflammation is along the line of a vein it is characteristic of thrombophlebitis. There may be an underlying sub-cutaneous worm-like thickening. If thrombophlebitis is the likely diagnosis, reassurance and treatment with topical anti-inflammatory medications may be indicated. When it is multifocal or recurrent, imaging to exclude an occult cancer may be indicated.
- When acute superficial inflammation overlies a bony promontory or is along the line of a tendon or fascia, it is likely to be caused by non-infective inflammation, such as bursitis, teno-synovitis or fasciitis. Rest and treatment with anti-inflammatory medications may be indicated.

When the superficial signs of inflammation are multi-focal, the cause is usually noninfective, being caused by a hypersensitivity or auto-immune reaction. The pattern of multi-focal superficial inflammation and associated signs may indicate a likely diagnosis. For example:

- An acute generalised pruritic rash, associated with breathlessness, tachypnoea and a wheeze are characteristic of a hypersensitivity reaction. Antihistamines and a salbutamol inhaler are indicated unless it is severe.
- A multifocal itchy blistering rash affecting the skin of the scalp and elbows is characteristic of dermatitis herpetiformis caused by coeliac disease. An anti-trans glutamase antibody test is indicated to confirm the diagnosis.

340

- A multifocal itchy flat blanching erythematous rash affecting the back of the face, the wrists, hands, knees and feet is likely to be eczema. Topical creams are indicated.
- A multifocal sore itchy red, slightly raised, scaly, non-blanching rash that typically affects the outside of the elbows, knees or scalp is characteristic of psoriasis. Topical creams and lotions are indicated unless it is severe.
- A multi-focal sore itchy red, slightly raised, blistering and crusty rash affecting the skin folds, face, neck and scalp is characteristic of pemphigus. A biopsy is indicated to confirm the diagnosis. Topical steroids are first-line treatment.
- Acute multifocal sores or ulcers on raised lumps with surrounding inflammation in a patient with a chronic inflammatory condition, such as rheumatoid arthritis or ulcerative colitis, are characteristic of pyoderma gangrenosum. A biopsy is indicated to confirm the diagnosis.
- Small firm, tender sub-cutaneous nodules, palpable purpura, blistering or ulceration, muscle and joint pains and tenderness are characteristic of polyarteritis nodosum. A biopsy may be indicated to confirm the diagnosis.
- Raised red patches in sun exposed areas, including a "butterfly" shape bridging the nose, is characteristic of systemic lupus erythematosus. There may be mouth ulcers, Raynaud's syndrome and joint swelling. Blood should be sent to measure auto-antibodies.
- A scaly erythematous rash associated with reduced power and tenderness of the trunk muscles would indicate dermatomyositis. Blood should be sent to measure creatine kinase and a punch biopsy may be indicated to confirm the diagnosis.

Occasionally, multi-focal superficial inflammation is caused by an infection. In which case, the location and the pattern of local signs are usually characteristic. For example:

- Multi-focal scaly blanching patches of erythema affecting the groin or perianal skin or under the breasts or skin folds is characteristic of a fungal infection.
- Multi-focal erythema with pitting, scarring, skin thickening, or small abscesses covering the cheeks is characteristic of acne.

Determining the cause of deep-seated inflammation is more challenging. The symptoms and signs together may be indicative but the diagnosis is usually based on probabilities and awaits the results of investigations. For example:

- An acute onset of joint pain within a slightly flexed joint is likely to be caused by septic arthritis. Joint swelling, warmth, overlying erythema and pain increased on minimal active or passive movement support the diagnosis. If there is no fever, the differential diagnosis includes arthritis or gout. Blood should be sent for a serum urate level and a joint aspiration or Xray may be indicated.
- Generalised muscle pain, tenderness and stiffness associated with reduced power and range of movement, worse in the morning, is characteristic of polymyalgia rheumatica. An ESR and CRP should be measured.
- An acute onset of right upper quadrant abdominal pain may be caused by local infection, such as from acute cholecystitis, hepatitis, appendicitis, diverticulitis, a duodenal ulcer or pyelonephritis (Figure 66). Localized tenderness and guarding confirm an inflammatory cause but an USS or CT scan, may be indicated.
- An acute onset of right lower quadrant abdominal pain may be caused by local infection, such as from acute appendicitis, salpingo-oophoritis or Yersinia, or from auto-immune inflammation, such as Crohn's disease (Figure 67). Localized tenderness and guarding confirm an inflammatory cause but an USS or CT scan, may be indicated.
- An acute onset of generalized abdominal pain may be caused by intra-abdominal infection, such as from a perforated appendicitis or diverticulitis, or from chemical inflammation, such as from a perforated peptic ulcer or acute pancreatitis, or from ischaemic inflammation, such as mesenteric ischaemia (Figure 68). Generalized tenderness and guarding confirms peritonitis but cannot discriminate between the different causes. A CT scan may be indicated.
- An acute onset of breathlessness and a cough are likely to be caused by pneumonia. Localized reduced air entry, a pleural rub, dullness to percussion and crepitations (crackles) are indicative of pulmonary consolidation caused by bacterial infection. A widespread wheeze without other chest signs is more characteristic of asthma, a hypersensitivity reaction. A CXR may be indicated.

Figure 66: Line diagram illustrating the differential diagnosis of right upper quadrant abdominal tenderness:

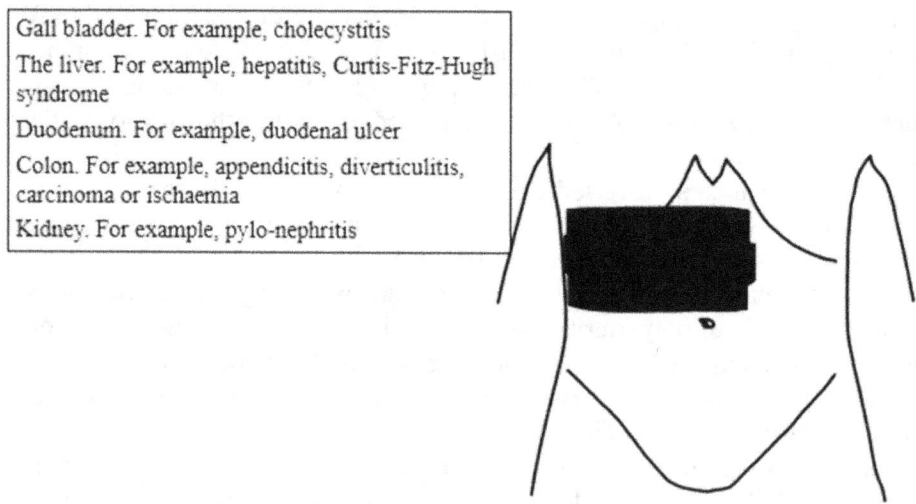

Gall bladder. For example, cholecystitis

The liver. For example, hepatitis, Curtis-Fitz-Hugh syndrome

Duodenum. For example, duodenal ulcer

Colon. For example, appendicitis, diverticulitis, carcinoma or ischaemia

Kidney. For example, pylo-nephritis

Figure 67: Line diagram illustrating the differential diagnosis of right lower quadrant tenderness

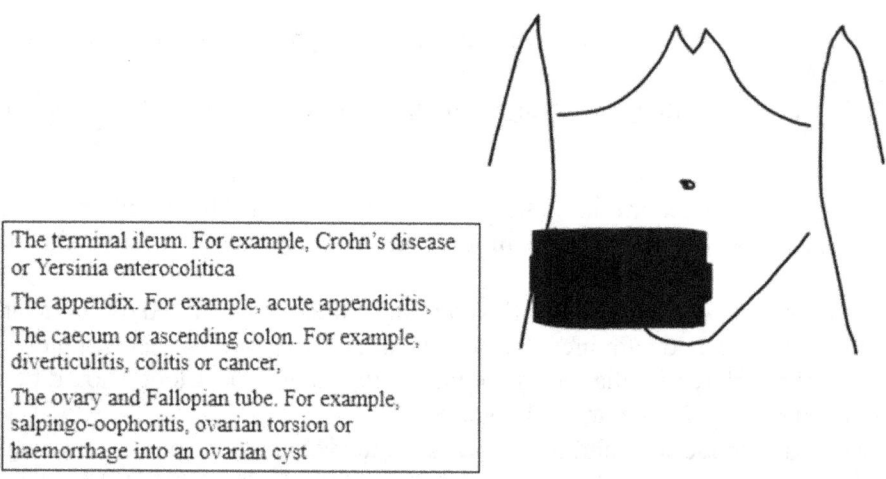

The terminal ileum. For example, Crohn's disease or Yersinia enterocolitica

The appendix. For example, acute appendicitis,

The caecum or ascending colon. For example, diverticulitis, colitis or cancer,

The ovary and Fallopian tube. For example, salpingo-oophoritis, ovarian torsion or haemorrhage into an ovarian cyst

Figure 68: Line diagram illustrating the differential diagnosis of generalized peritonitis

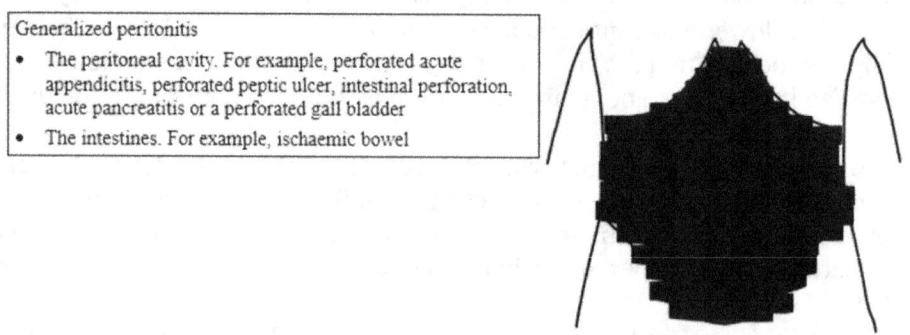

Generalized peritonitis
- The peritoneal cavity. For example, perforated acute appendicitis, perforated peptic ulcer, intestinal perforation, acute pancreatitis or a perforated gall bladder
- The intestines. For example, ischaemic bowel

When inflammation is suspected, the patient should be examined for signs of a fever. Signs of a fever are likely to be caused by infective inflammation. When a patient presents feeling ill with a fever, and there are no localizing symptoms, examining the patient may identify signs indicating a likely cause. For example:

- Loin tenderness from an asymptomatic UTI.
- Signs of a chest infection.
- Signs of a heart murmur caused by endocarditis.

When the type of problem is uncertain:

Ask yourself, is it a structural type of problem and how should it be managed?

When the patient presents with a visible or palpable mass, defect, scar or deformity there is a structural type of problem. The location and pattern of signs will indicate the likely diagnosis and management. For example:

- A firm circumscribed non-tender mass arising from within the skin on the head and back, sometimes with a punctum is likely to a sebaceous cyst. Usually, the patient can be reassured and discharged. Occasionally, when the sebaceous cyst gets infected, large, is tender or in the wrong place excision is indicated.
- A circumscribed non-tender sub-cutaneous soft mass is likely to be an uncomplicated lipoma. Usually, the patient can be reassured and discharged. Occasionally, when the lipoma is tender or large excision is indicated.
- A circumscribed non-tender hard mass arising from bone adjacent to a joint is likely to be an osteophyte, such as a Heberden's node. Usually, the patient can be reassured and discharged. Occasionally an X-ray is indicated to confirm the diagnosis.

When a patient presents with pain, deranged function or feeling ill the symptoms usually indicate when the problem is likely to be caused by a deep-seated structural type of problem and inform the local and associated signs to look for. Information about the person and the patient may inform the probability of structural problem. For example:

- Structural problems present since birth may be genetic or developmental. For example, kyphoscoliosis or pectus excavatum.
- Structural problems are more likely in the elderly.
- Manual jobs are associated with an increased risk of structural joint problems.
- A patient who has previously had an operation is more likely to have adhesions or scarring, a structural problem.
- Previous problems may increase the risk of recurrence of a structural problem, such as renal stones or a musculo-skeletal injury.
- The risk of Dupuytren's contracture is increased in patients who have DM or epilepsy, drink alcohol to excess or operate vibrating tools.

The pattern of symptoms and signs may indicate a structural type of problem. Determining the likely cause is often based on probabilities. Information about the person or the patient may indicate a likely cause but imaging investigations, such as an USS or a CT scan are often indicated. For example:

- When the symptoms indicate breathlessness is likely to be caused by a structural problem there are likely to be chest signs.
  - o Stridor or a wheeze indicate air turbulence caused by partial airway obstruction, such as bronchospasm, mucus or a tumour.
  - o Localized reduced air entry, dullness to percussion and vocal fremitus are likely to be caused by consolidation.
  - o Reduced air entry and dullness to percussion at the lung base without vocal fremitus is likely to be caused by a pleural effusion.
  - o Reduced air entry and hyper-resonance is likely to be caused by a pneumothorax.
  - o A barrel-shaped chest, peripheral cyanosis and clubbing and wide spread bilateral crepitations, would support a structural problem, such as COPD. A CXR may be indicated to exclude other diagnoses and spirometry to confirm the diagnosis.
    A CXR, CT scan or bronchoscopy, with or without a biopsy, may be indicated to determine the likely cause, formulate a diagnosis and assess severity
- When a patient presents with jaundice likely to be caused by a structural problem, there are likely to be abdominal signs.

- o Localised upper abdominal tenderness indicates the jaundice is likely to be caused by gallstones causing biliary tract obstruction.
- o A localized palpable non-tender sub-hepatic mass (Courvoisier's sign) likely to be a palpable gallbladder, associated with weight loss, would indicate malignant common bile duct obstruction.
    LFTs and an USS are indicated to confirm the diagnosis and assess severity.
- When the symptoms are typical of biliary colic, a non-tender mass in the region of the gallbladder confirms a structural type of problem. The differential diagnosis will include a mucocoele of the gall bladder, gall bladder or liver cancer or cancer of the head of the pancreas with sub-clinical jaundice. Measuring the LFTs and an USS or CT scan are indicated to formulate a diagnosis.
- When the symptoms indicate bowel obstruction, it is likely to be caused by a structural problem, such as adhesions or cancer.
  - o A scaphoid abdomen and a succussion splash are characteristic of gastric outlet obstruction likely to be caused by cancer or a peptic stricture. A CT scan, OGD or barium meal is indicated to formulate a diagnosis.
  - o Upper abdominal tympanic bloating and active bowel sounds indicates proximal intestinal obstruction. Generalised tympanic abdominal distension and active bowel sounds indicate distal small bowel obstruction. The presence of an irreducible slightly tender groin swelling indicates a hernia is the likely cause, whereas, the absence of a hernia and the presence of abdominal scars from previous surgery indicate adhesions are the likely cause. An absence of either increases the likelihood Crohn's disease or cancer is the cause. A CT scan is indicated to identify the cause and formulate a diagnosis.
  - o Right sided tympanic abdominal distension and right sided tenderness with normal bowel sounds indicate closed loop large bowel obstruction likely to be caused by a diverticular stricture or cancer. A CT scan is indicated to formulate a diagnosis.
- Recurrent episodes of lower abdominal discomfort with a variable bowel habit, mild tenderness and a tubular thickening in the left lower quadrant of the abdomen may be caused by a structural problem, such as diverticular disease. Investigations with a CT scan or a barium enema may be indicated to confirm the diagnosis.
- When the patient presents with a poor urinary stream, a palpable bladder and an enlarged prostate felt on rectal examination indicate bladder outflow obstruction. An USS and urodynamic studies are indicated to confirm the diagnosis and measurement of the creatinine and electrolytes to assess severity.
- A deep-seated knee pain and tenderness on one side of the joint line aggravated or precipitated by bending and straightening the knee joint both with and without rotational torque indicates a meniscal injury. An MRI or an arthroscopy will confirm the diagnosis.

Deformity, a structural abnormality, may be genetic or acquired. An acquired deformity may be caused by a neurological problem, such as a brachial plexus injury or chronic inflammation, such as ulnar deviation of the fingers at the metacarpophalangeal joints and "swan-neck" deformity of the fingers from chronic rheumatoid arthritis or phimosis from chronic balanitis.

When the type of problem is uncertain:

Ask yourself, could it be cancer and how should it be managed?

Cancer should be considered when there is a visible or palpable mass with the following characteristic features:

- A naevus or discoloured nodule may be a melanoma. Excision may be indicated to treat the problem and confirm the diagnosis.
- A small ulcer with raised irregular margins is likely to be an SCC or BCC. Excision may be indicated to treat the problem and confirm the diagnosis.
- "Peau d'orange" or nipple retraction in the breast may be caused by breast cancer. An urgent mammogram and biopsy of a mass may be indicated to confirm the diagnosis and plan treatment.
- A persistently hard or firm solitary deep-seated mass with irregular margins or feeling tethered. The location of the mass will indicate a likely cause.
  - o A palpable mass arising from the soft tissue or bone may be a sarcoma.
  - o A mass arising from the breast, salivary or thyroid glands or within the abdomen is likely to be an adenocarcinoma.
  - o A mass in a lymph node region is likely to be a primary lymphoma or secondary to a cancer elsewhere.

- An umbilical mass may be a "Sister Mary Joseph" nodule.
  A biopsy of the mass and a CT or MRI scan may be indicated to confirm the diagnosis and plan treatment.

The absence of a visible or palpable mass or naevus excludes a superficial cancer but not a deep-seated cancer. A deep-seated cancer usually presents with pain or deranged function and symptoms of a structural type of problem. Occasionally, it may present as a circulatory problem, such as emboli from an atrial myxoma, an inflammatory problem, such as when cancer causes a chest infection, a metabolic problem, such as hypercalcaemia caused by bone metastases, or a neurological problem, such as from a spinal cancer. Information about the person and the patient may indicate the increased probability of cancer. For example:

- Cancer is more likely in the elderly.
- Some occupations are associated with an increased risk of cancer.
- A patient who has previously been treated for cancer or is undergoing treatment may develop a recurrence or a metastasis.
- Chronic disease or radiotherapy many years previously increases the risk of cancer.

Cancer should be considered in the differential diagnosis when, there are associated signs of sarcopaenia, lymphadenopathy, hepatomegaly, ascites or an unexplained pleural effusion. When cancer is suspected, but the primary site is uncertain, proactively examine the sites of the common cancers. For example:

- Examine the chest for a localized wheeze, an area of consolidation or a pleural effusion.
- Examine the breasts in a female looking for an inverted nipple, peau d'orange or a mass.
- Examine the abdomen carefully to feel for a mass, organomegaly or ascites. Abdominal cancers need to be large and the patient thin to be felt.
- Perform a rectal examination to feel for a rectal or pelvic mass.
- Examine the lymph nodes, for lymphadenopathy.
- Examine the skin for a lesion, such as a melanoma.

When cancer is suspected an imaging investigation, such as a CT scan may be indicated to confirm or exclude the diagnosis.

When the type of problem is uncertain:

Ask yourself, is it a circulatory type of problem and how should it be managed?

A circulatory problem should be considered when there is a visible or palpable abnormality with the following characteristics:

- A red or purple naevus, patch or nodule that blanches under pressure. For example, a strawberry naevus, spider naevus, haemangioma or telangiectasia. The diagnosis is clinical, based on the appearance, and investigations are not usually indicated.
- Multiple 2-3mm diameter slightly raised non-blanching blue-red spots are likely to be "Campbell de Morgan spots". The patient can be reassured.
- Multiple red or purple non-blanching spots, petechiae, may be caused by thrombocytopaenia. Measuring the FBC will exclude thrombocytopaenia or leukaemia.
- Multiple red or purple non-blanching patches may be bruising or purpura.
  - Multi-focal unexpected bruising may be caused by a clotting abnormality, such as von Willebrand disease or haemophilia and petechial haemorrhages by thrombocytopaenia. A FBC and clotting studies are initially indicated to confirm the diagnosis.
  - The differential diagnosis of purpura includes thrombocytopaenia, such as idiopathic thrombocytopaenia purpura, autoimmune conditions, such as lupus erythematosus or Henoch-Schoenlein purpura, or infection, such as meningococcal septicaemia. Blood tests may include an FBC, clotting and auto-antibody tests to help formulate a diagnosis.
- A pale digit, that feels cold is ischaemic. A black anaesthetic digit is dead. A Doppler USS and echocardiogram may be indicated to determine the cause.

- A firm pulsating mass in the region of a named artery or when an artery is "too easily felt", may be aneurysmal. The differential diagnosis includes an ectatic artery or a mass closely associated with the artery. A Doppler USS may be indicated to confirm the diagnosis.
- A soft compressible mass in the region of a named vein may be a varicosity. A Doppler USS may be indicated to confirm the diagnosis.
- When there is a widespread change in skin texture.
  - o Smooth indentable subcutaneous swelling of the lower limbs, or of the lower back when the patient is confined to bed, is likely to be due to peripheral oedema. Heart failure is likely when there are associated signs of a raised JVP, basal pulmonary crepitations and an enlarged heart. Standard blood tests, an ECG and an echocardiogram may be indicated to confirm the diagnosis.
  - o Firm non-indentable subcutaneous swelling of a limb is likely to be due to be lymphoedema. Learning about the patient will indicate when it is likely to be secondary to a known problem, such as a previous axillary lymphadenectomy. The patient should be examined for a proximal mass. A CT scan may be indicated to confirm the diagnosis.
- When there is a widespread change in skin colour.
  - o Global pallor, including pallor affecting the conjunctiva, may be indicative of anaemia. The FBC should be measured to confirm the diagnosis.
  - o Single limb pallor may be indicative of ischaemia. The limb is likely to be cool with venous guttering and absent named pulses. Buerger's test is likely to be positive. Weak or absent named arteries and/or a bruit are characteristic of occlusive vascular disease. An enlarged expansile mass or easily palpable named arteries may be aneurysmal. Splinter haemorrhages, an arrythmia and/or a heart murmur may indicate emboli. Standard blood tests, an ECG, echocardiogram, Doppler USS or CT angiogram may be indicated to confirm the diagnosis.
  - o Single limb cyanosis may be indicative of superficial venous congestion, likely to be caused by deep vein thrombosis. A Doppler USS may be indicated to confirm the diagnosis.
  - o Peripheral cyanosis, particularly obvious in the fingers or, central cyanosis, around the mouth, is likely to be caused by hypoxia. Arterial blood gas measurement may be indicated to confirm hypoxia.
- When there is a widespread deep-seated tenderness affecting a large muscle or muscle group.
  - o When the calf is tender and swollen, and Homan's test positive a DVT is likely. A Doppler USS may be indicated to confirm the diagnosis.
  - o When a large muscle is very tender and swollen, and active or passive movement painful following trauma, compartment syndrome is likely. Measurement of compartment pressures may be indicated to confirm and monitor the pressures.

The absence of a visible or palpable peripheral abnormality makes significant peripheral vascular disease unlikely. When a patient presents with pain, deranged function or feeling ill the symptoms usually indicate when the problem is likely to be caused by a circulatory problem. This will inform the local signs to look for. Information about the person and the patient may inform the probability of a circulatory type of problem and a likely cause. For example:
- Circulatory problems are more likely in the elderly.
- Obesity, hyperlipidaemia, hypertension and smoking are recognised risk factors for atherosclerosis causing occlusive arterial disease.
- Previous TIA's and AF would increase the likelihood of another embolic circulatory problem.
- Collagen disorders, such as Marfan's syndrome increase the risk of an aneurysm.

The pattern of local and associated signs should support the symptoms and distinguish between occlusive, embolic or aneurysmal peripheral vascular disease, cardiac disease and a blood abnormality. Usually, however, investigations are indicated to determine the likely cause. For example:

- When the patient presents with a headache or a blackout, associated with unilateral facial, arm and leg weakness (hemiparesis), a stroke affecting the contra-lateral motor cortex is likely. Associated hyper-reflexia and upgoing planters, a positive Babinski response and a lateral visual field deficiency (hemianopia) support the diagnosis. There may be associated circulatory signs such as and an arrythmia, a carotid artery bruit or a heart murmur. Imaging investigations, such as an Echocardiogram, Doppler USS and a CT scan may be indicated to confirm the diagnosis.

- When the patient presents with central or left sided chest or shoulder pain and the symptoms indicate angina, signs may be absent unless there is a complication, such as heart failure. A resting ECG or an exercise ECG may be indicated to confirm the diagnosis.
- When the patient presents with widespread abdominal pain and the differential diagnosis includes mesenteric ischaemia, abdominal signs may be absent apart from mild tenderness on deep palpation. A CT angiogram is indicated to confirm the diagnosis.
- When a patient presents with unilateral blindness, a cherry red spot on fundoscopy may indicate retinal artery occlusion. A retinal artery CT angiogram is indicated to confirm the diagnosis.
- When a patient presents feeling ill with fatigue and weakness likely to be caused by anaemia, there are likely to be circulatory signs, such as pallor, a fast but weak pulse, a low blood pressure and tachypnoea. A FBC may be indicated to confirm the diagnosis.

When a circulatory problem is suspected, but the cause is uncertain, pro-actively examine the heart and peripheral vascular system. An absence of signs does not exclude a circulatory type of problem and investigations may be indicated. For example:

- A patient who presents following a transient blackout may have completely recovered from a TIA. A CT scan may be indicated.
- Breathlessness in the absence of chest signs may be caused by a PE. A CT angiogram may be indicated.
- Abdominal pain, progressive anorexia, weight loss and diarrhoea without any abdominal signs may be caused by mesenteric ischaemia. A CT angiogram may be indicated.

When the symptoms and signs indicate a circulatory problem, a checklist may inform the signs to look for to determine the likely cause:

- Look for signs of heart disease, such as a murmur.
- Look for signs of emboli, such as splinter haemorrhages.
- Look for signs of arterial occlusion, such as weak pulse or a bruit.
- Look for signs of thrombosis, such as swelling and tenderness.

When the type of problem is uncertain:

Ask yourself, could it be a neurological type of problem and how should it be managed?

A neurological problem may present as a visible or palpable abnormality. For example:

- A fusiform mass along the line of a nerve may be a neuroma.
- A deformity. For example:
  o Muscle weakness or wasting may be caused by a neurological problem. For example, unilateral facial muscle weakness is characteristic of Bell's palsy. When there is associated loss of taste and a pain in the ear it is called Ramsay Hunt syndrome.
  o A unilateral small pupil, drooping or the upper eyelid and absent sweating on the side of the face in Horner's syndrome.
- Abnormal movements. For example:
  o Loss of balance and coordination following a stroke.
  o A tremor.
- Signs of superficial injury, such as burn marks.

When the patient presents with pain or deranged function information learnt about the problem indicates the signs to look for, and the pattern of signs is likely to be diagnostic. For example:

- When the differential diagnosis includes migraine, depression, bipolar disorders or schizophrenia, an examination of the neurological system is undertaken to exclude signs in the expectation that none will be found. Investigations are not usually indicated and treatment is specific to the diagnosis.

- When the differential diagnosis of the headache or deranged function includes raised ICP the signs to look for include hypertension, bradycardia and slow breathing (Cushing's triad) and swelling of the optic disc (papilloedema) on fundoscopy. If raised ICP is suspected an urgent CT head is indicated to confirm the diagnosis.
- When a patient presents with atypical pain, paraesthesia or anaesthesia the site affected should be examined to determine whether it corresponds to a dermatome, a peripheral nerve or nerve root and associated signs sought.
  - A localized or "solitary" atypical pain affecting the thumb, index and middle fingers aggravated by extreme flexion or extension of the hand at the wrist is likely to be carpal tunnel syndrome. On examination, there may be wasting of the muscles of the thenar eminence, paraesthesia or numbness in the lateral part of the hand, a positive Tinel's or Phalen's test and apposition of the thumb and index finger is weak. It is likely to be caused by median nerve entrapment as it passes through the carpal tunnel. Proximal signs indicate a more proximal abnormality, such as a cervical C7 nerve entrapment or a brachial plexus injury. Carpal tunnel syndrome is initially treated symptomatically with rest and anti-inflammatory medications. When the diagnosis is uncertain nerve conduction studies may be indicated.
  - A deep-seated ache in one buttock and spreading down the back of a leg, worse on standing up straight is likely to be "sciatica". On examination, pain and paraesthesia in the distribution of the L5 or the S1 nerve root, pain increased by straight leg raising, an absent ankle tendon reflex and weakness in the foot or great toe on dorsi-flexion support the diagnosis. The course of the sciatic nerve, and in particular the lower back and buttock regions should be examined for signs of tenderness and to exclude a mass. Sciatica is initially treated symptomatically with rest and anti-inflammatory medications. Referral to a physiotherapist may be indicated. When severe, an MRI spine may be indicated.
- When a patient presents with global weakness, the examination should confirm the pattern of weakness, look for muscle wasting and assess power and the reflexes. For example:
  - Global weakness, without muscle wasting, together with slurred speech and eye lids drooping, that increases with repetitive activity, indicates myasthenia gravis. Anti-acetylcholine receptor antibody level should be measured to confirm the diagnosis.
  - Increasing global weakness associated with profound muscle wasting and brisk reflexes may be caused by motor neurone disease. Electromyography (EMG) and nerve conduction studies may be indicated to confirm the diagnosis.
  - Global weakness, associated with poor coordination and absent tendon reflexes may be caused by acute inflammatory demyelinating polyradiculopathy (Guillain-Barré syndrome). A lumbar puncture and nerve conduction studies may be indicated to confirm the diagnosis.
- When a patient presents with abnormal movements, such as a tremor, an abnormal gait or balance this should be observed and relevant associated signs sought. For example:
  - A fine tremor is likely to be physiological, such as when it is caused by anxiety or old age. Reassurance and lifestyle changes may be indicated.
  - A "pill-rolling tremor" at rest is characteristic of Parkinson's disease. Associated signs include bradykinesia, "cogwheel" rigidity and a shuffling gait: "marche a petit pas". A CT PET scan may be indicated to confirm the diagnosis.
  - An "intention" tremor, occurring when trying to undertake a purposeful movement, is characteristic of cerebellar disease. Associated signs include nystagmus, poor balance and ataxia, uncoordinated movements and dysarthria. A CT scan may be indicated to exclude a cerebellar lesion.
- When the differential diagnosis of deranged function includes an autonomic abnormality, such as achalasia, gastroparesis, malabsorption, slow transit constipation, faecal or urinary incontinence, postural hypotension or erectile dysfunction signs of autonomic neuropathy should be sought. The symptoms determine the signs to look for. For example:
  - A large dull supra-pubic mass, likely to be an enlarged bladder, may be caused by a neuropathic bladder. Blood tests to screen for deranged homeostasis, an USS, a urinary catheter and urodynamic tests may be indicated.
  - A patulous weak anal sphincter may be caused by a neurological problem. A spinal MRI to exclude a spinal lesion may be indicated.
  - A slow pupil reaction to light and postural hypotension may be caused by autonomic neuropathy. Symptomatic treatment, such as graduated compression hosiery may be indicated.
  - Upper abdominal bloating and a succussion splash may be caused by gastroparesis. An OGD to exclude gastric outlet obstruction and gastric emptying studies may be indicated.

o Abdominal bloating and faecal loading may be caused by slow transit constipation. A colonoscopy to exclude obstruction and symptomatic or lifestyle measures may be indicated.

When there is co-morbidity, such as DM or hypertension, management includes both optimising treatment and symptomatic or lifestyle measures. Specialist investigations, such as the tilt-table test or the thermoregulatory sweat test are rarely indicated.

When the symptoms and signs indicate a neurological problem, the examination should also focus on trying to determine the likely cause. A checklist may inform the signs to look for. For example:

* Look for signs of a central neurological abnormality.
* Look for a possible cause of nerve entrapment.
* Look for a possible cause of nerve damage.
* Look for signs of inflammation.
* Look for a mass.

When the type of problem is uncertain:

Ask yourself, could it be a metabolic type of problem and how should it be managed?

Metabolic problems should be considered in any patient who presents feeling ill with non-specific symptoms such as fatigue, poor concentration, global weakness and a change in weight, or with symptoms of deranged function. Frequently, metabolic conditions are only considered when other types of problem are unlikely or when the results of blood tests are known.

Information about the person and the patient may inform the probability of a metabolic type of problem and a likely cause. For example:

* Metabolic problems are more likely in the elderly.
* Metabolic problems may be a complication of medications, particularly when patients are taking multiple medications (polypharmacy).
* Metabolic problems may be a complication an ongoing illness, such as DM, haemolysis, cirrhosis, congestive cardiac failure, diabetes insipidus or the nephrotic syndrome.
* Metabolic problems may be a consequence of an unusual diet, such as a vegan diet.

Associated symptoms and signs may indicate a likely diagnosis based on probabilities or when there is a classic diagnostic pattern. For example:

* Some metabolic problems present because of an obvious change in colour.
  o Jaundice, associated with feeling ill, tired, itching, dark urine, pale stools and a tendency to bruise easily indicates liver failure. The differential diagnosis of jaundice includes, biliary obstruction, parenchymal liver disease, Gilbert's syndrome and drugs, such as chlorpromazine, carbamazepine, erythromycin, or rifampicin, haemolysis, ineffective erythropoiesis, blood transfusion or resorption of a haematoma. The signs to look for include a malar flush, spider naevi, palmar erythema, a liver flap, peripheral oedema, scratch marks, bruising, ascites, a tender liver, hepatomegaly, splenomegaly, and a caput medusae. Blood should be sent to the laboratory for measurement of liver function tests, electrolytes, urea and creatinine and an FBC and a liver US performed to confirm the diagnosis and assess severity.
  o Unexplained dark bronze skin pigmentation associated with feeling ill, fatigue, a change in behaviour, weight loss, widespread myalgia and arthralgia are characteristic of Addison's disease. The signs to look for would include measuring the blood pressure and muscle power. Investigations would include measurement of blood electrolytes, cortisol and adrenocorticotropic hormone to confirm the diagnosis.
* Associated symptoms of weight loss, polyurea, a dry mouth and polydipsia may be caused by DM. The examination should include looking for signs of weight loss and global weakness and measuring the vital signs. If there is a loss of skin turgor, tachycardia, hypotension and tachypnoea with Kussmaul breathing and sweet-smelling breath diabetic keto-acidosis is likely. Blood glucose level should be measured urgently.
* Coarse facial features with a prominent brow, nose and lower jaw, and widely spaced teeth may be caused by acromegaly. The patient should be asked if their hands are so swollen that rings no longer fit or the feet so

swollen that shoes are too small. Investigations such as an oral glucose tolerance test and measuring the level of insulin-like growth factor may be indicated to formulate a diagnosis.

- Associated weight gain, hoarseness and constipation would indicate hypothyroidism. The signs to look for include a dry skin, a puffy face and abdominal bloating. The throat should be examined for a goitre. Blood should be tested for TSH and thyroid hormones to confirm the diagnosis and assess severity.

- When a patient presents with hyperactivity, irritability and agitation, or a change in personality or with diarrhoea, associated with weight loss and a tremor they may be thyrotoxic. The signs to look for include a tremor, twitching, increased sweating, weight loss, an arrythmia, hyper-reflexia, exophthalmos, lid lag and a goitre. When a patient presents with exophthalmos and ophthalmoplegia, Graves' disease is likely. Blood should be sent for measurement of thyroid hormones and antibodies to confirm the diagnosis. The FBC and serum creatinine, urea and electrolytes, calcium, magnesium and phosphate should also be measured to screen for a secondary problem.

- Associated weight gain and a change in personality may be caused by long-term steroid use or Cushing's syndrome. The patient should be asked if they have an irregular menstrual cycle, reduced libido and erectile dysfunction, delayed healing and bruise easily. The signs to look for include a "Moon face" and a "buffalo hump", hirsutism, with baldness and brittle hair, thin skin and pink/purple striae and hypertension. Blood tests to measure steroid levels to confirm the diagnosis and to screen for an asymptomatic electrolyte abnormality may be indicated.

- When a patient presents with peripheral muscle cramps associated with paraesthesia or palpitations, they may have hypocalcaemia. The signs to look for include, uncontrolled movements, such as a tremor, muscle fasciculation, paraesthesia, scratch marks, coarse hair, brittle nails and dry skin, Chvostek and Trousseau's signs, and an arrythmia. If hypocalcaemia is suspected blood should be sent to the laboratory for measurement of calcium, magnesium and phosphate concentration and acid-base measurement to confirm the diagnosis and assess severity. The FBC and serum creatinine, urea and electrolytes should also be measured to screen for a secondary problem.

- When a patient presents with breathlessness but chest and cardiac signs are absent, it may be caused by a metabolic problem such as acidosis or uraemia. A sallow dry skin, scratch marks, abdominal bloating and peripheral oedema may indicate renal failure. Blood should be sent for a FBC and measurement of serum creatinine, urea and electrolytes, acid-base and blood gases to confirm the diagnosis and assess severity.

Metabolic problems do not usually cause pain. Notable exceptions include hypercalcaemia, gout or porphyria.

- When a patient presents with atypical abdominal or bone pain, associated with a dry mouth, polydipsia and polyurea, nausea, vomiting and constipation or confusion. it may be caused by hypercalcaemia. There may be few signs. If hypercalcaemia is suspected blood should be sent to the laboratory for measurement of calcium, magnesium and phosphate concentration to confirm the diagnosis. When the calcium concentration is raised the blood parathyroid hormone level should be measured to determine the cause.

- A sudden attack of joint pain, usually multi-focal and restricting movement, is occasionally caused by gout. There are signs of inflammation with erythema, swelling and tenderness. Blood should be sent to measure urate levels and joint fluid sent to be examined for urate crystals to confirm the diagnosis.

- When a patient presents with attacks of severe atypical widespread pains, in the chest, abdomen and limbs, associated with behavioural change, nausea, vomiting or a change in bowel habit it may be caused by acute porphyria. There may be blisters and erythema on sun exposed areas, weakness, arrythmia and hypertension. Blood tests depend on the likely type of porphyria.

A metabolic problem may be a secondary problem. For example:

- Deranged water and electrolyte balance may be secondary to:
  o The presenting problem. For example, fever, vomiting, diarrhoea or sweating, or weight loss.
  o An abnormal diet.
  o An ongoing condition, such as DM.
  o Medications, such as diuretics or insulin.
  Deranged water and electrolyte balance may cause a patient to feel ill, with fatigue, irritability or confusion, muscle weakness, spasms or cramps, palpitations, a tremor, a headache or seizures. The signs to look for are loss of skin turgor, tachycardia, hypotension, an arrythmia, a low JVP, bilateral basal crepitations and peripheral

pitting oedema. The serum and urine osmolality, blood haematocrit and serum electrolytes should be measured confirm the diagnosis.

- Hypocalcaemia may be secondary to:
  o The presenting problem. For example, acute pancreatitis, sepsis, renal failure, Vitamin D deficiency.
  o An abnormal diet.
  o A previous treatment, such as thyroidectomy or parathyroidectomy.
  o An ongoing condition, such as Crohn's disease or small bowel diverticulosis.
  o Medications, such as diuretics or ant-epileptic medications.

Hypocalcaemia may cause a patient to feel ill, with myalgia. The signs to look for include, a tremor, muscle fasciculation, paraesthesia, scratch marks, coarse hair, brittle nails and dry skin, Chvostek and Trousseau's signs. The blood electrolytes, including calcium, magnesium and phosphate and LFTs should be measured to confirm the diagnosis and assess severity and the urea and creatinine to screen for renal dysfunction.

When a metabolic problem is suspected a battery of tests are indicated to screen for abnormal homeostasis and organ function, in addition to more specific tests indicated by the pattern of symptoms and signs. The standard tests include (Appendix 2):

- Measuring the FBC.
- Measuring blood clotting.
- Measuring serum electrolytes, sodium, potassium, calcium, magnesium and phosphate concentration and urea and creatinine.
- Measuring serum LFTs.
- Measuring pO_2, pCO_2, pH, base excess and lactate in the arterial blood to assess gas transfer and acid-base homeostasis.
- A 12 lead ECG.

While examining the site of the abnormality:

Ask yourself, how severe is the problem and how should it be managed?

Local signs of severity include:

- The size of a mass, an aneurysm or an ulcer.
- Tenderness.
- Local colour change, such as pallor or gangrene.
- The extent of a wound, cellulitis or a burn.
- The range of movement of a joint.
- Leg length or circumference.
- Limb, joint or abdominal girth.
- The extent of a deformity, such as leg length or scoliosis.
- Visual acuity or hearing.
- The involvement of important nearby structures. For example:
  o When cellulitis involves or is close to a susceptible part of the body, such as the eye or a prosthesis, such as a pacemaker.
  o When a cancer is close to an organ, such as the eye, or a structure, such as a named blood vessel or nerve.
- Future risk may be a measure of severity. For example, when an infection is close to a prosthesis.

When a sign is measurable it is objective so is a reproducible measure of severity that can be reliably used to assess change. other signs are subjective and could be influenced by other variables and lack reproducibility. For example:

- The size of a deep-seated swelling or fullness, or the internal depth of a mass is subjective when the deep margins are difficult to feel.
- Tenderness is subjective, because, as with an assessment of pain it is affected by many variables. A visual analogue score when the site is palpated: 0 = no tenderness to 10 = exquisitely tender may help increase the objectivity.

351

When a sign is subjective, severity is usually described. For example, "pale" appearance, "poor" air entry, a "weak" pulse, "mild" tenderness, "weak" power, or a "loud" bruit.

Some diagnoses should always be considered severe. For example:

- Severe pain and tenderness, signs of cellulitis with blue/purple or black patches indicating necrotizing fasciitis or Fournier's gangrene in the scrotum. Urgent treatment with intravenous antibiotics, a CT scan and surgical debridement may be indicated.
- A swollen leg with tender calf muscles is likely to be caused by a DVT. Bursting calf pain on walking and a cyanosed and swollen limb with prominent superficial veins and deep calf tenderness indicates "phlegmasia caerulea dolens" caused by extensive deep venous thrombosis; a severe local problem with a risk of venous infarction. Urgent venous imaging, with, for example, an USS or a venogram, is indicated to confirm the diagnosis and assess severity and anticoagulation to reduce the risk of deterioration.
- Claudication on walking is characteristic of an ischaemic limb. A pale limb with venous guttering, weak or absent arterial pulses and a positive Buerger's test would support the diagnosis. When the limb is cold, the calf muscles tender or there is peripheral numbness or paraesthesia, the diagnosis is critical limb ischaemia and the limb is at risk of becoming gangrenous if untreated or developing the complication of a compartment syndrome when treated. Additional questions should be asked to exclude symptoms of "rest pain". A critically ischaemic limb should be managed as a medical emergency.
- In an at-risk patient, such as following a limb crush injury or a burn, severe pain, swelling and tenderness in a muscle aggravated by active or passive movement may indicate compartment syndrome. Compartment syndrome should be managed as a medical emergency. Urgent decompression may be indicated.

When there are signs of a local complication the problem is likely to be severe. For example:

- An irreducible inguinal hernia becoming tender or being associated with signs of small bowel obstruction or ischaemia. Urgent referral to a surgeon is indicated.
- Ulceration complicating varicose eczema. Treatment of the varicose veins should be reviewed and the ulcer dressed.
- Infection of an ischaemic foot. Antimicrobial treatment should be started urgently and referral to a vascular surgeon considered.
- When the patient presents with a pulsatile midline abdominal swelling likely to be a AAA it is likely to be severe when:
  o It is tender.
  o There is back pain.
  o Absent lower limb pulses indicating the AAA is complicated by downstream peripheral vascular disease, thrombosis or an occluding intimal flap.
  o Splinter haemorrhages or ischaemic toes indicating the AAA is complicated by downstream emboli.
  It may be appropriate to refer the patient urgently to a vascular surgeon.

The severity assessment should also include an assessment of risk of a future problem. For example:

- The risk of a mole or in-situ dysplasia becoming cancer. A specialist opinion may be indicated.
- The risk of cancer developing when there is carcinoma-in-situ, such as anal intraepithelial neoplasia. Referral to a colo-proctologist may be indicated.
- The likelihood of an aneurysm rupturing. Serial scans are likely to indicate the rate of change and predict the risk of rupture.
- The risk of a hernia obstructing. Femoral hernia and irreducible hernia are at increased risk of obstruction.
- A young patient with a tender testicle, likely to be caused by torsion, is at risk of testicular infarction. Emergency referral to a urologist is indicated.

Local severity may inform:

- The choice of investigation. For example, anal stenosis is a relative contraindication for a colonoscopy.

- Whether to treat or not and the choice of treatment. For example, a soft subcutaneous smooth, well-defined non-tender swelling likely to be a lipoma is often left untreated or removed under a local anaesthetic. When the lipoma is deep-seated, close to important structures or the diagnosis is uncertain investigations may be indicated prior to excision under a general anaesthetic.
- Management priority. For example, when a patient is very breathless from a suspected PE, a CT angiogram is indicated, rather than wait for a ventilation-perfusion scan.

Occasionally, the local severity assessment will inform the diagnosis. For example:

- The severity of the pain, tenderness and the local signs will distinguish between cellulitis, an abscess and necrotizing fasciitis. Necrotizing fasciitis is a life-threatening emergency.
- Right upper abdominal colic may be severe, but the abdominal tenderness mild indicating biliary colic. Mild right upper abdominal pain with "severe" tenderness is likely to be cholecystitis. When a tender mass is palpable, the diagnosis includes an empyema or localized perforation. An empyema or perforation is a serious problem to be managed urgently.

Severity not only refers to the severity of the problem locally but also to the impact on the patient. Information about the person, the patient, the problem and from an examination of the site of the problem may indicate the need to examine the patient to look for associated or systemic signs.

While examining the site of the abnormality:

Ask yourself, what associated or systemic signs are likely?

Usually, the symptoms will indicate whether or not associated or systemic signs are likely. In addition, while examining the site of the problem consider whether an examination to look for associate or systemic signs is indicated and determine the aims. The aims may include formulating or confirming a diagnosis, determining the likely cause or to inform management. The aims and nature of the problem will determine the signs to look for. For example:

- To formulate a diagnosis. For example, when a patient presents with a fusiform firm swelling, likely to be a neuroma, look for other swellings elsewhere and café au lait spots to diagnose neurofibromatosis.
- To confirm a diagnosis. For example, when a patient presents with unilateral signs of weakness, look for associated signs including, hyper-reflexia and upgoing planters, a positive Babinski response and a lateral visual field deficiency (hemianopia).
- To determine a likely cause. For example, when a patient is jaundiced, look for signs that will indicate a likely cause, such as:
  o Pallor, a tachycardia and splenomegaly indicting haemolytic anaemia.
  o A liver flap, spider naevi, palmar erythema hepatomegaly, ascites and a caput medusae indicating liver cirrhosis.
  o A pyrexia, tachycardia, and tender hepatomegaly indicating hepatitis.
- To assess severity. For example, when a patient has a breast lump, look for signs of cancer, such as supra-clavicular or axillary lymphadenopathy, a pleural effusion and hepatomegaly indicating metastatic spread.
- To determine the likely location of the abnormality. For example, when a male patient presents with a palpable bladder, examine the back and perform a rectal examination to palpate the prostate and check anal sphincter tone and contraction and perineal sensation to identify a possible cause.
- To plan management. For example, when an operation is the treatment of choice it may be appropriate to examine the chest and peripheral vascular system to assess fitness for an anaesthetic.

Examine the Patient for Associated Signs

Information about the person, the problem, the patient and from an examination of the site of the problem/abnormality will indicate the associated signs to look for. For example:

- When a patient presents with breathlessness and anaemia is suspected, look for pallor and tachypnoea and palpate the pulse for a tachycardia.

- When heart failure is suspected, look for a raised JVP, basal crepitations, an enlarged heart and peripheral oedema.
- When a patient presents with petechial haemorrhages and a coagulopathy is suspected, look for bruising and for signs of hepato-splenomegaly.

Before examining the patient to look for associated signs it is good practice to explain to the patient why you want to examine elsewhere and to check that they give their consent. Usually, the aims of examining the patient for associated signs are to look for signs to complete a diagnostic pattern or to exclude a diagnosis, to determine the location of the abnormality or the type of problem, to assess severity and to plan management. Occasionally, it is appropriate to look for associated signs to inform management. In summary, associated signs may influence:

- The diagnosis.
- The likely location of the abnormality or the type of problem.
- An assessment of severity.
- The management plan:
  o The priority.
  o The choice of investigation.
  o The choice of treatment.
  o The timing of a follow up consultation.

While examining the patient for associated signs, ask yourself:

What is the likely diagnosis or the differential diagnosis?

When the diagnosis is uncertain, ask yourself:

What is the location of the abnormality?
What is the type of problem?

Throughout the examination, ask yourself:

How severe is the problem?
What is the management plan?

While examining the patient:

Ask yourself, what is the likely diagnosis and how should it be managed?

The pattern of symptoms, local and associated signs may be diagnostic. This will then inform management. For example:

- When a patient presents with skin rash likely to be caused by an auto-immune problem:
  o Associated tender swollen muscles is characteristic of dermatomyositis.
  o Associated small tender sub-cutaneous nodules is characteristic of polyarteritis nodosum.
  o Associated mouth ulcers, Raynaud's syndrome and joint swelling is characteristic of systemic lupus erythematosus.
  o A skin biopsy of the rash may be indicated to confirm the diagnosis.
- Associated pruritus, swollen eyes, lips, tongue or face, breathlessness, a wheeze, a cough and constricted throat, watery eyes, a runny nose and a sore throat and a tachycardia are characteristic of a hypersensitivity reaction. Removing or stopping the antigen and treatment with an antihistamine or a steroid are indicated.
- When a patient presents with jaundice, associated with itching, dark urine and pale stools indicating "obstructive" jaundice, it is likely to be caused by choledocholithiasis. On examination.
  o Upper abdominal tenderness and an absence of other signs would indicate choledocholithiasis.
  o Associated spider naevi, palmar erythema, a liver flap, peripheral oedema, ascites and a caput medusae would indicate alcoholic liver cirrhosis.

o   Tender hepatomegaly and a fever would indicate the jaundice may be caused by hepatitis or choledocholithiasis is complicated by infection: ascending cholangitis.

o   A well-defined non-tender palpable sub-hepatic mass may be a palpable gallbladder (Courvoisier's sign) caused by cancer obstructing the common bile duct. There is likely to be associated weight loss and may be ascites or lymphadenopathy.

Blood tests to measure the LFTs, viral titres and an upper abdominal USS may be indicated.

The more complete the clinical picture, the greater the likelihood the diagnosis is true, and conversely, although an absent associated sign does not exclude a diagnosis, it may signpost that other diagnoses should be considered again. For example:

*   When a patient presents with breathlessness, likely to be caused by heart failure, local signs of bilateral basal crepitations and basal dullness associated with a raised JVP, an enlarged heart and pitting oedema of the lower limbs would support the descriptive diagnosis. The diagnosis becomes more likely when there are symptoms or signs to indicate a likely cause. For example:
    o   A heart murmur may indicate an abnormal heart valve is the likely cause of the heart failure. The nature of the murmur will indicate the likely valvular abnormality.
    o   Hypertension, absent or weak peripheral pulses and bruit may indicate atherosclerotic disease of the arteries.
    o   A rubbing or squeaking sound in time with each heart-beat, particularly on leaning forward is characteristic of pericarditis.
    o   The absence of cardiac symptoms and pitting oedema would suggest a primary pulmonary problem may be possible. Breathlessness and pitting oedema without any cardiovascular signs would suggest hypalbuminaemia.

    Blood tests, a CXR to assess the lungs and heart, an ECG to exclude an electrical abnormality, an echocardiogram to assess cardiac structure or an angiogram to assess the arterial circulation may be indicated to confirm the diagnosis and assess severity.
*   When the patient presents with an acute headache, it is likely to be caused by stress or migraine.
    o   Associated signs, such as unilateral weakness, a visual field deficiency and swelling of the optic disc (papilloedema) on fundoscopy, slurred speech, hypertension, bradycardia and slow breathing (Cushing's triad) would indicate raised ICP, likely to be caused by a structural intracranial abnormality. The absence of signs of Cushing's triad would not exclude a raised ICP.
    o   Associated neck and spinal pain, aggravated by spinal movement would raise concern it could be meningitis. Meningitis becomes more likely if there are signs of a fever, associated papilloedema, a mild weakness or abnormal sensation, or a purpuric rash: signs that may only be found if specifically sought. An absence of these signs does not exclude the diagnosis.

    Careful and early review or a CT scan may be indicated to formulate a diagnosis.
*   When the patient presents with a tremor, it may be caused by Parkinson's disease, particularly if it appears to be a "pill rolling" tremor. Associated signs of bradykinesia, impaired balance and coordination, "cogwheel" rigidity and muscle stiffness are diagnostic. However, if these signs are absent, Parkinson's disease has not been excluded but other diagnoses should be considered, such as a physiological tremor, hyperthyroidism or hypercalcaemia, drug or alcohol abuse/withdrawal or an intention tremor due to a cerebellar abnormality. It may be appropriate to ask specific questions and look for other associated signs.

    Screening blood tests may be indicated.

Occasionally, when a diagnosis is unlikely, but is common or important, it may be appropriate to examine the patient for associated signs to ensure the diagnosis has been excluded. For example:

*   When the symptoms and signs indicate breathlessness is caused by a primary pulmonary problem, such as a chest infection, examining for associated cardiovascular signs may be indicated to confidently exclude a cardiac abnormality. A CXR may be indicated.
*   When a patient presents because they are passing small volumes of urine likely to be caused by bladder outflow obstruction a palpable dull symmetrical suprapubic mass arising from pelvis is likely to be a very full bladder caused by chronic urinary retention. On rectal examination an enlarged prostate would indicate a likely cause.

Nevertheless, it may be appropriate to exclude associated signs of autonomic neuropathy or a spinal problem. Urodynamic studies may be indicated.

- When the symptoms indicate groin and upper thigh pain is caused by a hip problem, the hip is examined first. It may be appropriate to examine the back or contralateral hip to exclude a problem elsewhere or other joints to exclude a multifocal abnormality, such as rheumatoid arthritis or juvenile arthritis. An Xray may be indicated.

- When a patient presents with elbow pain aggravated by making a fist or gripping an object such as a door handle, pain and tenderness centred on the lateral epicondyle of the humerus and aggravated by extending the hand at the wrist against resistance would support the diagnosis of "tennis elbow". The examination should also be used to exclude medial epicondylitis, radial tunnel syndrome, inflammatory or degenerative arthritis or biceps or triceps tendinitis. Topical anti-inflammatory medication, rest, splinting and physiotherapy may be indicated.

Ask yourself, what is the likely location of the abnormality and how should it be managed?

Associated signs may help determine the location of the abnormality causing the problem. This information, together with information about the person, the problem, the patient and the local signs will inform management. Although most problems are caused by an abnormality at the index site, when the differential diagnosis includes a condition that may be caused by an abnormality elsewhere it may be appropriate to examine for relevant associated signs. For example:

- When a patient presents with a marble sized non-tender jugulo-digastric mass likely to be caused by an enlarged lymph node, it may be caused by primary abnormality, such as lymphoma, but it is more likely to be secondary to, for example, infection or a cancer elsewhere.
  - o If the swelling is tender and has been present for a few days and the patient has recently had a sore throat and the neck has felt uncomfortable it is likely to be an inflamed, reactive, lymph node secondary to a throat infection. It would then be appropriate to examine the mouth, head and neck for an infection.
  - o If the swelling is minimally tender, has been persistent and increasing in size for several weeks and the patient denies having had a recent infection, it may be cancer. Nearby parts of the body, such as the face, mouth, head and neck should be examined looking for an abnormality. Other lymph node regions, including the neck, axillae, groins, liver and spleen, should be examined to determine whether it is part of a multi-focal problem, such as metastatic disease from a primary elsewhere. The absence of signs elsewhere does not exclude a primary elsewhere and imaging investigations may be indicated.
- When a patient presents with a black toe, it is obviously ischaemic. It is likely to be secondary to an embolus or occlusive peripheral vascular disease elsewhere. The rest of the cardio-vascular system should be examined.
  - o Splinter haemorrhages may be caused by multiple emboli. A murmur, a bruit or a proximal aneurysm may indicate a source of emboli. An echocardiogram and a Doppler USS may be indicated.
  - o Hypertension, absent or weak named pulses or a bruit would indicate occlusive vascular disease. A Doppler USS may be indicated.

  The absence of signs elsewhere does not exclude vascular disease.
- When a patient presents with thoraco-lumbar back pain, likely to be referred from a retro-peritoneal abnormality, abnormal signs, such as a mass or tenderness in the back are unlikely. Abdominal examination may reveal deep-seated epigastric tenderness, such as from pancreatitis or a posterior duodenal ulcer. A fusiform pulsatile expansile midline mass is likely to be an AAA. Imaging with a CT scan may be indicated.

When the problem is likely to be caused by an abnormality elsewhere, such as a circulatory or neurological problem, the associated signs may indicate the likely location of the abnormality. For example:

- When a patient presents with symptoms and signs of an ischaemic limb, the signs are likely to indicate the location of the occlusion. As a rule, the occlusion is distal to the most distal palpable arterial pulse. For example, pulses absent beyond a palpable common femoral artery pulse indicates superficial femoral artery occlusion or pulses absent beyond the aorta indicate aorto-iliac artery occlusion. A bruit may indicate the site of a stricture. Imaging with a Doppler USS or angiogram may be indicated.
- When a patient presents feeling breathless and chest signs are absent, associated signs of:
  - o Pallor, pale conjunctiva and tongue and a weak fast pulse and low blood pressure would indicate anaemia. An FBC is indicated.

o   Sallow sweaty skin, loss of skin turgor, a weak fast pulse, low blood pressure and peripheral oedema would indicate renal failure. Blood tests are indicated to confirm the diagnosis, exclude anaemia and assess homeostasis.

o   Laboured breathing and sweet-smelling breath would indicate diabetic ketoacidosis. The blood glucose should be measured urgently to confirm the diagnosis and blood tests are indicated to assess homeostasis and exclude a secondary abnormality.

o   Associated swelling and tenderness in a calf would indicate a likely PE caused by an embolus from a DVT. Anticoagulation should be started while awaiting the result of blood tests including an arterial blood gas measurement and a CT PA to assess severity and confirm the diagnosis.

- When a patient presents with atypical pain, paraesthesia or anaesthesia in the distribution of innervation by a named peripheral nerve, associated signs, such as a mass, inflammation or scarring proximally, along the line of the afferent nerve, would indicate a location for the abnormality. When the distribution corresponds to a dermatome, deep-seated tenderness in the region of the dorsal root, spinal deformity or limited movement of the spine would support the likely location of the abnormality.

Ask yourself, what is the likely type of problem and how should it be managed?

When the diagnosis is uncertain, associated signs may help distinguish between different types of problem (Figure 69).

Figure 69: Illustrating the questions to ask yourself when the type of problem is uncertain.

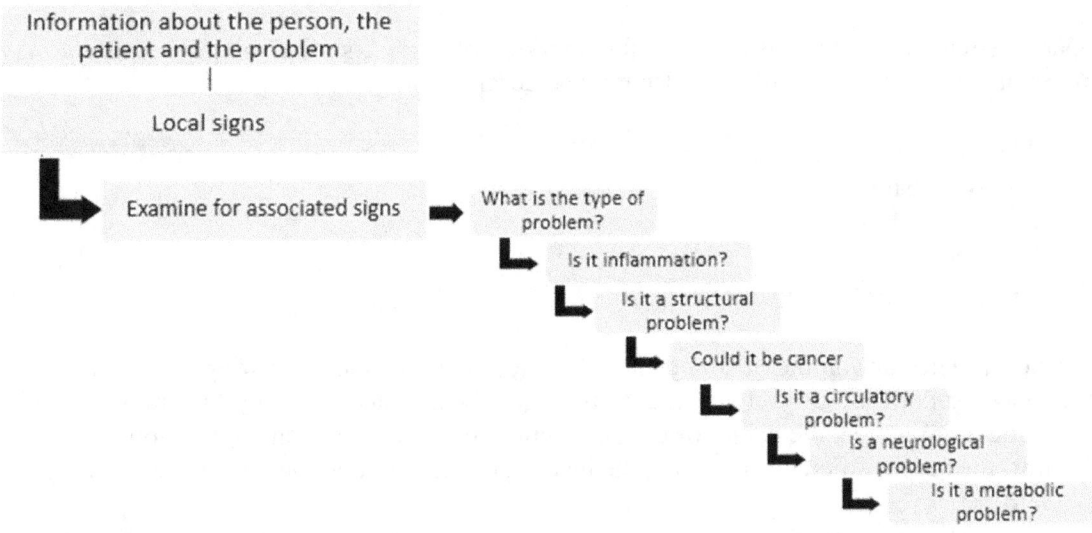

Information about the problem and from an examination of the location of the problem will indicate the signs to look for. For example:

- Generalized abdominal pain and tenderness is likely to be caused by a perforated appendicitis, diverticulitis, peptic ulcer or acute pancreatitis. However, if mesenteric ischaemia is likely, there may be associated signs, such as a heart murmur, weak peripheral pulses and bruits, or splinter haemorrhages. A CT scan is usually indicated to formulate a diagnosis.

- A headache is likely to be caused by a neurological problem, such as a tension headache or migraine. However, it may be caused by a structural problem, such as a meningioma, a circulatory problem, such as an AV malformation or a haemorrhage or inflammation, such as encephalitis if there are associated neurological signs, such as weakness or paraesthesia. Signs of a fever would support an infective inflammatory problem.

Ask yourself, how severe is the problem and how should it be managed?

Associated signs inform not only the diagnosis but also the severity assessment, i.e. the impact on the patient. Occasionally associated signs are specifically sought to assess severity. Associated signs that may be used to assess the impact on the patient include:

- Observing the patient may be a proxy severity assessment. For example:
  o When a patient cannot finish a sentence due to their breathlessness, it is severe.
  o When a patient cannot be distracted from their pain, it is likely to be severe.
  o A patient with colic who is bent double or continuously moves around trying to find a comfortable position and is grimacing and sweating has severe pain.
  o When a patient avoids or refuses to use a part of the body, the problem is likely to be severe. For example, a child with a forearm fracture.
  o When the patient can only walk a short distance before stopping to rest due to the pain, such as claudication or angina or is unable to walk properly because of the pain, an antalgic gait, the problem is severe.
- Measuring the JVP or the cardiac apex may be used as a measure of the severity of heart failure.
- Tachypnoea may be used to assess the severity of a primary pulmonary problem as well as an assessment of the systemic impact on the patient.

Measurable signs, such as respiratory rate or heart rate, are objective, so are reproducible measures of severity. They can be reliably used to assess change. However, many signs are subjective, and are influenced by many variables. Therefore, inter-observer or over-time variability is likely and the sign lacks reproducibility. For example:

- The apparent strength of a pulse is an unreliable measure of cardiac stroke volume because it may be affected by many variables. The strength of the pulse may be described as:

  0   = Absent
  1   = Barely palpable
  2   = Easily palpable
  3   = Full
  4   = Aneurysmal or bounding

- The presence/absence or volume of sounds heard on auscultation, such as during ventilation, a heart murmur, a bruit or bowel sounds are subjective because they may be affected by many factors including the timing or duration of the examination, the nature of the obstruction, the size of the lumen, the flow velocity, the patient's body habitus, the quality of the stethoscope, the hearing of the examiner and extrinsic noise.
- Percussion to assess resonance is subjective.
- The assessment of power is subjective except when normal or profoundly reduced. An assessment using a scale of 0 = no contraction to 5 = normal power is affected by many factors, including the motivation of the patient, the circumstances and the opinion of the examiner.

The clinical significance of signs to assess severity is increased when signs are considered together. For example:

- Measuring the height and weight and calculating the body mass index (BMI) or calculating the lean body mass (body weight minus body fat) using a formula, such as the Boer formula, the James Formula or the Hume Formula to assess the severity of anorexia or obesity.
- When bleeding is suspected the patient should be examined both to diagnose bleeding when occult, and to assess severity. When the patient appears ill, confused and drowsy, peripherally cold and sweaty, with a tachycardia, hypotension and tachypnoea blood loss is likely to be severe: >1L.
- The respiratory rate in a breathless patient assesses severity locally, at the index site, whereas the use of accessory muscles of respiration, impaired concentration, drowsiness, a tachycardia and cyanosis are associated signs indicating severity. A severely breathless patient should be managed as a medical emergency.
- Breathlessness due to bronchospasm is likely to be severe when there is tachypnoea, RR >20 breaths/minute, associated with a quiet generalised wheeze and breathing is strenuous and expiration is forced using accessory muscles of respiration. Associated signs of impaired concentration, drowsiness, fatigue, a tachycardia,

hypotension and cyanosis indicate hypoxia. Bronchodilators and humidified oxygen may be indicated while awaiting the results of an ABG to assess the impact on gas transfer and acid-base balance, blood tests to exclude anaemia and screen for deranged homeostasis and a CXR to exclude a chest abnormality.

- When a raised ICP is suspected, the patient should be examined both to diagnose a raised ICP and to assess severity. When the patient appears ill, confused and drowsy, hypertensive BP >160/100, the pulse slow, HR <60bpm, with a widened pulse pressure, the breathing slow, RR < 8/min, and irregular with periods of rapid breathing followed by absent breathing (Blot's respiration), papilloedema is present ("Cushing's triad") severe ICP is likely and the patient should be managed as a medical emergency. An urgent CT scan may be indicated to confirm the diagnosis.
- When there is mass, likely to be caused by cancer, looking for associated signs of sarcopaenia, lymphadenopathy, hepatomegaly, ascites or a pleural effusion can indicate "severity", i.e., metastatic spread. A CT scan may be indicated to confirm the diagnosis and stage the cancer.
- When a patient has cardio-vascular disease, impalpable or weak named arterial pulses and a bruit elsewhere indicate widespread disease, a measure of severity. A Doppler USS or angiogram may be indicated to confirm the diagnosis.
- Determining the Glasgow coma score to assess the level of consciousness. An urgent CT scan may be indicated to formulate a diagnosis.

For some problems the signs together with the results of investigations inform a severity assessment score. For example:

- Heart failure score to estimate severity and the risk of death.
- CURB (Confusion, Urea, Respiratory rate, Blood pressure) score to estimate the risk of death from infection.
- Pneumonia severity index to estimate the morbidity and mortality risk.

Occasionally, associated signs are sought to look for a secondary problem or a complication. For example:

- When a patient has reflux oesophagitis and waterbrash, an associated wheeze may indicate occasional aspiration.
- When a patient has varicose veins, there may be signs of lipo-dermatosclerosis above the medial malleolus.
- When a patient has had rheumatic fever or septicaemia, there may be a new murmur indicating endocarditis.

When examining the site of the problem, the local signs, the likely diagnosis or possible diagnoses, the severity assessment or management options may indicate the need to look for systemic signs.

Examine the Patient for Systemic Signs

Information about the person, the patient or the problem, or from examining the site of the problem or the associated signs will indicate whether the patient should be examined for systemic signs and what signs to look for. For most patients, the aim of examining the patient for systemic signs is to assess the impact the problem is having on the patient, i.e., severity, and to inform management. Occasionally, systemic signs will inform the type of problem and the diagnosis.

Examining and measuring systemic signs is not always indicated. However, a decision not to examine, measure and record systemic signs should be a deliberate decision because, sometimes appearances are misleading so that, although the patient may appear well, they are not, and the systemic signs may be abnormal. In addition, measuring and recording systemic signs may be of value as a baseline for comparison in the future even when they are not relevant to the current problem. Before examining the patient to look for systemic signs it is good practice to explain to the patient why you want to examine them and to check they give their consent.

A systemic examination usually starts with the global assessment of the patient and then the vital signs are measured.

- Look at the patient. Ask yourself:

    Do they look ill?
    Are they flushed, pale, cyanosed or "grey"?
    Do they appear sweaty?

Are they breathless or struggling to breathe?
Have they lost weight?

When a patient is systemically ill, they may have a "grey" complexion with sunken eyes, dry lips and tongue. The cheeks may be flushed, breathing rapid and shallow. They may be peripherally cold and slightly sweaty. They may have a hunched appearance with evidence of weight loss and muscle wasting.

- Assess their higher brain function and behaviour. Ask yourself:

Do they respond normally to questions?
Do they appear drowsy, lethargic, listless or apathetic?
Are they confused or disorientated?
Is their recall normal?
Can they think logically and make appropriate decisions?

When a patient is systemically ill, there may be a change in their behaviour or functional performance. They may appear listless and lack energy, become apathetic and disinterested, and work and everyday tasks become difficult. There is a change in their thought processes and conversation. Thinking, decision making and response times become slow, conversation may be confused or monosyllabic.

- Measure the vital signs. Although the reference range for most vital signs is influenced by age, gender, height, weight and fitness, a patient is severely ill when the vital signs deviate significantly from the reference range.
  - o Measure the core body temperature.
    - Oral temperature reference range: 35.7-37.4°C
    - Tympanic temperature reference range: 35.6-37.6°C
    - Axillary temperature reference range: 35-37°C
    - Rectal temperature reference range: 36.3-37.8°C
  - o Feel the pulse to measure the heart rate and to assess the rhythm and strength.
    - A normal resting heart rate is 60-80 beats per minute (bpm). In general tachycardia is when the heart rate is persistently >100bpm at rest and a bradycardia when it is <50 bpm.
    - A normal pulse has a regular rhythm. There are many causes of an irregular rhythm including, ectopic beats or AF.
    - A normal pulse can be felt with mild pressure on the artery.
    - When it is difficult to feel it may signify a narrow pulse pressure caused by a low cardiac output or an arrythmia, such as AF.
    - When it is very strong it may be bounding due to increased cardiac output, such as following exercise, anaemia or thyrotoxicosis, or due to low peripheral resistance caused by fever.
    - The apparent strength of a pulse is an unreliable measure of cardiac stroke volume because it may be affected by many factors including, skin thickness, arterial vessel depth and size, wall calcification and the sensitivity of the examiner's fingers.
  - o Measure the BP. The reference range is 80-120mmHg.
    - Mild hypertension is when the BP is in the range 130/90-160/100mmHg.
    - Hypertension is moderate in the range 160/100-180/110 mmHg
    - Hypertension is severe when the systolic BP is >180mmHg or the diastolic >110mmHg.
  - o Measure the respiratory rate. The reference respiratory rate is 12-16 breaths per minute.
    - Tachypnoea is when the rate is >21/min.
    - Bradypnoea is when the rate is <8/minute.
- Assess the work required to breathe. An increased work of breathing occurs when the airway resistance is increased or the lung compliance decreased. The associated signs indicating an increased work to breathe include:
  - o The patient uses accessory respiratory muscles (principally the sternomastoid muscles).
  - o There is nasal flaring.
  - o There is a tracheal tug.
  - o There is intercostal retraction on inspiration and paradoxical abdominal movements.

In general, the greater the deviation from the reference range and the faster the rate of change, the more severe the problem and the greater the risk of a complication. For example:

- A very fast or very slow heart rate risks a stroke or heart failure.
- A very high blood pressure risks a brain haemorrhage or heart attack, a very low blood pressure organ damage.
- A very fast respiratory rate risks causing heart failure or an arrythmia, a very slow respiratory rate risks hypoxia and hypercapnia.
- A very high temperature risks a seizure, hypothermia heart failure.

While examining the patient for systemic signs, ask yourself:

What is the likely diagnosis or the differential diagnosis?

Systemic signs are, frequently non-specific, so are unlikely to help determine the location of the abnormality causing the problem. However, the systemic signs may indicate the type of problem. Therefore, when the diagnosis is uncertain, ask yourself:

What is the type of problem?

Throughout the examination, ask yourself:

How severe is the problem?
What is the management plan?

While examining the patient:

Ask yourself, what is the likely diagnosis or the differential diagnosis?

Systemic signs are generic; meaning that the same signs change in response to many different problems. Individually, a sign is unlikely to indicate a particular diagnosis but, in conjunction with other symptoms and signs, it may indicate or exclude a likely diagnosis or type of problem. For example:

- When a deep-seated infection is suspected, signs of a fever would support the diagnosis. The absence of a fever would not exclude the diagnosis.
- When a patient presents with left lower quadrant abdominal pain and tenderness, signs of a fever may help distinguish between diverticulitis and diverticular disease. The absence of a fever would not exclude diverticulitis.
- When the patient presents with bleeding, such as a haematemesis, a tachycardia and hypotension are likely to be caused by reduced circulating blood volume. The absence of these signs would exclude significant blood loss.

While examining the patient:

Ask yourself, what is the likely type of problem?

When the diagnosis is uncertain, systemic signs may help distinguish between different types of problem. Information about the problem and from an examination of the problem will indicate the signs to look for. For example:

- When a patient is peripherally hot and sweaty with a temperature >38 °C, the pulse fast, but weak and difficult to palpate with a tachycardia >120 bpm, they have a fever likely to be an infective inflammatory type of problem, such as a bacterial or viral infection.
- When a patient is peripherally pale, cold and sweaty, with a tachycardia, a fall in the mean arterial pressure, tachypnoea and a reduced urine output, hypovolaemia, such as from haemorrhage is likely: a metabolic or circulatory type of problem.

While examining the patient:

Ask yourself, how severe is the problem?

Severity not only refers to the problem locally, but also to the impact on the patient. The impact on the patient, or on a part of the patient is increased when there is an underlying abnormality or morbidity. For example:

- The elderly are less able to tolerate an infection.
- The impact of a chest infection is greater in a patient with COPD.
- The impact of hypovolaemia is greater in a patient with IHD.
- The signs of sepsis are masked in patients taking steroids or who are immunosuppressed.

Therefore, severity assessment should be considered together with information about the person and the patient. Systemic signs that assess the impact on the patient and are an important part of the severity assessment include:

- Impaired mental state, feeling ill, drowsy or confused may be used to assess the severity of a primary brain problem or indicate a systemic illness is severe.
- A change in weight is a measure of severity. When rapid or profound the problem is severe. In addition to weight, measures include the body mass index (BMI): a BMI of 18.5-24.9 is "ideal", skin fold thickness or waist circumference. For some patients it is appropriate to calculate the lean body mass (body weight minus body fat) using one of the formulae available: such as the Boer formula, the James Formula or the Hume formula.
- A change in colour: looking flushed, pale, or cyanosed. Colour alone is an unreliable sign for the diagnosis of a fever, anaemia or cyanosis because it may be affected by many factors including lighting in the room and the opinion of the examiner. However, when overt the problem is severe.
- Perspiration is an unreliable sign for the diagnosis of a fever.
- Core body temperature, heart rate, blood pressure and the respiratory rate. A change in heart rate may be in response to a cardiac arrythmia when it assesses the local problem or in response to a systemic problem, such as sepsis, hypovolaemia or thyrotoxicosis when it can be used as a measure of the impact on the patient. Similarly, tachypnoea may be used to assess the severity of a primary pulmonary problem or a systemic illness.

Frequently, the pattern of signs determine severity. For example:

- A gradual loss of blood, causing anaemia, can be compensated for by water redistribution without reducing circulating volume or eliciting a significant physiological response until the anaemia is severe, <8g/dL. Signs of pallor, tachycardia, hypotension and tachypnoea indicate the anaemia is severe.
- When a patient presents with acute haemorrhage, which may be overt, such as from penetrating trauma, haematemesis or melaena, or occult, such as from blunt trauma, an ectopic pregnancy or a ruptured abdominal aortic aneurysm or spleen, a rapid loss of blood reduces the circulating volume and quickly elicits a physiological response. The initial response to an acute haemorrhage is to increase cardiac work and peripherally vasoconstrict to prioritise circulating blood flow to the vital organs: the brain, and the heart at the expense of the periphery, the muscle beds, the kidneys and the gastro-intestinal tract. Clinically this is manifest as tachycardia, a fall in the mean arterial pressure, cold and sweaty skin, tachypnoea and a reduced urine output. The physiological responses can indicate the volume of blood lost: a systolic BP <90 mmHg, HR >120 bpm, and a RR >20 breaths/minute, indicate the patient is in shock suggesting 1-1.5L of blood loss, representing about 30% of circulating volume (the adult blood volume is 70mL/kg, or about 5L for a 70kg man). Fit patients can tolerate such a loss, and, if they are very fit, may manifest little change in heart rate, blood pressure or respiratory rate. On the other hand, patients with significant co-morbidity such as vascular or respiratory disease may be in extremis with profound hypotension, angina at rest or symptoms of hypoxia. Profound hypotension, MAP <60 mmHg, a paradoxical bradycardia (the Bezold-Jarisch reflex) and loss of consciousness, indicate cardiovascular collapse.
- When a patient is peripherally hot and sweaty with a temperature >38°C or is peripherally cold and sweaty with a temperature <35°C, the pulse fast, but weak and difficult to palpate with a tachycardia >120 bpm, hypotension with a systolic BP <90 mmHg and tachypnoea with a RR >20 breaths/minute or a slow (<8 breaths/minute) weak and a shallow respiratory rate with shallow mouth breathing ("panting"), they are likely to be in septic shock. Associated signs may include confusion, delirium or drowsiness.

Occasionally, systemic signs are sought to diagnose or exclude a complication. For example:

- When a patient presents with symptoms of ureteric colic, signs of a fever will indicate obstruction is complicated by uro-sepsis.
- When a patient presents with persistent profuse vomiting and/or diarrhoea, a dry mouth, loss of skin turgor, a tachycardia with a weak pulse, hypotension and anuria would indicate hypovolaemia is a secondary problem and it is likely to be complicated by renal failure.

Occasionally, the aim of looking for systemic signs is to assess the risk of a complication. For example:

- The risk of harm is increased in proportion to the severity of hypertension. When the hypertension is severe, the patient is at risk of a complication such as a heart attack, a stroke or heart failure.
- For a patient with paroxysmal AF the risk of a stroke is <1.5% per year, whereas when the AF is permanent the risk of a stroke is almost 2% per year.
- A BMI <15 is severely underweight whereas a BMI of 15-18.5 is underweight. Severely underweight people have increased mortality. A BMI of >40 is severely obese with an increasing risk of metabolic syndrome and other medical conditions.

It should be noted that finding the systemic signs are within the reference range may not exclude a severe problem. Early in an illness, in a young fit patient or when the problem is longstanding systemic signs may be within the reference range even though the patient is seriously ill. For example:

- A septic patient may have vital signs in the reference range but can rapidly deteriorate into multi-organ failure.
- A young adult may have a pulse and blood pressure in the reference range even though they have a very low haemoglobin.
- A patient who is breathless from severe heart failure may have a respiratory rate in the reference range at rest even though the cardiac output is very low.
- A patient with an apparently normal urine output could have severe renal failure.
- A patient with ischaemic bowel may "look well" but could have severe metabolic acidosis and impending shock.

A further deterioration may reach a tipping point when the signs rapidly deteriorate.
While examining the patient:

Ask yourself, what is the management plan?

A severely ill patient should be managed in the right environment, with the right staff and the right facilities. For other patients, the severity will influence the management plan and may determine the priority and choice of investigations or treatment.

Tests are often indicated to assess the severity of the problem or to screen for an asymptomatic secondary abnormality or complication (Appendix 2). Initial investigations may include:

- Measuring blood haemoglobin to diagnose anaemia and assess the severity of anaemia.
- Measuring blood WBC count, the CRP level or the ESR to diagnose and assess the severity of a systemic inflammatory response.
- Measuring blood platelet count, prothrombin time and blood clotting factors to diagnose and assess the severity of a coagulopathy.
- Measuring serum urea, creatinine and electrolytes, calcium, magnesium and phosphate concentration to assess the impact on homeostasis.
- Measure blood glucose to assess glycaemic control.
- Measure serum LFTs to diagnose liver disease.
- Measure pO_2, pCO_2, pH, base excess and lactate in the arterial blood to assess gas transfer and acid-base homeostasis.
- Insert a bladder catheter to monitor urine output hourly to assess renal function.

- A 12 lead ECG to measure the frequency, pattern, and magnitude of the electrical depolarization/ repolarization cycle to diagnose and assess the severity of abnormalities in the electrical activity of the heart.
- Imaging with an X-ray, USS, CT or MRI scan depending on localizing symptoms or signs to formulate a diagnosis and assess severity.
- Specialist investigations may be indicated for some problems. For example:
  - An echocardiogram to image cardiac structure and assess function.
  - An exercise ECG or cardiac or pulmonary exercise testing (CPET) to measure the effect of exercise on blood pressure, heart rate and rhythm and oxygen uptake to assess cardio-pulmonary performance and capability.
  - Spirometry to measure pulmonary function including forced expiratory volume in one second (FEV_1), tidal volume (TV), forced vital capacity (FVC), inspiratory capacity and expiratory reserve volume.
  - Urodynamic studies to assess bladder capacity and micturition.

Examine for Signs of a Secondary Problem or a Complication

When there are symptoms of a complication or a secondary abnormality, this will indicate the signs to look for. For example:

- When a patient develops heart failure or palpitations following a viral infection, it may be appropriate to auscultate for a pericardial rub indicating pericarditis.
- When a patient presents with rectal bleeding caused by straining to pass hard stools, the anus should be examined for a haemorrhoid or fissure.
- When a patient has sustained a lower leg crush injury, it would be appropriate to examine for compartment syndrome.
- When a patient presents feeling unwell with symptoms of a UTI, there may be signs of a fever.
- When a patient has had profuse vomiting and diarrhoea, there may be signs of hypovolaemia.

For some patient's the examination is undertaken to screen for another problem, a secondary abnormality or a complication. This could be related to the presenting problem, such as when a patient includes a red flag symptom, to a previous or ongoing co-morbidity or a known risk factor. Usually, information about the patient and the problem will indicate whether an examination is indicated. For example:

- In a patient with a known AAA, it may be appropriate to examine the lower limbs for signs of emboli.
- In a diabetic patient, it may be appropriate to examine for autonomic neuropathy or retinopathy.
- In a paraplegic patient, it may be appropriate to examine for a neuropathic "pressure" ulcer.

The signs and likely diagnosis inform the investigations indicated to confirm or formulate a diagnosis, to assess severity or to screen for a problem.

Use Available Information to Formulate a Diagnosis or a List of Possible Diagnoses and Inform Management

Linking the available information will bridge the divide between the presenting problem, the diagnosis and management. The signs should be understood and interpreted together with information about the person, the patient and the problem to determine the likely cause. In the absence of pathognomonic signs or a recognised diagnostic pattern, the available information should be used to refine a differential diagnosis and determine a management plan so that each piece of information is additive. When the information is consistent and fits a pattern, the likelihood of a diagnosis is increased and management more likely to be appropriate. When a diagnosis is likely, treatment may be started, when uncertainty remains investigations may be indicated. For example:

Presenting problem	A skin lesion
Examine the site	A 5mm dark brown smooth-edged firm nodule skin on the face
Ask yourself, what is the likely location of the abnormality?	Superficial, skin
Ask yourself, what is the likely type of problem?	Cancer
Provisional diagnosis	Melanoma
Provisional management plan:	Urgent excision biopsy
Learn about the problem	Increasing in size over several months. No
Learn about the person:	65-year-old farmer
Learn about the patient	No other medical problem
Working diagnosis:	Malignant melanoma
Provisional management plan:	Urgent excision biopsy
Ask yourself, how severe is the problem?	
Examine for associated signs	Several firm nodules, likely to be lymph nodes, are palpable in the neck. No abdominal mass or chest sign
Examine for systemic signs	No abnormal signs
Working diagnosis	Malignant melanoma with metastases
Management plan	FNA of a cervical mass for cytology to confirm the diagnosis

Presenting problem:	An increasingly painful knee
Learn about the person:	56-year-old builder
Learn about the patient	Using a moisturizing cream, Vitamin D3 ointment and topical steroids for psoriasis
Learn about the problem	Increasing pain, swelling and stiffness, with a reduced range of movement over several months.
Ask yourself, what is the likely location of the abnormality?	Right knee joint
Ask yourself, what is the likely type of problem?	Non-infective inflammation
Learn more about the person	Played football until 10 years previously
Provisional diagnosis	Osteoarthritis
Diagnoses to exclude	Psoriatic arthritis, other auto-immune conditions
Provisional management plan	An Xray
Examine the site	A warm tender knee with widespread "boggy" swelling. A reduced range of movement. Pain on active and passive movement
Ask yourself, what is the likely location of the abnormality?	Right knee joint
Ask yourself, what is the likely type of problem?	Non-infective inflammation
Provisional diagnosis	Osteoarthritis
Provisional management plan:	An Xray
Diagnoses to exclude	Psoriatic arthritis, other auto-immune conditions
Examine for associated signs	Multifocal patches of psoriasis Minor swelling of other joints, including the fingers and toes. Nail pitting
Examine for systemic signs	N/A
Working diagnosis	Psoriatic arthritis
Management plan	An Xray. Start NSAID treatment. Referral to a rheumatologist.

Chapter 10
Concluding the Consultation

Abstract

The concluding conversation is important because it not only signals the end of the consultation but also because it may be all that the patient remembers. A good finish should leave the patient and the HCP happy and give the patient hope going forward. It should also ensure the patient is fully informed both about their problem and future care, and establish a reservoir of goodwill, laying the foundations for a successful working relationship increasing the likelihood of adherence and compliance with future care.

A consultation is more likely to have been successful if it has been meaningful and met the wishes, needs and expectations of both the patient and the HCP. The concluding conversation is the opportunity to ensure all relevant information has been exchanged, a management plan agreed and the patient is happy. It should include a summary of what has been discussed and include an opinion and information relevant to the patient, such as the diagnosis or cause of the problem and an outline of the agreed management plan. The agreed management plan then needs organising. When this includes prescribing a treatment this is usually done before the patient leaves. When management involves organising an investigation, a follow up appointment or a referral, this may be done before the patient leaves or later. The information exchanged during the consultation, an opinion and the evidence for the opinion, then need to be documented.

In conclusion, the importance of the concluding conversation is out of proportion to the time spent.

Introduction

All consultations start with introductions and learning the headline information and finish with a concluding conversation. A good finish is important because it may be all that the patient remembers from the consultation and may influence compliance and adherence with future care. When the consultation is finished, documentation needs to be completed and the management plan implemented.

Concluding a consultation is an art. There are many different ways a consultation can be concluded and it is for the HCP to find the best way that suits them and their patient. Most consultations reach a natural conclusion when information exchange is complete and a management plan agreed. There are then recognised local and national conventions for saying goodbye.

The aim of this chapter is to discuss how to conclude the consultation.

"A consultation that ends well is likely to be a successful consultation."

Adam Widdison

Determine the Aims of the Concluding Conversation

The principal aims of the concluding conversation are to end the consultation in a way that leaves the patient happy and informed and to record a summary of the information learnt, the opinion of the HCP, including a working diagnosis or differential diagnosis and a management plan. Meeting these aims should ensure the consultation ends with a good working relationship and facilitate adherence and compliance with future care. For some patients and some consultations there may be additional aims, including:

- To check that all information relevant to meeting the aims of the consultation has been learnt and correctly understood.
- To share relevant information with the patient and to check that the information is understood by the patient.
- To ensure the patient agrees with the recommended management plan and knows what is going to happen in the future.

Determine Whether a Concluding Conversation Is Indicated

A concluding conversation is always indicated before the patient leaves.

Unfortunately, rarely, a patient walks out of a consultation preventing a concluding conversation. In such circumstances, relevant information should be documented.

Determine the Focus and Format of the Concluding Conversation

The focus and format will vary between patients depending on the aims, the context, the patient and the information learnt during the consultation. For example:

- When a patient presents with a new problem the initial focus of the concluding conversation will be on checking all relevant information has been learnt and understood. Then the focus will be on explaining the working diagnosis or differential diagnosis and recommending a management plan.
- When a patient has attended the consultation following a diagnostic investigation the focus of the concluding conversation will be on checking all relevant information has been understood and explaining the recommended management plan.

Check that Relevant Information Has Been Learnt and Understood Correctly

It may be appropriate to summarise what has been discussed to check that relevant information has been learnt and understood correctly and signals to the patient the consultation is about to end. If the patient's permission is sought first, the patient will know that this is a final conversation and is likely to listen more carefully. The questions to ask could include:

Would it be OK if we finished by summarising what we have talked about?
Before we finish, can I check I have correctly understood what you have said?

Summarizing the information is also an opportunity to organise your thoughts, check the information is correct and internally consistent and ask another question if indicated. It also demonstrates to the patient that you have listened to them and gives them an opportunity to add additional information. It may be appropriate to ask:

Is there anything you think I have missed?
Is there anything else I should know?

Before information is recorded at the end of the consultation it may be necessary to check certain facts with the patient to ensure they are correctly recorded.

Share Relevant Information with the Patient

The concluding conversation is an opportunity to share relevant information, such as an explanation of their symptoms, the results of a test, what you think is wrong with them, the implications or prognosis, what you recommend, what is involved and what will happen next to ensure the patient is informed, help establish a good relationship and lay the foundation for a successful pathway of care. Before sharing information with the patient, it may be appropriate to ask:

Would you like to hear what I/we think/know?
Can I explain what I/we think is going on?
Can I tell you what I/we think/recommend?

Some information will be new to the patient and some may have been shared during the consultation. Some information may need to be repeated because it is important, to ensure understanding, as part of a summary or to introduce other new information. The information should be shared in a way that the patient understands: some patients want detailed information and others very little.

Some information can be explained to the patient and some is best provided in other ways, such as by an information leaflet, a video or referral to an on-line resource and some needs the specialist knowledge of another HCP. It is important to document the information shared with the patient.

When you are uncertain regarding, for example, the diagnosis, it is often helpful to demonstrate you understand their problem and the impact it is having on them before describing the uncertainties, difficulties or issues and then provide reassurance that you will do everything you can to help them. Reassurance is important because it will give the patient hope going forward.

Occasionally, it is inappropriate to share some information. Deliberately withholding information is fraught with risk and should always be done in the best interests of the patient and having considered the possible consequences.

Recommend and Agree a Management Plan

Before the consultation ends it is important to have agreed an outcome with the patient; a management plan. The management to recommend should be determined during the consultation based on the information learnt. The management plan recommended should not be a surprise to the patient at the end of the consultation; it should have been discussed, if only briefly, during the consultation. Management may include a treatment, lifestyle advice or reassurance and the patient discharged. For many patients, investigations are indicated and for some patients a follow up consultation recommended to assess change, following an investigation, or to assess the response to treatment, to monitor a problem or treatment or to plan a treatment. Occasionally, admission to hospital or referral to another HCP is indicated.

There are many factors to consider before recommending a management option. Firstly, the management aims should be compatible with the aims of the consultation. Then it is important to ensure the management planned is indicated, appropriate, meeting the needs and wishes of the patient, and the benefits outweigh the risks. A recommendation should include an explanation of the management aims when these are unclear, the alternatives, the benefits and risks, the limitations and what the management involves for the patient. When there is choice, the options should be discussed with the patient. When the choice is in the balance, there are significant risks or the patient is likely to have a firm opinion, a more detailed discussion may be indicated. Information exchange is necessary for informed consent.

A recommendation remains a recommendation until it has the agreement of the patient, although usually it is appropriate simply check they are in agreement. For example:

I am going to organise/start [investigation/treatment]. Is that OK?
I recommend [outcome], is that alright with you?

Although, increasingly guidelines and the recommendations from an MDT are available, the responsibility for deciding management rests with the HCP and the patient. Once agreed, the management plan is a form of contract. When a treatment is agreed, the HCP is proposing a likely outcome and risk and the patient is agreeing to comply and adhere with the treatment. When an investigation is agreed, the HCP is giving an undertaking to organise a test or a procedure and the patient is agreeing to comply with the instructions and to turn up.

End the Consultation

The consultation should be ended according to recognised local social and cultural convention. For example, stand up and shake hands and wish the patient goodbye. Occasionally, concluding a consultation is difficult. For example:

- When a patient is very talkative.
- When a patient remains unclear or confused.
- When a patient wants more reassurance or is dis-satisfied with the consultation.

Each HCP develops their own way of managing such situations.

For the HCP, the consultation does not end with the concluding conversation. After the consultation the HCP needs to ensure:

- All relevant information is documented.
- The agreed management is organised.
- Reflect on the consultation and, when indicated, debrief with a colleague.

Document Relevant Information

A record of relevant information should always be recorded either during the consultation or at the end of the consultation. The aim is to ensure there is a lasting contemporaneous account of the consultation. Information such as the patient's name, date of birth and a unique number, the date and time of the consultation and the name, signature and unique identifier of the HCP should be associated with every patient record.

The traditional proforma format using headings may be indicated when it is important to simply document all information. For example, when first meeting a patient. However, a standardised format using pre-determined headings does not enable important information to be highlighted or relevant information to be co-located and the reasoning for an opinion or for excluding an opinion is frequently unclear.

> **The content, focus and format of the record is not only a record of what was learnt and discussed but also is a record of the evidence and reasoning for an opinion and management plan**

More experienced clinicians record the information using a narrative format and only occasionally use headings, such as when it is important to highlight information. When using a narrative, one format does not meet all needs. For example:

- When a patient is known to the HCP and presents with a visible or palpable abnormality, the signs on examination and information about the problem are presented together as evidence for a diagnosis or list of possible diagnoses. Information about the person and the patient relevant to planning management should then be included.
- When a patient is seen following an investigation, a summary of key information about the problem, the results the investigation and the signs on examination should be presented together as evidence for an opinion. Information about the person and the patient relevant to planning management should then be included.
- When a patient presents with a new problem and has a risk factor, information about the problem, the signs on examination and the risk factor(s) should be recorded together as evidence for an opinion.
- When the aim is to assess the patient, such as for an operation, this should be stated at the start of the record. Information about the person, the patient and the signs on examination, including important negative information, should be recorded as evidence for an opinion.

The headings to use for a complete record of information exchanged during the consultation

---

Main headings used when recording information from the consultation

Identification information

Headline information

Information about the person

Information about the patient

Information about the problem

Information from the examination

Opinion

Usually, the aims of the consultation are implied, such as when a patient presents with a new problem and the aims are to formulate a diagnosis and plan management. However, in some patients, the aims should be specified. In which case, they are usually included with other headline information and associated with the context. For example, Mr Smith is a 57-year-old man seen for a pre-operative assessment (the aim) prior to an inguinal hernia repair (the context). Usually, the aims of the examination are self-evident, but if there is uncertainty, or the examination is limited, the aims should be specified. For example, the patient was examined to screen for cardiovascular disease. Similarly, the aims of management are usually implied and can be assumed. However, when there is uncertainty or potential for confusion the aims should also be specified. For example, the FBC was measured to exclude anaemia or blood cholesterol was measured as a screening test. The focus of the record should then be on information relevant to meeting the aims.

When recording information, facts should be distinguished from opinion and important facts highlighted, such as safety concerns or when the opinion of the patient impacts on management. It should be clear to a third party what information is fact and what an opinion. There should be sufficient information included to evidence an opinion and, in particular, the diagnosis and management planned. Relevant negative information should be included, particularly when it is the reason for excluding an important or possible diagnosis or management option. The content, focus and format of the record should ensure evidence is linked with the opinion so that the clinical reasoning is apparent. For example:

- When the patient presents with a new problem and the aims of the consultation are to formulate a diagnosis and plan management, information about the problem and relevant signs should be linked with the recommended working diagnosis and management plan.
- Information about the person or the patient, such as risk factors, that influences the differential diagnosis or working diagnosis should be linked with the diagnosis and management plan.
- Important safety concerns that influence management should be linked with the management plan.

When information is co-located with evidence it may be appropriate to repeat it to highlight it, such as when medications are listed. When information is shared with the patient, the record should include the content of the discussion. It should be an accurate record of what was said, such as an explanation of the benefits and risks of a procedure or the influence of a patient's opinion or a safety concern and linked with the diagnosis or management plan.

Record the headline information

The record should always start with headline information. It is usually summarised in a simple statement that includes the patients name and demographic information, such as the age, the context of the consultation, first impressions and a headline summary of the presenting problem or the information already known. This naturally leads onto the record of relevant information. For example:

- "Mr F S is a 47-year-old male who presented with a new rash. On examination…"
- "Mr P S is a fit and well 33-year-old married man who was referred by his GP with a suspected inguinal hernia. On examination there was…"
- "Miss S J is 22-year-old single lady who presented as an emergency with acute breathlessness. The breathlessness started…"
- "Mrs S S is a 63-year-old lady who was referred from the breast cancer screening service because of an abnormality on her mammogram. The mammogram had shown…"

When the aim of the consultation is unclear or limited it should be stated to avoid any future confusion as to the purpose of the consultation. For example:

- "Mrs R J is an 83-year-old widow who lives in a care home and was referred by her GP for physiotherapy to help treat her shoulder pain (aim). This was a constant…"
- "Miss N S is a 19-year-old university student who wanted contraceptive advice (aim). She is a …"

Record relevant information about the person

For most patients, learning detailed information about the person is unnecessary and any information about them is limited to information from the introductory conversation, such as their occupation or close relations and should be documented with other headline information. For example:

- "Miss S J is 22-year-old computer gamer who presented as an emergency with acute breathlessness."
- "Mr P S is a fit and well 33-year-old self-employed builder who was referred by his GP with a suspected inguinal hernia."

When there is additional information that influences the understanding or interpretation of other information about the patient, the problem or from the examination, or when formulating a diagnosis or planning management this is often recorded in context or highlighted. For example:

- "Mr F S is a 47-year-old married nurse who presented with a new rash. She was recently swimming in a river while on holiday when she was bitten by an insect."
- "Mrs S S is a 63-year-old cleaner who recently developed severe back pain, radiating down the back of her legs. Clinically the diagnosis is a central disc prolapse. She is very anxious and has agoraphobia, so rarely leaves her home. She does not think she could tolerate an MRI scan but will try to cope with a CT scan if she can be accompanied by a friend."

When a patient has expressed the wish not to be treated this should be clearly documented. For example:

- "Mrs PR is a 93-year-old who presented with a fungating breast cancer. She lives alone having recently lost her husband, who died peacefully from cancer. She does not want any investigations or treatment despite knowing that the cancer is likely to spread or get worse without treatment."

Record information about the person as a patient

It is important to document all relevant background medical information including important negatives. When first meeting a patient, headings may be indicated for completeness and to highlight relevant background medical information. When information about the patient is relevant to the problem, the diagnosis or the management it should be co-located with information about the problem or with the signs found even if this information is duplicated. For example:

- When a patient who presents with headaches is found to be hypertensive information such as whether or not they smoke, are obese or are being treated for hypercholesterolaemia should be recorded as risk factors together with information about the problem.
- When a young patient who presents with a change in bowel habit and rectal bleeding is found to have several first-degree relatives who have been diagnosed with bowel cancer, this information should be linked to the problem as a hereditary colo-rectal cancer is likely to be a diagnosis to exclude.

When the patient is well known to the HCP or information about the patient has been previously recorded and is unlikely to have changed, it is only necessary to record that there has been no change.

The headings to use for recording information about the patient:

Information about the patient

- o **Safety information**
  - ▪ Previous allergic reactions
  - ▪ Previous adverse reactions
  - ▪ Infection risk to others
  - ▪ Susceptibility to infection
  - ▪ Bleeding or thrombosis risk
  - ▪ Other safety concerns

- o **Ongoing morbidity and treatment**

- o **Past-morbidity and treatment**

- o **Potential morbidity and treatment**
  - ▪ Medical risk factors and treatment
  - ▪ Genetic risk factors
  - ▪ Lifestyle risk factors
  - ▪ Other risk factors

- o **Medications**

Record information about the problem

When the patient presents with a new problem, a record of relevant information about the problem usually follows the headline information and precedes the examination findings and the working diagnosis or a list of possible diagnoses. Information that indicates or excludes a likely diagnosis should be linked. When the patient is seen as a follow up consultation, it may be sufficient to state the underlying problem within the headline information and then to include a statement about any change or about the results of a test. For example:

- "Mr F T is a 75-year-old man who was seen as a follow up to assess the response to fluoxetine started 3 months ago to treat depression. He reported…"
- "Mrs L E is a 30-year-old lady with a goitre was seen following recent thyroid function blood tests. The tests showed…"

When a patient is seen by a second HCP it may be sufficient to state that the symptoms were confirmed or the same as previously recorded. When the patient is seen following a screening test, they may be asymptomatic. In which case, this should be recorded.

Record information from the examination

It is not usually necessary to state the aims of the examination as the aims of the examination are often the same as the aims of the consultation. Frequently, they can be implied within the record. However, when the aims or indications for the examination are unclear, they should be documented. For example: "The breasts were examined to look for signs of an asymptomatic primary."

When a patient presents with a new problem, the symptoms and signs should be linked because together they provide the evidence for the diagnosis and for excluding some diagnoses. When the examination is to assess severity or to plan management it may be more appropriate to link the examination findings with other information about severity or the management plan. For example:

- There was no evidence of paraesthesia in the digits caused by chemotherapy.
- The sub-cutaneous lump had not changed.
- In a female with hepatomegaly, it would be appropriate to examine the breasts to look for a possible primary cancer. In which case, the record may include:
- A hard left upper quadrant breast lump palpated may be a primary cancer.
- There was no evidence of a rectal mass making rectal cancer unlikely.

When a patient presents following a screening test, there may not be any relevant symptoms or signs. Nevertheless, important negatives should be recorded.

Frequently, the examination record includes a diagram. This can be more informative than using words to describe the signs (Figure 70a, 70b, 70c).

Figure 70a: To illustrate the findings on a breast examination

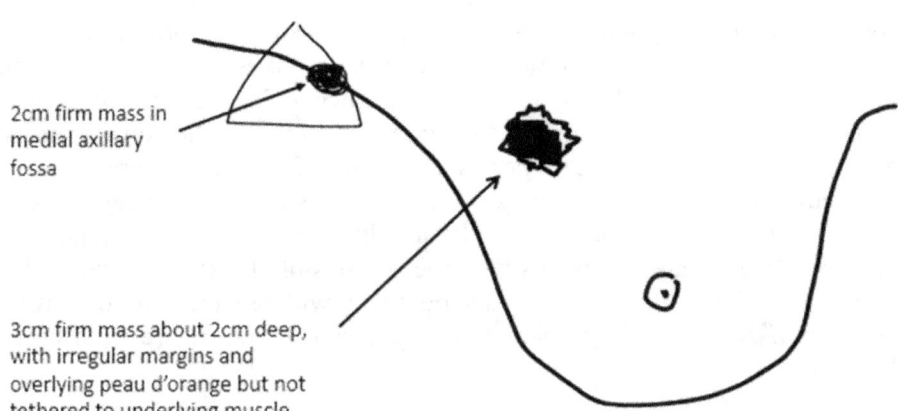

2cm firm mass in medial axillary fossa

3cm firm mass about 2cm deep, with irregular margins and overlying peau d'orange but not tethered to underlying muscle

Figure 70b: To illustrate the findings on examination of the chest.

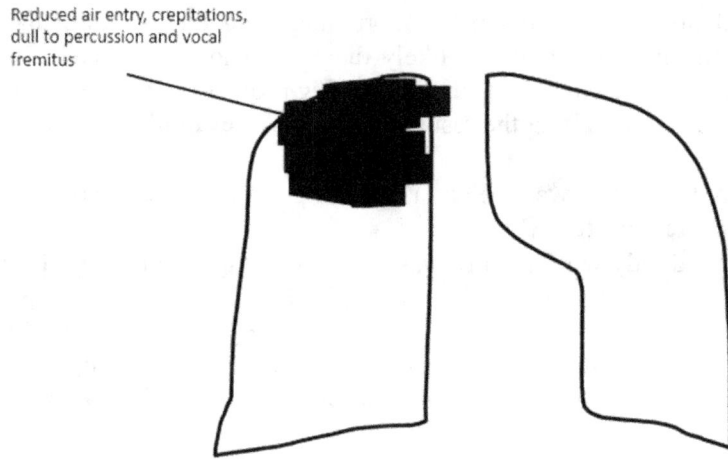

Reduced air entry, crepitations, dull to percussion and vocal fremitus

Figure 70c: To illustrate the findings on an abdominal examination.

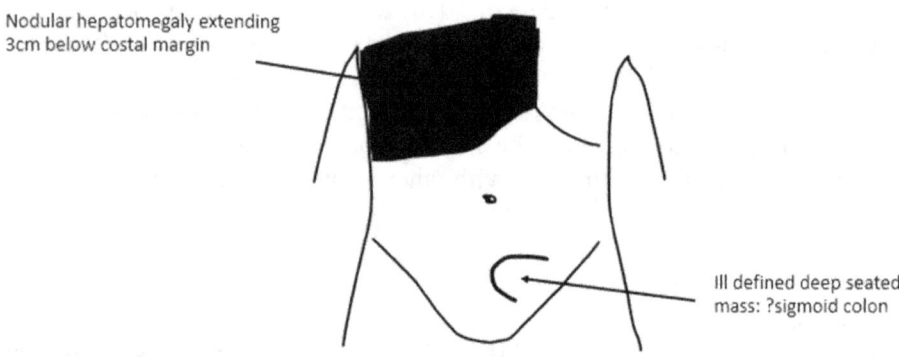

Nodular hepatomegaly extending 3cm below costal margin

Ill defined deep seated mass: ?sigmoid colon

When an examination was not possible or incomplete, the reasons for this should be recorded.

Document an opinion

The opinion usually includes a working diagnosis or a list of possible diagnoses and a management plan. There should be a clear link between the presenting problem, the symptoms and signs, and the opinion. The opinion should be supported by the information documented.

Implement a Management Plan

Patient care does not end when the consultation is over. When management includes investigations, specialized treatment, a follow up or another HCP, ongoing care needs to be organised and coordinated.

A clinician with suitable training, authority and experience usually takes overall responsibility for managing the care pathway. On occasions they need to lead, to delegate, to influence and persuade. They must be prepared to make decisions, to act in the best interests of the patient and then be responsible for the consequences. Although one HCP carries overall responsibility for managing the patient's care, an HCP rarely works alone. Most are part of a multidisciplinary team. Members of the team have different roles within a pathway, and different professional responsibilities. A good working relationship between HCPs and different teams will help patient care.

Responsibility for planning management remains with the responsible HCP but responsibility for adherence and compliance rests with the patient. For all patients a management plan will be successful only if it is adhered to and the instructions are complied with. A successful consultation and a good working relationship make adherence and compliance more likely.

Reflect on the Consultation and Debrief if Indicated

Every consultation is an opportunity for learning and self-development. Reflecting on the consultation will ensure this opportunity is taken. For example, it may highlight a learning need or signpost when a change is indicated.

There are many rewards to be gained from practicing medicine, few greater than saving someone's life, improving someone's quality of life or seeing someone get better following an illness. On the other hand, life can be very hard for some people and medical illnesses can cause terrible suffering. This inevitably will affect the HCP. Having emotional thoughts and feelings is natural. It is necessary for the HCP to understand patient suffering, to be compassionate, sensitive, tender and caring. It is also necessary to maintain a professional detachment, to be able to think objectively without allowing emotions or personal opinions to be an inappropriate influence affecting thought processes or performance and to not allow someone else's distress become your own personal distress. Doing the best that you can to help the patient is a pre-requisite for a clear conscience. Talking to other people, colleagues and friends helps manage the stress and emotions associated with providing health care.

Being an HCP is not just a job, it is a way of life, but it should not be a lonely one

---

Appendix 1:
Examples of Checklists

A checklist to help determine the likely location of the abnormality and the differential diagnosis of a mass or tenderness in the abdomen.

- Midline pain and tenderness or a mass.
  - In the upper abdomen (T6-9) is likely to be from an embryological foregut structure:
    - The stomach. For example, gastritis, a gastric ulcer, localized perforation, a gastric volvulus, or acute gastric dilation.
    - The duodenum. For example, duodenitis, a duodenal ulcer, or a localized perforation.
    - The pancreas. For example, pancreatitis or cancer of the body of the pancreas.
    - Biliary tract. For example, cholangitis, biliary colic or bile duct obstruction.
  - In the mid- or central abdomen (T9-11) is likely to be from an embryological midgut structure:
    - The small bowel. For example, inflammation, a localized perforation, obstruction, adhesions or ischaemia.
    - The caecum, ascending and proximal two thirds of the transverse colon. For example, intestinal obstruction, adhesions or colitis.
    - The aorta and retroperitoneal tissues. For example, AAA, aortitis or lymphadenopathy.
  - In the lower abdomen (T11-12 and L1) is likely to be from an embryological hindgut or pelvic structure: the left colon and upper rectum. For example, diverticular disease, colitis, cancer or ischaemia.
  - Suprapubic pain and tenderness are likely to arise from:
    - The bladder. For example, acute retention of urine or cystitis.
    - The ovaries, For example, an ovarian cyst, salpingo-oophoritis or a cancer.
    - The uterus. For example, pregnancy, endometriosis, a large or involuting fibroid, a pyometrium or endometrial cancer.
- Unilateral pain and tenderness or a mass.
  - In the right upper quadrant is likely to be from:
    - The liver. For example, hepatitis, trauma or a tumor.
    - The biliary tract. For example, biliary colic or cholecystitis.
    - The duodenum. For example, a peptic ulcer.
    - The hepatic flexure of the colon. For example, diverticulitis, colitis or a cancer.
  - In the right lower quadrant is likely to be from:
    - The terminal ileum. For example, Crohn's disease or Yersinia enterocolitica.
    - The appendix. For example, acute appendicitis.
    - The caecum or ascending colon. For example, diverticulitis, colitis or cancer.
    - The ovary and Fallopian tube. For example, salpingo-oophoritis, ovarian torsion or hemorrhage into an ovarian cyst.
  - Flank pain is likely to arise from a retroperitoneal structure on that side. For example:
    - The ureter. For example, ureteric colic.
    - The kidney. For example, pyelonephritis, cancer, trauma or infarction.
    - The gonads. For example, testicular torsion.
- The retroperitoneum. For example, a retroperitoneal hematoma from a ruptured abdominal aortic aneurysm or retroperitoneal inflammation from acute pancreatitis. When the pain is felt in the back and there are no visible or palpable signs or tenderness at the site, the pain may be referred from a retroperitoneal structure. The location of the back pain indicates the likely structure affected and this will be confirmed if a mass or localized tenderness is felt. For example:
  - Lower thoracic back pain may be referred from acute pancreatitis or pancreatic cancer.
  - Lumber back pain may be referred from an expanding abdominal aortic aneurysm, pancreatitis, a retroperitoneal hematoma or from para-aortic lymphadenopathy.

A checklist to help determine the location of the abnormality of a circulatory type of problem.

- Heart abnormalities including:
  - Coronary artery disease
  - Valvular heart disease
  - Cardiomyopathy
  - Ventricular aneurysm
  - Arrhythmia
  - Mural thrombus
  - Pericarditis
- Abnormalities affecting the circulating blood include:
  - Hypovolaemia
  - Anaemia
  - Polycythaemia
  - Deranged clotting
  - Hyper viscosity
  - Hypoxia caused by respiratory failure
  - Carbon monoxide poisoning
- Abnormalities affecting the circulation including:
  - Atherosclerosis
  - Thrombosis
  - Intimal flap
  - Embolism
  - Aneurysm
  - Shunting
  - Vasculitis

A checklist to help determine the likely type of problem and the list of possible diagnoses when the location is a primary brain abnormality

- Neurological type of problem. For example:
  - Migraine
  - Depression
  - Bipolar disorders
  - Schizophrenia
  - Parkinson's disease
  - Autism
  - Cerebral palsy
  - Seizures
- Personality or challenging behavioural disorders. For example:
  - Anxiety
  - Paranoia
  - Panic attacks
  - Obsessive-compulsive
  - Body dysmorphic disorder
  - Eating problems
- Disorders of sensory processing. For example:
  - Chronic pain syndromes
  - Phantom pains
  - Irritable bowel syndrome
  - Fibromyalgia
- Structural type of problem. For example:
  - Traumatic brain injury
  - Dementia
  - Hydrocephalus
  - Cysts and pseudocysts
  - Abscess
- Benign tumours. For example:
  - Meningioma
  - Astrocytoma
- Cancer: primary or secondary
- Inflammatory type of problem. For example:
  - Meningitis
  - Encephalitis
  - Abscess
- Circulatory type of problem. For example:
  - Intra-cerebral vascular abnormalities. For example:
  - Arteritis
  - AV malformation
  - Berry aneurysm
  - Intra-cranial haemorrhage. For example:
  - Sub-dural haemorrhage
  - Epi-dural haemorrhage
  - Sub-arachnoid haemorrhage

A checklist to help determine the likely cause of a structural abnormality

- Tumours or "swellings"
  - Benign.
    - Solid
    - Cyst
    - Pseudocyst
  - Malignant
- Trauma. For example, haematoma, seroma, scarring, rupture, hemarthrosis or fracture.
- Foreign body.
- Degenerative changes affecting:
  - A solid structure. For example, osteoarthritis.
  - A hollow organ, duct or tube. For example, calculi, bezoar, a stricture, scar tissue or adhesions.
- Hernia
  - Superficial. For example, inguinal, umbilical, incisional, femoral or Spigelian hernia.
  - Internal. For example, hiatus hernia or mesenteric hernia.
- Deformity
  - Congenital. For example, haemangioma, AV malformation, Riedel's lobe or horseshoe kidney.
  - Acquired. For example, Dupuytren's contracture or swan-neck deformity.

A checklist to help determine the likely cause of a circulatory abnormality.

- A local or regional problem. For example:
  - A stenosis
  - An embolus
  - Thrombosis
  - An aneurysm or varix
  - An AVM
- A systemic, multifocal or widespread problem. For example:
  - A cardiac abnormality. For example:
  - IHD
  - Valvular heart disease
- Peripheral vascular disease. For example:
  - Atherosclerosis
  - Aneurysm
  - Vasculitis
  - Vasospasm
- Blood problems. For example:
  - Anaemia
  - Hypovolaemia
  - Clotting abnormality
  - Thrombotic abnormality

When the symptoms indicate the patient feels ill because of chronic systemic inflammation and the location of the abnormality and the cause are uncertain, the differential diagnosis includes:

- Cancer, such as lymphoma or renal cell cancer or a paraneoplastic syndrome
- An unusual bacterial infection. For example,
  - Osteomyelitis
  - Endocarditis
  - TB
  - An occult abscess
  - Brucellosis
  - Coxiella burnetti (Q fever)
  - Rickettsia
- A viral infection. For example,
  - HIV
  - Herpes zoster
  - EBV
- An unusual infection. For example,
  - Malaria
  - Toxoplasmosis
  - Fungal infection
  - Sarcoidosis
  - Histoplasmosis

Appendix 2:
Frequently Undertaken Investigations

> Measure the FBC count when a patient is suspected of anaemia or is bleeding
>
> An FBC is indicated when a patient is suspected of anaemia to confirm or exclude the diagnosis, to assess severity and to identify a likely cause. An FBC is also indicated in patients presenting with overt or suspected occult bleeding, palpitations, angina or heart failure, intermittent claudication, or with pigmented gallstones, jaundice or splenomegaly, to screen asymptomatic high-risk patients, such as patients > 65 years, patients who are ill, septic, or on a restrictive diet, or in patients who have renal, liver or gastro-intestinal tract disease, patients taking NSAIDs or anticoagulants or who are having an invasive procedure or an operation; or for assessment or monitoring purposes, such as the response to treatment.
>
> The number of circulating red blood cells (reference range 5-6 million/uL in men, 4-5 million/uL in women), blood haemoglobin concentration (reference range 140-175 g/L in males and 125-155 g/L in females), the mean red blood cell haemoglobin concentration (MCHC reference range 33.4-35.5 g/dL), the mean corpuscular haemoglobin (MCH reference range 27-31 pg/cell), the mean cell volume (MCV reference range 80-96 fL/red cell) are measured together with the WBC count and platelet count. The fraction of the whole blood composed of red blood cells (the haematocrit) is 40-54% in males and 36-46% in females. Circulating blood cells, haematocrit and blood haemoglobin concentration vary according to age, sex, ethnic origin and altitude.
>
> A Hb of >110 g/L in women and >120 g/L in men has a 5% false negative rate for diagnosing anaemia. In other words, anaemia is excluded in 95% of patients. The higher the Hb level the lower the false negative rate. Point of care testing with a haemoglobinometer is more unreliable: the specificity is >80% for diagnosing anaemia when the Hb is <110 g/L and >99% when Hb <60g/L. The critical difference is >15%. In other words, a change of >15% is likely to be significant.
>
> Anaemia can be caused by excessive blood loss, chronic disease, haemolysis, haematinic deficiency or a production abnormality. In patients with anaemia, the red cell indices (MCV, MCH and MCHC) may indicate the likely cause:
>
> - A low MCV, MCHC and MCH (microcytic hypochromic anaemia), indicates low iron stores caused by excessive blood loss, or iron deficiency, such as due to diet or coeliac disease.
> - Anaemia associated with a high MCV, MCH and MCHC (megaloblastic anaemia) is indicative of Vitamin B12 deficiency (usually pernicious anaemia) and/or folate deficiency, such as from coeliac disease. Other causes include liver disease, thyrotoxicosis and cancer.
> - Anaemia associated with a normal MCV and MCHC (normochromic, normocytic anaemia) is indicative of "anaemia of chronic disease", such as cancer, chronic inflammation, liver and kidney failure.
> - Anaemia associated with reduced numbers of blood cells indicates either hemolysis, such as Sickle cell disease, hereditary spherocytosis or autoimmune hemolytic anaemia, or production failure, such as aplastic anaemia, myelofibrosis, leukemia and bone marrow metastases. The red cell indices can be variably affected.

Measure the WBC count when a patient has an unexplained tendency to infections.

WBCs, a key part of the immune defence system, originate in the bone marrow and circulate through the blood stream, tissues and lymphatics. Measuring the WBC count is indicated to diagnose or exclude haematological disorders such as leukaemia or myelodysplasia, in addition to being used to diagnose, screen for, or assess the severity of inflammation.

There are 4-11,000 WBCs per mL of blood. The major types of WBC are neutrophils (granulocytes, 55-75%), lymphocytes (T and B cells, and natural Killer cells, 20-40%), eosinophils (1-4%), monocytes (2-8%) and basophils (0.5-1%). Abnormal WBCs, such as pro-genitor white cells may not be identified correctly by the cell counter leading to abnormal results.

An increased neutrophil count is likely to be in response to bacterial or fungal infection and an increased lymphocyte and monocyte count a response to a viral infection or TB.

A very high WBC count may be caused by:

- An auto-immune disorder such as SLE or rheumatoid arthritis
- Myelofibrosis
- Cancer, such as polycythaemia, leukaemia or lymphoma.

A low WBC count may be caused by:

- Infection, such as HIV
- An autoimmune disorder, such as SLE
- A bone marrow disorder, such as myelodysplasia
- A haematological cancer, such as lymphoma or leukaemia
- Disease of the liver or spleen, such as hypersplenism
- Medications, such as immuno-suppression medications

When the WBC count is abnormal, an examination of a blood film may be indicated

Measure the platelet count and request tests of blood clotting when a patient is suspected of having a bleeding risk

An FBC is not only indicated when a patient has overt or occult bleeding or anaemia, but also when a patient has a bleeding risk. An FBC measures the number of circulating red blood cells (reference range 5-6 million/μL in men and 4-5 million/μL in women), blood haemoglobin concentration (reference range 140-175 g/L in males and 125-155 g/L in females), the mean red blood cell haemoglobin concentration (MCHC, reference range 33.4-35.5 g/dL), the mean corpuscular haemoglobin (MCH reference range 27-31 pg/cell), the mean cell volume (MCV reference range 80-96 fL/red cell) together with the WBC count (reference range 4-11000/μL) and platelet count (reference range 150-400,0000/μL). Some types of abnormal cells, such as microcytes, schistocytes and spherocytes, may be misidentified as platelets by the laboratory analyser causing spuriously high platelet counts.

An increased risk of bleeding may be caused by thrombocytopaenia or thrombocytosis, when there are too few or too many platelets in the blood.

- Thrombocytopaenia (platelet count <150,000/μL) may be idiopathic or caused by Vitamin B12 and folate deficiency, cancer, such as myeloma, myelodysplasia, or aplastic anaemia, HIV or auto-immune disease or by medications, such as heparin.
- Thrombocytosis (platelet count >400,000/μL) may be idiopathic or caused by inflammation, trauma, cancer, including polycythaemia vera, myelofibrosis or leukaemia, iron deficiency, haemolysis or hypersplenism or by medications, such as furosemide or ranitidine.

An increased risk of bleeding may be caused by a clotting abnormality. When a clotting abnormality is suspected, measurement of prothrombin time, thrombin time and activated partial thromboplastin time is indicated.

- The prothrombin time (PT reference range 8.4-12.5 seconds), usually presented as the International Normalised Ratio (INR) to reduce variability, measures the rate of conversion of prothrombin to thrombin (requiring factors II, V, VII, and X) within the extrinsic clotting pathway. A prolonged PT can be caused by, impaired synthesis in liver disease due to warfarin use or because of Vitamin K deficiency, increased loss in disseminated intravascular coagulopathy (DIC), dilution after a massive blood transfusion, or the presence of an inhibitor to factors VII, X, II/prothrombin, V, or fibrinogen.
- The thrombin time (TT reference range 12-19 seconds) measures the rate of conversion of fibrinogen into fibrin. A prolonged TT can be caused by liver disease, consumption in DIC or medications such as heparin or dabigatran.
- The activated partial thromboplastin time (aPTT reference range 25-35 seconds) measures the rate blood clots to assess the intrinsic clotting pathway (clotting factors XII, XI, IX, VIII, X, V, prothrombin, fibrinogen, pre-kallikrein and kininogen). Increase may be caused by medications such as unfractionated heparin, Vitamin K deficiency, DIC and clotting factor deficiencies, such as haemophilia.

Additional specialist investigations may be indicated, such as the measurement of:

- Clotting factors, such as Factor VIII
- Fibrinogen level
- Fibrin degradation products
- Anti-thrombin III level

Measure the CRP to assess the inflammatory response

The blood concentration of CRP is a surrogate marker of circulating proinflammatory cytokines, and as such is a "non-specific" marker of inflammation. Inflammation, from any cause, stimulates the liver to synthesize and secrete "acute phase proteins", including CRP, mannose-binding protein, complement factors, ferritin, and caeruloplasmin, all of which have different functions. CRP is an opsonin, it binds to lyso-phosphatidyl choline expressed on dead and dying cells and phosphocholine on some microorganisms, including pneumococcus, to trigger complement activation and phagocytosis (CRP was named because it is a protein that binds, "reacts", to the C-polysaccharide antigen of pneumococcus). CRP (and fibrinogen) is synthesized in the liver and released into the blood within 6 hours of a rise in circulating cytokines. This can mean there is a delay of up to 12 hours before the blood CRP level starts to increase and 48 hours before the CRP peaks. Therefore, a normal CRP does not exclude inflammation, including sepsis, early in the course of the illness. CRP is frequently measured to diagnose inflammation, to exclude inflammation, to screen for complications, or for assessment or monitoring purposes. For example, to assess a change in the severity of the inflammatory response or the response to treatment. However, CRP lacks diagnostic specificity; it increases in both infective and non-infective inflammatory conditions, including cardio-vascular disease, cancer, inflammatory bowel disease and auto-immune condition rheumatoid arthritis, so an abnormal CRP should be interpreted in the context of the clinical picture and in conjunction with other tests depending on the clinical context.

The normal blood CRP concentration is 0.8-3 mg/dL. In general, mild inflammation leads to increases to the range 10 to 40 mg/dL, while more severe inflammation leads to serum levels >40 mg/dL. The sensitivity and specificity for the diagnosis of sepsis is 65-75%. If inflammation is clinically suspected the likelihood CRP will be high, LR+ = 2.5, and the likelihood it will exclude inflammation, LR- = 0.5. Therefore, a normal test does not exclude sepsis. On the other hand, a normal CRP does exclude some chronic inflammatory conditions such as polymyalgia, giant cell arteritis, or myeloma, and, conversely, a high CRP excludes scleroderma, polymyositis, dermatomyositis and SLE.

CRP is often used to monitor the response to treatment, such as the response to antimicrobial treatment in bacterial infections, and immunosuppressants in colitis. However, CRP has a long plasma half-life of 19 hours, so there is a long delay before CRP falls. In general, if CRP is being used for monitoring, tests should not be repeated within 24 hours. The inter-individual variation is 75% and the intra-individual variation >40%, so a significant change is needed to reflect a real difference in CRP concentration.

Measure the ESR to assess the inflammatory response

The ESR, a measure of the rate at which red blood cells settle to the bottom of a vertical tall thin tube, is a non-specific marker of inflammation. ESR, is a measure of physical characteristics of blood and is affected by many variables including the shape, size and number of RBCs and plasma levels of proteins, such as alpha-1 antitrypsin, haptoglobin, caeruloplasmin, complement, CRP, fibrinogen and immunoglobulins. It is essentially a surrogate marker of circulating blood fibrinogen and immunoglobulin levels. Measuring the ESR is not routinely indicated to diagnose or exclude inflammation, to assess the inflammatory response, or to screen asymptomatic patients because the risk-benefit ratio of investigating a raised result in the absence of corresponding signs or symptoms is uncertain. CRP is generally considered to be a more sensitive and responsive measure of the inflammatory response. However, measuring the ESR is indicated when an auto-immune condition, such as polymyalgia rheumatica, rheumatoid arthritis, systemic lupus erythematosus, De Quervain's thyroiditis, or a chronic infection, such as tuberculosis and infective endocarditis is suspected. It is can also be used to differentiate giant cell arteritis from other causes of headache or Takayasu's arteritis from Kawasaki disease. The maximum normal ESR for men is the (age in years)/2 and for women the (age in years+10)/2. A normal ESR has a high negative predictive value for many auto-immune inflammatory conditions, but the sensitivity and specificity is unclear, because it is affected by many variables.

Microbiological test

Microbiological tests are indicated when a patient is likely to be an infection risk to others, to screen asymptomatic high-risk patients, such as MRSA screening, in addition to formulating a diagnosis, to exclude an infection, to screen for infection as a complication, such as a post-operative fluid collection, or for assessment or monitoring purposes, such as the response to treatment.

A representative sample should be collected aseptically and sent for microscopic examination, culture in a growth medium, and serology testing (MC&S) or for toxin testing, such as for C. difficile toxin. Frequently, when screening, several different sites are sampled.

The sensitivity and specificity of microbiological testing is variable: a false positive result may be from contamination or a false negative result from a sampling or processing error. A negative test result does not exclude an infection.

Measure the blood sugar level.

Glucose is an essential fuel for the brain. Hypoglycaemia can occur in any patient being treated for DM, or in patients with sepsis, anorexia, liver, heart, or renal disease, causing confusion, disorientation and seizures. When the blood glucose level (BGL) is high (reference range 4-8 mmol/L), glucose is excreted in the urine, causing polyuria, dehydration and thirst. Fat is broken down to fatty acids, which are oxidised to ketones (aceto-acetone, and beta hydroxybutyrate) in the liver, causing metabolic acidosis and weight loss. Any patient suspected or at risk of hyper- or hypo-glycaemia should have their BGL measured. A random BGL of >7 mmol/L, confirmed on repeated tests, or a BGL of >11.1 mmol/L 2 hours after a 75g oral glucose load (Glucose tolerance test) is generally considered sufficient to diagnose DM. DM is the most common cause of hyperglycaemia but the differential diagnosis includes Cushing's syndrome or a glucagonoma. Hypoglycaemia is usually caused by treatment for DM but it can occur in sepsis, excess alcohol, liver, heart, or renal dysfunction, and anorexia. If these diagnoses are excluded and the hypoglycaemia is persistent then an insulinoma is likely. BGL is also used to monitor treatment. The critical difference is about 18%. In other words, a change of >18% in the BGL is likely to be significant.
Glycated haemoglobin (HbA1c) can also be used to exclude a diagnosis of DM. The HbA1c blood level correlates with average concentration of blood glucose over the preceding 2-3 months. If the blood HbA1c is <48 mmol/L (6.5%) DM is unlikely, but if it is in the range 42-48 mmol/L it may be considered "pre-diabetes".

Measure the serum sodium and potassium chloride concentrations.

Serum sodium and potassium chloride concentration are frequently measured to screen for secondary abnormalities in salt and water homeostasis. Sodium, potassium and water freely move between the circulation and tissue fluid along diffusion gradients, whereas the intra-cellular concentration of sodium and potassium is maintained by the Na/K ATPase membrane channel pump. In an average 70kg man there is approximately 3000 mmol of sodium, of which 95% is extracellular and 3500 mmol of potassium, of which 98% is intracellular (where the concentration is maintained at about 140 mmol/L). Muscles contain 40% of the total body potassium. Sodium, potassium, chloride and water are continually lost in urine, sweat, vomit and faeces. Of these, only urinary losses can be regulated. We need a maintenance intake of >1L of water/day and 1.5-2.5 mg of salt/day (>150 mmol sodium/day and >50 mmol potassium/day) to maintain normal serum concentrations. The electrolytes sodium (reference range 135-145 mmol/L), potassium (reference range 3.5-5.5 mmol/L) and chloride (reference range 96-106 mmol/L) are the main determinants of blood and tissue fluid osmolarity, which is principally regulated by the kidneys. The critical difference is >10%. In other words, a change of >10% in the serum concentration is likely to be significant. Reference ranges assume that 93% of the serum volume is water and 7% lipid and protein. The measured sodium concentration is inversely affected by changes to the water, lipid or protein concentration.
The commonest causes of hyperkalaemia are acute and chronic kidney disease and diuretics. Isolated, hyperkalaemia can be caused by cell death such as haemolysis, thrombocytosis, leucocytosis, tumour

389

lysis syndrome or rhabdomyolysis (including crush injury or compartment syndrome) acidosis, acute kidney injury and medications, such as spironolactone, heparin, and proton pump inhibitors. Severe hyperkalaemia (>6.5 mmol/L) can cause life threatening arrythmia. Unexpected and unexplained hypernatremia can be caused by diabetes insipidus, and hyperkalaemia by Addison's disease.

Hyponatraemia and hypokalaemia can be caused by excess loss, such as diarrhoea or vomiting, diuretic medications, excess water intake or organ failure such as cirrhosis, congestive cardiac failure or the nephrotic syndrome. Intracellular potassium buffers changes in serum potassium so that a decrease in serum potassium concentration of about 1 mmol/L indicates a total potassium deficit of 200-400 mmol.

Measure serum creatinine concentration.

Creatine is absorbed from the diet and is synthesized in the liver, pancreas and kidneys. It circulates in the blood and is taken up by cells where it is phosphorylated by creatine kinases in the mitochondria. Phosphocreatine is the partner in a high-energy phosphate shuttle with ADP, acting as a rapidly available energy source during intense demand. It is an essential intracellular energy reservoir and source. Creatinine is the soluble nitrogenous waste product of creatine. Creatinine is transported in the blood to the kidney where it is filtered and excreted in urine. Measurement of serum creatinine is indicated to screen for deranged salt or water balance or deranged renal function. The reference range for creatinine is 62-115 μmol/L in men, and 53-97 in women (due to their lower muscle mass). The critical difference is >20%. The wide reference range and analytic variation mean that large changes may not be abnormal, and conversely significant deterioration of renal function can occur without the result exceeding the upper limit of the reference range. Repeat tests, and change over time are important. Clinically, creatinine is often used to assess the severity of kidney injury:

Stage 1: Serum creatinine 1.5-1.9xbaseline creatinine or urine output <0.5mL/kg/hour for 6 hours
Stage 2: Serum creatinine 2-2.9xbaseline creatinine or urine output <0.5mL/kg/hour for 12 hours
Stage 3: Serum creatinine >3xbaseline creatinine or urine output <0.5mL/kg/hour for 24 hours

The "glomerular filtration rate" (eGFR, expressed in mL/min/1.73 m^2), is estimated from the plasma creatinine concentration using equations which vary between laboratories. eGFR is frequently used as a measure of renal function:

Stage 1: eGFR > 90. "Normal" kidney function
Stage 2: eGFR 60 to 89. Mildly abnormal kidney function
Stage 3: eGFR 30 to 59. Moderately abnormal kidney function
Stage 4: eGFR 15 to 29. Severely abnormal kidney function
Stage 5: GFR < 15. "Acute kidney injury" possibly needing dialysis

The eGFR is affected by age, gender, race and size. Many elderly patients (40% of patients aged >75 years) have an eGFR 30-59 mL/min/1.73 m^2, i.e., stage 3 CKD and many die with CKD not because of their CKD. In the absence of albuminuria, there is no reduction in life expectancy. eGFR can decrease at a rate of 13 mL/min/1.73 m^2/decade after 50 years of age.

Tests of liver function and damage.

Measure the blood bilirubin concentration.

Macrophages of the reticulo-endothelial system, including the Kupffer cells of the liver, breakdown haem from old and damaged RBCs into bilirubin. Bilirubin is converted to a more soluble bilirubin glucuronate by glucuronyl transferase and excreted in the bile, together with bile salts, phospholipids, fatty acids, lecithin and cholesterol. The threshold serum bilirubin is normally 25% and analytical variation 15% so a 25% change is needed before it is clinically significant.

Measure serum enzymes.

The transaminases, aspartate (AST) and alanine aminotransaminase (ALT), alkaline phosphatase (ALP) and gamma glutamyl transferase (GGT) are released into the blood when the liver cells are damaged. ALT and AST are intra-cellular enzymes found in the liver, cardiac and skeletal muscle, kidneys, brain, pancreas, lungs, leucocytes, and red cells. GGT is found in the cell membranes of hepatocytes and biliary epithelial cells, kidneys, spleen, heart, brain and seminal vesicles. ALP is also an intracellular enzyme concentrated mostly in the bile canaliculi of the liver and in bone, but can also be from the intestine, kidney, placenta, and leucocytes. The reference range for ALT and AST is 0-45 Iu/L, for GGT 0-30 Iu/L, and for ALP 30-120 Iu/L. The release of these enzymes into the circulation occurs with hepatocellular injury, including biliary tract obstruction. The causes of raised aminotransaminases include alcohol, medications, such as paracetamol, non-steroidal anti-inflammatory drugs, antibiotics, HMG Co-A-reductase inhibitors, antiepileptic drugs, antituberculosis drugs, herbal medications, illicit drug use, non-alcoholic steatohepatitis (NASH), sepsis, cholecystitis or obstructive jaundice, hepatitis, autoimmune diseases, haemochromatosis, Wilson's disease, congestive cardiac failure, ischaemic hepatitis, α1-Antitrypsin deficiency, coeliac disease, DM, hypothyroidism, or Addison's disease, and glycogen storage diseases. Very high aminotransferase levels (>10 times normal) occur in ischaemic liver injury, acute viral hepatitis, drug or toxin induced liver injury, and occasionally in chronic bile duct obstruction. Raised levels of GGT may occur in obesity, pancreatic disease, myocardial infarction, AKI, COPD, DM, and alcoholism, and drugs including carbamazepine, phenytoin, and barbiturates. Raised levels of ALP may occur in the third trimester of pregnancy, in adolescents, bile duct obstruction, primary biliary cirrhosis, primary sclerosing cholangitis, drug induced cholestasis, liver or bone metastases, and bone disease, such as Paget's disease. If there is uncertainty, whether or not an ALP increase is from the liver or bone, the GGT concentration can be used to discriminate: GGT rises in liver but not bone disease.

Measure serum albumin concentration.

The liver synthesises non-essential amino acids, creatine, and most of the plasma proteins, including albumin and haem, the clotting factors, and the acute phase proteins, including CRP and fibrinogen. Albumin (reference range 35-50 g/L) accounts for about 55% of the total protein concentration (reference range 35-55 g/L), which also includes globulins, such as alpha 1 antitrypsin, haptoglobin, caeruloplasmin, transferrin, gamma globulins and C reactive protein (35%, 20-35g/L), fibrinogen (6.5%), hormones, enzymes and precursors. Albumin is an important transport protein and significantly contributes to the plasma oncotic pressure. It is synthesised by the liver at a rate of about 10g/day to compensate for catabolism and losses in the urine and gastrointestinal tract. Synthesis, dependent on amino acids in the diet and intestinal absorption, is increased in response to a fall in colloid oncotic pressure and decreased by cytokines. Albumin lacks sensitivity and specificity as a measure of liver function, because the half-life is long, about 20 days, and the blood concentration is affected by hydration, capillary permeability and loss. The inter-individual variation is 9% and the intra-individual variation 3%, so the critical difference is 12%, i.e., a change of >10% reflects a real difference in the albumin concentration.

Measure prothrombin time.

The synthesis of coagulation factors (except factor VIII) is an important function of the liver. The prothrombin time (reference range 8.4-12.5 sec) measures the rate of conversion of prothrombin to thrombin (requiring factors II, V, VII, and X) and thus reflects a vital synthetic function of the liver. Vitamin K is required for post-translational gamma carboxylation to activate factors II, VII, IX and X. The half-life of the clotting factors is <24 hours so serial measurement can be used to monitor liver function.

Measure blood glucose concentration.

Gluconeogenesis in the liver generates glucose from lactate, pyruvate, aceto-acetyl CoA, oxaloacetate and alphaketoglutarate, glycerol and odd-chain fatty acids. Glucose is stored in the liver (1-200g) and muscles (3-400g) as glycogen, and used to maintain blood glucose levels (reference range 4-8 mmol/L).

Imaging investigations.

Imaging investigations frequently used include, USS, CT scan, MRI scan, endoscopic retrograde cholangio-pancreatography (ERCP). Additional tests may be indicated:

- If hepatitis is suspected, blood should be screened for virus serology and autoimmune serology: circulating immunoglobulins, antinuclear antibodies, antibodies to smooth muscle, anti-microsomal antibodies and antibodies to the soluble liver antigen.
- Ferritin to screen for haemochromatosis
- Tests of caeruloplasmin and copper in the blood to screen for Wilson's disease
- Measure alpha1-antitrypsin

Request a liver USS.

A B-mode ultra-sound scan (USS), performed either trans-cutaneously, endoscopically, during open surgery or laparoscopically, is frequently used for the diagnosis of gallstones and bile duct stones, to investigate the liver, an upper abdominal mass, or to assess the anatomy of the liver and biliary tract. The ultrasound transducer creates high frequency (2-20MHz) pressure waves and detects waves reflected back. The amplitude of the waves returning to the detector are converted to shades of grey in "B-mode" ("brightness mode") USS. The picture is affected by the transmission properties of the tissues, and the depth, and the proportion of the wave reflected back is determined by the tissues at boundary zones, the contour of the boundary zone, and the angle the wave hits the boundary zone. The waves are not transmitted by bone and the image is compromised by obesity or if intra-abdominal gas is interposed. All USSs are operator, patient and tissue dependent. A transabdominal USS is >95% sensitive, and >90% specific for diagnosing gallstones >2mm in diameter. Endoscopic USS is more sensitive at detecting and assessing microlithiasis (stones <0.5 mm in diameter) and stones in the common bile duct. USS can distinguish echo-free cysts from echogenic solid lesions <1cm in diameter. Cystic lesions include simple cysts, cyst-adenoma's, choledochal cysts and echinococcus infection. Solid lesions can be benign or malignant. USS can assess the size, shape, internal and peripheral architecture to distinguish between benign and malignant liver lesions and biliary strictures.

Doppler USS are used to assess portal blood flow, to diagnose or assess the extent of portal vein thrombosis, vascular hepatic malformations, and to assess the patency of porta-caval shunts. Doppler mode uses the difference in transmitted and received wave frequency to produce a spectral or colour image. Flow in the tissues changes the wave frequency. The colour image reflects the flow rate which can also be calculated. Doppler USS is sensitive (>90%) at detecting portal vein thrombosis. USS elastography can be used to assess the severity of hepatic fibrosis in patients with chronic hepatitis or cirrhosis and a contrast enhanced USS can distinguish a haemangioma from a metastasis.

Measure the Arterial blood gases (ABGs) to assess gas transfer and acid base homeostasis.

ABG concentrations and acid-base are important measures of homeostasis. Most oxygen is transported in the blood bound to haemoglobin in the red blood cells: 1g of haemoglobin can combine with up to 1.35mL of oxygen. The number of red blood cells, their haemoglobin concentration and their saturation (oxygen content divided by oxygen capacity) determine the oxygen delivery capacity. The uptake of oxygen by haemoglobin is proportional to the pO2. As blood passes through the peri-alveolar capillaries it is exposed to a high pO2 in the alveoli and rapidly becomes fully saturated (>95% saturation). In metabolically active tissues, oxygen is consumed, pO2 in the interstitial fluid falls, oxygen dissociates from oxy-haemoglobin in the capillary RBCs and diffuses into the tissues. The rate and extent of the dissociation is proportional to the pCO2 and 2,3 DPG, and the temperature, and inversely proportional to the pH. Oxygen delivery is an example of "just-in-time logistics", because the tissue reserves are limited, and delivery failure will rapidly lead to hypoxia and the need for anaerobic respiration in actively metabolising tissues.

Carbon dioxide is a waste product of cellular respiration that needs to be excreted. Carbon dioxide rapidly diffuses from the tissues and dissolves in the capillary blood. It freely crosses the plasma membrane into the red blood cells where intracellular carbonic anhydrase catalyses the formation of bicarbonate from carbon dioxide and water. Bicarbonate then freely diffuses between the intracellular and extracellular compartments in exchange for chloride ions. Most carbon dioxide (70%) is carried as bicarbonate, and a small quantity carried in solution in direct proportion to the pCO_2, and combined with proteins, particularly deoxyhaemoglobin, as carbamino compounds. In the lungs carbon dioxide dissociates from carbonic acid, facilitated by circulating carbonic anhydrase, to diffuse along a partial pressure gradient into the alveoli to be expired. In the renal tubules of the kidneys, bicarbonate is actively reabsorbed from the glomerular filtrate and hydrogen ions are actively secreted in exchange for sodium ions. As a consequence, expired air contains a high partial pressure of carbon dioxide and urine is acidic.

Metabolic processes continually produce acids, such as lactic acid, ketones, phosphoric acid, uric acid, sulphuric acid, and hydrochloric acid in addition to carbonic acid, so that intracellular pH is about pH 7. Proteins and phosphate are intracellular buffers whereas bicarbonate, proteins, inorganic phosphates and ammonia are extra-cellular buffers. Flux across the cell membrane is both passive along concentration gradients and active by carriers or through channels such as the sodium-potassium ATPase channel. These acids are temporarily buffered in the blood while they are carried to the lungs or kidneys to be excreted, or to the liver to be metabolised. The hydrogen ion excretory capacity of the kidneys is reached at a urinary pH of 4 so any additional acid accumulates within the blood. When acid production exceeds buffering or excretory capacity the pH falls. This is metabolic acidosis. The fall in the blood pH is detected by pH sensing chemoreceptors on the ventrolateral surface of the medulla oblongata increasing the depth and rate of ventilation so that more carbon dioxide is excreted compensating for the fall in pH. Acid-base balance is tightly regulated because deviations can profoundly affect proteins (charge, configuration and function), and consequently enzyme and receptor function. Any significant change in pH will have widespread effects.

ABG measurement is indicated to assess gas transfer or acid-base balance in any ill patient, such as a septic or bleeding patient, or if the functional abnormality, such as organ failure, is severe or prolonged, or if they have serous ongoing illnesses, such as DM, or renal, liver, heart or respiratory failure, or are taking certain medications, such as insulin or metformin. The ABG cannot be used to formulate a diagnosis, nor does it necessarily indicate the impact of an abnormality on the patient: a normal pO_2 does not indicate normal tissue oxygenation, nor does a low pO_2 necessarily indicate tissue hypoxia.

pO_2, pCO_2 and blood pH, are measured in an analyser, whereas bicarbonate, lactic acid and base excess are derived and are therefore estimated. The arterial pO2, reference range 10.6-13.3 kPa (80-100 mmHg), is a measure of the pressure exerted by the 1-2% of oxygen dissolved in blood plasma. The pCO_2, reference range 4.77.45 kPa (35-45 mmHg), is a measure of the amount of CO_2 dissolved in blood. Only 5% of CO_2 is dissolved, most, 90%, is transported as bicarbonate. The reference range for arterial blood pH is 7.38-7.42. In most patients, pH is a function of both pCO2 and bicarbonate: pH is inversely proportional to pCO_2 and directly proportional to bicarbonate. Blood lactic acid concentration can also influence pH. Base excess (reference range -2 to +2 mEq) is a measure of the metabolic component of acid-base balance: a negative BE indicates excess acid. Therefore, serum pH, pCO_2, lactic acid, bicarbonate and base excess should be interpreted together. If a venous blood sample is analysed the pH, pCO_2 and bicarbonate values are similar to the arterial values, whereas the pO_2 is less than half that in an ABG.

The causes of hypoxia include, reduced inspired pO_2, such as at high altitude, when alveolar ventilation is reduced, such as airway obstruction, drugs or neuromuscular weakness, when there is ventilation-perfusion mismatch caused by consolidation or a PE, when the resistance to gas diffusion is increased, such as pulmonary oedema or fibrosis, or in circulatory failure, such as haemorrhage, anaemia, cardiac failure, or arterial occlusion. Hypercapnia is associated with respiratory acidosis and occurs when there is alveolar hypoventilation, such as asthma or COPD, severe lung disease, including consolidation or pulmonary oedema, central respiratory depression caused by drugs, typically opioids or anaesthetic agents and neuromuscular diseases or weakness affecting the respiratory muscles, such as motor neurone disease or myasthenia gravis.

The causes of acidosis include increased blood acid concentration due to either raised carbonic acid concentration ("respiratory" acidosis), or another acid ("metabolic" acidosis), usually lactic acid caused by impaired perfusion, such as sepsis, or ischaemia, or impaired carbohydrate metabolism, such as liver failure, by excessive bicarbonate loss, such as profuse diarrhoea (hyperchloremic acidosis) or a high output pancreatic or intestinal fistula or by insufficient renal excretion of acid as can occur in hypovolaemia, acute tubular necrosis or chronic kidney injury or ketoacidosis in diabetics or following starvation.

Respiratory alkalosis is invariably caused by hyperventilation, such as when a patient is very anxious, hypoxic, caused by a PE, a pneumothorax, asthma or COPD, or due to hyperthyroidism or following a brain injury, such as a stroke, or head injury, or due to drugs and toxins, such as salicylates or theophylline. Metabolic alkalosis, is usually caused by excess loss of acid through vomiting. Other rare causes include cystic fibrosis, milk-alkali syndrome or excess bicarbonate, or hyperaldosteronism.

Measure the blood oxygen saturation to assess hypoxia

The oxygen saturation (SaO2) of the blood is often measured using a "point of care" pulse oximeter that computes arterial haemoglobin oxygen saturation from the relative absorption of two wavelengths of light trans-illuminating an extremity (usually the finger-tip or an ear lobe). The absorption varies with the amount of blood in the tissue bed and the relative amount of oxygenated and de-oxygenated haemoglobin. Pulse oximetry is solely a measure of oxygen saturation and gives no indication of pCO2, pH or bicarbonate concentration. The SaO2 reading is affected by skin pigmentation, low perfusion states, motion artefact, anaemia and polycythaemia, and abnormal haemoglobin.

The pulse oximeter reference range of SaO2 95-98% is a measure of the 98-99% of the total oxygen in arterial blood that is bound to haemoglobin in red blood cells. For most oximeters the reading is +/-2% of the true value, but they can overestimate saturation if the level of SaO2 <80%. The oxygen-haemoglobin dissociation curve is sigmoid shaped so that the SaO2 is >95% if the pO2 is >10.6 kPa, but the SaO2 is >91% until the pO2 falls below 8kPa. Oxygen saturation is also a measure of oxygen carrying capacity if the haemoglobin concentration is in the reference range. In an anaemic or bleeding patient, the SaO2 may be normal but the oxygen carried is significantly reduced.

Measure the serum calcium

The intra- and extra-cellular concentration of calcium is very low because 99% of the calcium is in the form of calcium phosphate in the skeleton. Calcium metabolism is normally controlled by parathyroid hormones, calcitonin and Vitamin D. Ionized calcium is the biologically active form affecting the function of enzymes, including the clotting factors, and plasma membrane channels; in particular the voltage gated sodium ion channels. Hypercalcaemia reduces the flux through these channels making them less excitable causing lethargy and muscle weakness. On the other hand, a reduced concentration of serum ionized calcium causes sodium ions to leak into nerve cells making them hyper-excitable causing paraesthesia and muscle spasms. Serum calcium concentration should be measured in any patient suspected of hyper- or hypo-calcaemia. Symptoms may include feeling unwell, tired, and irritable, myalgia, abdominal pain, paraesthesia or pruritis and signs such as coarse hair and dry skin or uncontrolled movements (tremor or fasciculation). In addition, measurement is indicated in patients with heart failure, osteoporosis and fractures, acute pancreatitis, peptic ulcers, renal stones and unexplained ileus or constipation:

Serum calcium (reference range 2.2-2.6 mmol/L) includes both ionized calcium (reference range 1.3-1.5 mmol/L) and calcium bound to albumin and other circulating proteins. Ionized calcium is usually an estimate, in which serum albumin concentration is used to "correct" total serum calcium concentration using a formula. Direct measurement of serum ionized calcium from an uncuffed blood sample is more representative. Serum calcium measurements do not reflect total body calcium.

The sensitivity for hypercalcaemia is approximately 25% and specificity 90%. The likelihood serum calcium will diagnose hypercalcaemia (LR+) is about 2.5, and exclude a diagnosis of hypercalcaemia (LR-) about 0.75. The false positive rate for hypocalcaemia is >10% and the false negative rate about 75%. If calcium levels are being monitored a change of 8% reflects a real difference in concentration. Small changes in serum calcium should be confirmed by repeating the test.

A new diagnosis of hypercalcaemia may be caused by hyperparathyroidism, osteolytic bone metastases, multiple myeloma, paraneoplastic syndromes, such as from small cell cancers, or chronic kidney injury. Hypocalcaemia can occur in sepsis, acute pancreatitis, deranged acid-base homeostasis or hypoparathyroidism. It can also be caused by medications, such as anti-epileptic drugs, thiazide and loop diuretics, bisphosphonates and long-term lithium use, by a low calcium diet, hypervitaminosis A and D, milk-alkali syndrome or malabsorption due to chronic diarrhoea or alcoholism. Hypocalcaemia is often associated with, and may be caused by, hypomagnesaemia. Calcium is usually measured together with ALP, sodium, potassium, magnesium and phosphate, and the acid-base balance. The serum calcium concentration should be interpreted in the context of the clinical picture and additional tests, such as serum parathyroid hormone concentration, a bone scan, blood immunoglobulin assay or urinary analysis for "Bence-Jones" proteins, may be indicated to formulate a diagnosis.

Measure the serum magnesium

Serum magnesium concentration is frequently measured to screen for secondary electrolyte abnormalities in conjunction with sodium, potassium, calcium, and phosphate. Serum magnesium is maintained by a normal dietary intake of 12 mmol/day, and tightly regulated by the balance between renal excretion and internal distribution (principally bone metabolism). Renal losses are influenced by serum magnesium, calcium and phosphate concentrations (hypo-phosphataemia is associated with increased loss), and the hormones parathyroid hormone (PTH), calcitonin, anti-diuretic hormone (ADH), insulin and glucagon. Serum magnesium is present as free ionised magnesium, bound to albumin, and complexed with anions such as phosphate and bicarbonate. As with calcium >80% of the 1000 mmol of magnesium in the body is present in bone, and less than 1% in the extracellular fluid. Serum magnesium affects the electrical properties and permeability of membranes and particularly the electrical activity of the heart and its conducting systems and is an intra-cellular co-factor in more than 300 cellular enzymatic processes.

Measurement of serum magnesium concentration is indicated to screen for an abnormality in any patient feeling ill, with deranged function, in pain, with neurological symptoms, such as seizures, paraesthesia, dizziness, tremor and tetany, cardiac arrhythmias, with gastrointestinal symptoms, such as vomiting and diarrhoea, in renal disease, endocrine disease, such as DM, hypothyroidism, and Addison's disease, in alcoholism; acute pancreatitis and during refeeding after starvation and if serum sodium, calcium or phosphate are abnormal.

Serum magnesium (0.7-1.1 mmol/L) is the fourth most common cation. The critical difference is >15%.

Low serum magnesium indicates a deficiency but, because most is intracellular, normal serum magnesium does not exclude a negative total body magnesium. Hypomagnesaemia may result from reduced intake, reduced absorption, increased gastrointestinal loss, from vomiting or diarrhoea, increased urine loss from renal failure, redistribution, such as refeeding syndrome and "hungry bone" syndrome or sequestration in fat necrosis in acute pancreatitis and may be caused by medications, such as diuretics, mannitol, aminoglycosides and chemotherapy medications. Hypermagnesemia is uncommon but may be caused by acute kidney injury, lithium, hypothyroidism, Addison's disease, milk-alkali syndrome and familial hypocalciuric hypercalcaemia.

Measure the serum phosphate

Phosphorus is the most abundant anion in the body accounting for 1% of body mass. Most, 85%, of total body phosphate is in bones and teeth and <1% is extracellular. Phosphorylated metabolites include adenosine triphosphate, 2-3 diphosphoglycerate, and glucose-6-phosphate. In addition, phosphate is a constituent of bio-membranes, nucleic acids and hydroxyapatite crystals in bone. Phosphorus is an essential element and plays an important role in multiple biological processes: energy metabolism, cell signalling, cell differentiation and proliferation and bone metabolism, particularly during growth. The maintenance of extra- and intra-cellular phosphate levels is important for cell function. Serum phosphate concentration is dependent on the balance between intestinal absorption, renal excretion (normally about 13mg/kg/day) and internal distribution (principally bone metabolism). Increasing serum phosphate or 1,25-dihydroxyvitamin D stimulates fibroblast growth factor 23 production, which reduces serum phosphate levels and vice versa. Regulation is complex and poorly understood involving numerous hormones including parathyroid hormone, calcitriol, 1,25dihydroxyvitamin D and phosphotonin peptides including fibroblast growth factor 23 (produced by osteocytes and osteoblasts). Feedback loops, acid-base balance and serum calcium are important.

Measurement of serum phosphate is indicated in any patient feeling ill, with deranged function caused by gastrointestinal disease, such as vomiting, diarrhoea, malnutrition or malabsorption, as part of the refeeding syndrome or following treatment for diabetic ketoacidosis, alcoholism, respiratory alkalosis, sepsis and insulin treatment, by renal disease, endocrine disease, such as hyper- or hypoparathyroidism; bone metastases; rhabdomyolysis, Vitamin D excess or deficiency, or medications, such as glucocorticoids, cisplatin, pamidronate and phospho-soda laxative abuse.

The extracellular concentration of phosphate (reference range 0.8-1.5mmol/L) is 100 times less than the intracellular concentration. The critical difference is >20%.

Hyper-phosphataemia can result from increased phosphate intake, such as phosphosoda laxative abuse, Vitamin D intoxication, hypoparathyroidism, decreased phosphate excretion (acute kidney injury) or a disorder of phosphate distribution, such as bone metastases, or rhabdomyolysis. Hypo-phosphataemia can be caused by increased renal excretion, hyper-parathyroidism, Fanconi's syndrome or "oncogenic osteomalacia" (bone metastases causing increased fibroblast growth factor 23 production), decreased intake, Vitamin D deficiency, vomiting, diarrhoea, malnutrition or malabsorption (including chelation of dietary phosphate by antacids), medications, such as glucocorticoids, cisplatin, pamidronate, or intracellular shift, such as part of the refeeding syndrome, following treatment for diabetic ketoacidosis or alcoholism, respiratory alkalosis, sepsis, and insulin treatment.

Abbreviations

μg	microgram
μL	microliter
μmol	micromole
2,3 DPG	2-3 diphosphoglycerate
AAA	Abdominal aortic aneurysm
ABG	Arterial blood gas
ABV	Alcohol by volume
ACS	Acute coronary syndrome
ADH	Anti-diuretic hormone
ADP	Adenosine diphosphate
AF	Atrial fibrillation
AFP	Alpha feto protein
AI	Artificial intelligence
AKI	Acute kidney injury
ALP	Alkaline phosphatase
ALT	Alanine aminotransaminase
AMI	Acute myocardial infarction
ANP	Atrial naturetic peptide
APACHE	Acute physiology and chronic health evaluation
APC	Adenomatous polyposis coli
aPTT	Activated partial thromboplastin time
AST	Aspartate aminotransaminase
ARDS	Adult respiratory distress syndrome
ATP	Adenosine triphosphate
ATPase	Adenosine triphosphatase
AVM	Arterio-venous malformation
BCC	Basal cell cancer
BGL	Blood glucose level
BMI	Body mass index
BP	Blood pressure
BPH	benign prostatic hypertension
bpm	Beats per minute
BRCA 1 or 2	Breast Cancer gene
C.difficile	Clostridium difficile
CEA	Carcino embryonic antigen
CFS	Chronic fatigue syndrome
Cl	Chloride
CMV	Cytomegalovirus
CO_2	Carbon dioxide
COPD	Chronic obstructive pulmonary disease
COVID	Corona virus infection
CPET	Cardiac or pulmonary exercise testing
CRP	C reactive protein
CT	Computed tomogram scan

CT PA CT	Pulmonary angiogram
CVA	Cardio-Vascular Accident
CXR	Chest radiograph
DIC	Disseminated intravascular coagulopathy
DM	Diabetes mellitus
DVT	Deep vein thrombosis
EBV	Epstein Barr Virus
ECG	Electrocardiogram
eGFR	Estimated glomerular filtration rate
EMG	Electromyography
ERCP	endoscopic retrograde cholangio-pancreatography
ESBL	Extended spectrum beta lactamase
ESR	Erythrocyte sedimentation rate
FAP	Familial adenomatous polyposis
FBC	Full blood count
FEV$_1$	Forced expiration volume in one second
fL	Femtoliter
FVC	Forced vital capacity
g	Gram
GGT	Gamma glutamyl transferase
GMC	General Medical Council
GORD	Gastro-oesophageal reflux disease
H2RA	Histamine 2 Receptor Antagonist
HbA1c	Haemoglobin A1c
hCG	Human chorionic gonadotrophin
HCP	health care practitioner
HIV	Human immunodeficiency virus
HLA	Human leukocyte antigen
HR	Hazard ratio
IBS	Irritable bowel syndrome
IgG	Immunoglobulin G
IHD	Ischaemic heart disease
INR	International normalised ratio
ITP	Idiopathic thrombocytopaenia
iu	International units
IVU	Intravenous urogram
IVU	Intravenous urogram
JVP	Jugular venous pressure
K	Potassium
kg	Kilogram
L	Liter
LFT	Liver function test
LR	Likelihood ratio
LVH	Left ventricular hypertrophy
m	Meter
MAP	Mean arterial pressure
MC&S	Microscopy, culture and serology
MCH	Mean corpuscular haemoglobin
MCHC	Mean red blood cell haemoglobin concentration
MCV	Mean cell volume
MDT	Multidisciplinary team
ME	Myalgic encephalopathy
mEq	Milli equivalents

mg	Milligram
MHC	Major histocompatibility complex
mHz	Mega Hertz
mL	Millilitre
mmHg	Millimeters of mercury
mmol	millimole
MRI	Magnet resonance image
MRSA	Methicillin resistant Staphylococcus aureus
MS	Multiple sclerosis
MSOF	Multi-system organ failure
Na	Sodium
NASH	Non alcoholic steatohepatosis
NHS	National Health Service
NSAIDs	Non steroidal anti-inflammatory drugs
O_2	Oxygen
OGD	Oesophago-gastro-duodenoscopy
Pa	Pascals
PCI	Percutaneous coronary intervention
PCOS	Polycystic ovary syndrome
PE	Pulmonary embolus
pg	Picograms
PID	Prolapsed intervertebral disc
pL	Pico liter
PND	Paroxysmal nocturnal dyspnoea
pO2	Partial pressure of oxygen
PPIs	Proton pump inhibitors
PPV	Positive predictive value
PSA	Prostate Specific Antigen
PT	Prothrombin time
PTH	Parathyroid hormone
RBC	Red blood cell
RR	Respiratory rate
SAH	Sub-arachnoid haemorrhage
SaO_2	Arterial oxygen saturation
SBO	Small bowel obstruction
SCC	Squamous cell cancer
SLE	Systemic lupus erythematosis
TB	Tuberculosis infection
TCC	Transitional cell carcinoma
TFTs	Thyroid function tests
TIA	Transient Ischaemic Attack
TNM	Tumour, lymph node status, metastases
TT	Thrombin time
UC	Ulcerative colitis
UK	United Kingdom
USS	Ultrasound scan
UTI	Urinary tract infection
VDRL	Venereal disease research laboratory
VQ scan	Ventilation perfusion scintiscan
WBC	White blood cell count